Role of NO in Disease: Good, Bad or Ugly

Role of NO in Disease: Good, Bad or Ugly

Editors

Mats B. Eriksson
Anders O. Larsson

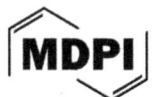

Basel • Beijing • Wuhan • Barcelona • Belgrade • Novi Sad • Cluj • Manchester

Editors
Mats B. Eriksson
Uppsala University
Uppsala
Sweden

Anders O. Larsson
Uppsala University
Uppsala
Sweden

Editorial Office
MDPI AG
Grosspeteranlage 5
4052 Basel, Switzerland

This is a reprint of articles from the Special Issue published online in the open access journal *Biomedicines* (ISSN 2227-9059) (available at: https://www.mdpi.com/journal/biomedicines/special_issues/NO_in_Disease).

For citation purposes, cite each article independently as indicated on the article page online and as indicated below:

Lastname, A.A.; Lastname, B.B. Article Title. *Journal Name* **Year**, *Volume Number*, Page Range.

ISBN 978-3-7258-1563-0 (Hbk)
ISBN 978-3-7258-1564-7 (PDF)
doi.org/10.3390/books978-3-7258-1564-7

© 2024 by the authors. Articles in this book are Open Access and distributed under the Creative Commons Attribution (CC BY) license. The book as a whole is distributed by MDPI under the terms and conditions of the Creative Commons Attribution-NonCommercial-NoDerivs (CC BY-NC-ND) license.

Contents

About the Editors . . . . **vii**

Anders O. Larsson and Mats B. Eriksson
Role of NO in Disease: Good, Bad or Ugly
Reprinted from: *Biomedicines* 2024, *12*, 1343, doi:10.3390/biomedicines12061343 . . . . **1**

Jenny Ericson, Michelle K. McGuire, Anna Svärd and Maria Hårdstedt
Total Nitrite and Nitrate Concentration in Human Milk and Saliva during the First 60 Days
Postpartum—A Pilot Study
Reprinted from: *Biomedicines* 2024, *12*, 1195, doi:10.3390/biomedicines12061195 . . . . **5**

**Tomas Weitoft, Johan Rönnelid, Anders Lind, Charlotte de Vries, Anders Larsson,
Barbara Potempa, et al.**
Exhaled Nitric Oxide Reflects the Immune Reactions of the Airways in Early
Rheumatoid Arthritis
Reprinted from: *Biomedicines* 2024, *12*, 964, doi:10.3390/biomedicines12050964 . . . . **13**

**María Varela, Miriam López, Mariana Ingold, Diego Alem, Valentina Perini,
Karen Perelmuter, et al.**
New Nitric Oxide-Releasing Compounds as Promising Anti-Bladder Cancer Drugs
Reprinted from: *Biomedicines* 2023, *11*, 199, doi:10.3390/biomedicines11010199 . . . . **24**

**Marieann Högman, Andreas Palm, Johanna Sulku, Björn Ställberg, Karin Lisspers,
Kristina Bröms, et al.**
Alveolar Nitric Oxide in Chronic Obstructive Pulmonary Disease—A Two-Year Follow-Up
Reprinted from: *Biomedicines* 2022, *10*, 2212, doi:10.3390/biomedicines10092212 . . . . **42**

**Achini K. Vidanapathirana, Jarrad M. Goyne, Anna E. Williamson, Benjamin J. Pullen,
Pich Chhay, Lauren Sandeman, et al.**
Biological Sensing of Nitric Oxide in Macrophages and Atherosclerosis Using a
Ruthenium-Based Sensor
Reprinted from: *Biomedicines* 2022, *10*, 1807, doi:10.3390/biomedicines10081807 . . . . **53**

Weiwei Kong, Yixin Liao, Liang Zhao, Nathan Hall, Hua Zhou, Ruisheng Liu, et al.
Kidney Renin Release under Hypoxia and Its Potential Link with Nitric Oxide:
A Narrative Review
Reprinted from: *Biomedicines* 2023, *11*, 2984, doi:10.3390/biomedicines11112984 . . . . **72**

**Juan Agustín Garay, Juan Eduardo Silva, María Silvia Di Genaro
and Roberto Carlos Davicino**
The Multiple Faces of Nitric Oxide in Chronic Granulomatous Disease: A Comprehensive Update
Reprinted from: *Biomedicines* 2022, *10*, 2570, doi:10.3390/biomedicines10102570 . . . . **85**

Christoph V. Suschek, Dennis Feibel, Maria von Kohout and Christian Opländer
Enhancement of Nitric Oxide Bioavailability by Modulation of Cutaneous Nitric Oxide Stores
Reprinted from: *Biomedicines* 2022, *10*, 2124, doi:10.3390/biomedicines10092124 . . . . **100**

Andy W. C. Man, Yawen Zhou, Ning Xia and Huige Li
Endothelial Nitric Oxide Synthase in the Perivascular Adipose Tissue
Reprinted from: *Biomedicines* 2022, *10*, 1754, doi:10.3390/biomedicines10071754 . . . . **120**

Nikolay O. Kamenshchikov, Lorenzo Berra and Ryan W. Carroll
Therapeutic Effects of Inhaled Nitric Oxide Therapy in COVID-19 Patients
Reprinted from: *Biomedicines* 2022, *10*, 369, doi:10.3390/biomedicines10020369 . . . . **137**

About the Editors

Mats B. Eriksson

Mats B. Eriksson, MD and PhD, is an Associate Professor at the Department of Surgical Sciences, Section of Anaesthesiology and Intensive Care Medicine at Uppsala University, Uppsala, Sweden, and an Affiliated Professor of Critical Care at Nova Medical School, New University of Lisbon, Portugal. He has been the principal tutor of two PhD students, who have completed their theses and contributed scientifically to several additional graduations. His research has focused on sepsis and septic conditions, from both clinical and experimental aspects. Special interest has been paid to the interface between inflammation and coagulation. He has been an invited speaker at several international conferences and presented research at scientific meetings in all five major continents. He also has considerable experience in clinical trials, both as an organizer and as an investigator.

Anders O. Larsson

Anders O. Larsson, MD and PhD, is Professor at the Department of Medical Sciences, Section of Clinical Chemistry, Uppsala University, Sweden. He has been the principal tutor of seven PhD students that have presented their theses. His main research field is laboratory technology. A focus area within this field has been kidney function markers, especially glomerular filtration markers and tubular damage markers. Another area has been proinflammatory cytokines and cardiovascular risk. He has been involved in both clinical and experimental studies. Several of the studies have been intensive care-related, looking for improved markers for acute kidney injury and infectious diseases including COVID-19. He has been participating in international collaborations such as the Global Burden of Disease consortium and determination of glomerular filtration rate consortia.

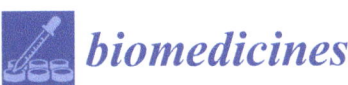

Editorial

Role of NO in Disease: Good, Bad or Ugly

Anders O. Larsson [1] and Mats B. Eriksson [2,3,*]

1 Department of Medical Sciences, Section of Clinical Chemistry, Uppsala University, 751 85 Uppsala, Sweden; anders.larsson@akademiska.se
2 Department of Surgical Sciences, Section of Anaesthesiology and Intensive Care Medicine, Uppsala University, 751 85 Uppsala, Sweden
3 NOVA Medical School, New University of Lisbon, 1099-085 Lisbon, Portugal
* Correspondence: mats.b.eriksson@uu.se; Tel.: +46-761333818

Citation: Larsson, A.O.; Eriksson, M.B. Role of NO in Disease: Good, Bad or Ugly. *Biomedicines* 2024, 12, 1343. https://doi.org/10.3390/biomedicines12061343

Received: 30 May 2024
Revised: 14 June 2024
Accepted: 17 June 2024
Published: 18 June 2024

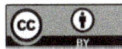

Copyright: © 2024 by the authors. Licensee MDPI, Basel, Switzerland. This article is an open access article distributed under the terms and conditions of the Creative Commons Attribution (CC BY) license (https://creativecommons.org/licenses/by/4.0/).

This Special Issue of *Biomedicines* (https://www.mdpi.com/journal/biomedicines/special_issues/NO_in_Disease), accessed on 30 May 2024, focuses on the role of nitric oxide in disease, attempting to demonstrate some of its "Good, Bad, or Ugly" effects. The Editors wish to thank the authors for their valuable contributions, and we are happy to present valuable studies on nitric oxide (NO) from multiple perspectives. NO is present in the airways, and its relationships with both chronic obstructive pulmonary disease and rheumatoid arthritis are highlighted. NO donations may also have therapeutic potential in bladder cancer. Furthermore, the biological sensing of NO using a ruthenium-based sensor may have great utility in atherosclerosis. NO in human breast milk, as determined via total nitrite and nitrate concentrations, is more abundant in the first 30 days than at day 60 postpartum; this may have implications for successful and unsuccessful breastfeeding. This Special Issue also contains five review articles, three of which indicate the importance of NO in various tissues and its relation to diseases; the potential effects of NO are reviewed in this context. Due to the SARS-CoV-2 pandemic, considerable interest has been paid to inhaled NO (iNO) and its ability to reduce inflammatory lung injury, lower pulmonary vascular resistance, and enhance ventilation/perfusion matching.

This Special Issue emphasizes the importance of NO and presents new data through various overviews that collate recent updates on NO.

In 1998, Robert Furchgott, Louis Ignarro, and Ferid Murad were awarded the Nobel Prize in Physiology or Medicine for their significant discovery of nitric oxide (NO) as a signaling molecule in the cardiovascular system. According to Alfred Nobel's will, a maximum of three persons can share the prize [1]. Therefore, Salvador Moncada was not awarded the Nobel Prize (a decision that has been criticized, even by Robert Furchgott) [2].

This highly potent two-atom radical containing an unpaired electron exhibits a wide range of physiological activities. NO has played a crucial role in evolution, from fungi to mammals, acting as both an intercellular and intracellular messenger in invertebrates [3].

NO is an essential biological mediator in the living organism that is biosynthesized from L-arginine using NADPH and molecular oxygen, a reaction catalyzed by enzymes termed nitric oxide synthases, consisting of different subtypes depending on the tissue type. Nitrite can act as a substrate for NOS-independent generation of NO in vivo, and such reduction can occur systemically in both blood and tissues [4,5]. NO has a short biological lifetime that can be counted in seconds (or even less) depending on its presence in intravascular/extravascular tissues [6]. In blood, NO rapidly reacts with oxygenated hemoglobin, forming its metabolites, nitrate and nitrite. The reaction rate of NO in aqueous solutions of with oxygen and hemoglobin follows second-order kinetics, i.e., the rate of NO's disappearance is proportional to the square of the concentration of NO. Thus, NO is not likely to act as a circulating humoral substance [7]. NO produced in the endothelial cells of blood vessels signals the surrounding smooth muscle to relax, leading to vasodilation and allowing for the biological activity of endothelium-derived relaxing factor and a subsequent increase in blood flow [8,9]. NO is also an important messenger in the central nervous system, where it facilitates cell communication. Glutamate, a neurotransmitter, starts a reaction that forms NO. NO regulates several important functions in the central nervous system, including processes associated with mood disorders [10,11].

Since NO among several other options is a vasodilator able to reduce both systemic and pulmonary blood pressure [12], various drugs have been designed to activate NO signaling and enhance NO bioavailability as beneficial cardiovascular effects; alternatively, by contrast, they may attenuate NO inactivation through reactive oxygen species exerting antioxidant effects. More recently, the products of NO oxidation, nitrite and nitrate, have been acknowledged as sources of NO after recycling back to NO. Activation of the nitrate–nitrite–NO pathway may generate NO from both anions and induce antihypertensive effects. Interestingly, human arterial blood added to a ruthenium-based NO sensor complex may be utilized as a point-of care test for early detection of unstable coronary plaque and monitoring of NO-related cardiovascular disease [13].

Furthermore, endogenous NO continuously regulates pulmonary and systemic circulations in several species (including humans), as evidenced by the fact that NOS inhibition increases pulmonary and systemic vascular resistance. Additionally, endogenous NO modifies hypoxic vasoconstriction. Inhaled NO is a selective pulmonary vasodilator; it rapidly diffuses across the alveolar–capillary membrane into the pulmonary vessels, where NO activates guanylate cyclase. Since inhalation of NO is a prerequisite for such an effect on the pulmonary vascular bed, the risk of ventilation/perfusion mismatch and pulmonary shunting is diminished. NO may decrease pulmonary arterial pressure and improve oxygenation and has therefore been approved by the FDA for treatment of hypoxic newborns affected by persistent pulmonary hypertension. More recently, the outbreak of SARS-CoV-2, a respiratory infectious disease that causes both pulmonary and cardiovascular complications, has exposed new indications for NO therapy. Endothelial dysfunction, increased pulmonary vascular permeability, and the formation of pulmonary venous thrombi frequently accompany SARS-CoV-2 infection and contribute to the development of pulmonary artery hypertension. Inhaled NO has the ability to counteract several of these deleterious effects of COVID-19. In a multicenter phase II trial, high-dose inhaled nitric oxide improved arterial oxygenation in adults with acute hypoxemic respiratory failure due to COVID-19. Whether inhaled NO may serve as an adjunct therapy against bacterial, viral, and fungal infections remains to be elucidated [14–18].

NO is synthesized during sepsis and septic shock, conditions that feature increased levels of NO and lowered blood pressure, the latter leading to subsequent impairment of organ perfusion. Several clinical trials have attempted to modulate the formation of inducible nitric oxide synthase (iNOS) from NO through treatment with nitric oxide synthase (NOS) inhibitors, of which L-NAME has been the most extensively studied. Contrary to what could be expected, L-NAME turned out to increase mortality in sepsis patients by increasing the number of cardiac and pulmonary adverse events. Asymmetric dimethylarginin (ADMA) is a direct endogenous NOS inhibitor that exerts microvascular dysfunction and proinflammatory and prothrombotic conditions in the endothelium, and there is a relationship between plasma levels of ADMA and mortality in sepsis patients. Hence, the lowering of ADMA has been suggested as a potential therapeutic approach to reduce organ damage and mortality in sepsis. NO may cause methemoglobinemia, a potentially life-threatening condition, since this form of hemoglobin cannot bind oxygen. This condition can be treated with methylene blue, which acts by blocking the enzyme guanylate cyclase, thereby reducing excessive nitric oxide production, counteracting its vasorelaxant effect, and increasing blood pressure during sepsis. Patients with sepsis and septic shock treated with methylene blue exhibit reduced time until vasopressor discontinuation, reduced length of stay in the intensive care unit, and reduced days on mechanical ventilation as compared to placebo. In a retrospective study evaluating the effect of methylene blue in shock, reduced 28-day mortality in critically ill patients was noted when methylene blue was administered as a bolus followed by a continuous infusion [19–21].

NO is a free radical that along with other free radicals contributes to the body's defense against micro-organisms. NO may also scavenge other free radicals and reacts in vivo with superoxide, thereby forming peroxynitrite, a highly reactive compound that can generate nitrogen dioxide and carbonate radicals upon reaction with carbondioxide. Excessive formation of peroxynitrite may contribute to numerous adverse events, including DNA damage and the disruption of cell membranes. Peroxynitrite is involved in several diseases but may also, at high concentrations, protect against microbes. At low concentrations, peroxynitrite exerts protective mechanisms in several organ systems [22]. Abundant production of NO can induce the release of inflammatory cytokines and also trigger oxidative stress, factors involved in the pathogenesis of several immunopathologies including diabetes, graft-versus-host reaction, rheumatoid arthritis, systemic lupus erythematosus, experimental autoimmune encephalomyelitis, and multiple sclerosis [23].

Thus, due to the multiple physiological and pathophysiological roles of NO, this Janus-faced molecule can act as a double-edged sword, exerting good, bad, and ugly effects.

Author Contributions: All authors contributed equally to the writing and editing of this Editorial. All authors have read and agreed to the published version of the manuscript.

Funding: This research received no funding.

Conflicts of Interest: The authors declare no conflicts of interest.

References

1. Facts on the Nobel Prize in Physiology or Medicine. Available online: https://www.nobelprize.org/prizes/facts/facts-on-the-nobel-prize-in-physiology-or-medicine/ (accessed on 30 April 2024).
2. de Berrazueta, J.R. The Nobel Prize for nitric oxide. The unjust exclusion of Dr. Salvador Moncada. *Rev. Esp. Cardiol.* **1999**, *52*, 221–226. [CrossRef]
3. Cristino, L.; Guglielmotti, V.; Cotugno, A.; Musio, C.; Santillo, S. Nitric oxide signaling pathways at neural level in invertebrates: Functional implications in cnidarians. *Brain Res.* **2008**, *1225*, 17–25. [CrossRef] [PubMed]
4. Lundberg, J.O.; Weitzberg, E. NO generation from nitrite and its role in vascular control. *Arterioscler. Thromb. Vasc. Biol.* **2005**, *25*, 915–922. [CrossRef] [PubMed]
5. Aktan, F. iNOS-mediated nitric oxide production and its regulation. *Life Sci.* **2004**, *75*, 639–653. [CrossRef] [PubMed]
6. Thomas, D.D.; Liu, X.; Kantrow, S.P.; Lancaster, J.R., Jr. The biological lifetime of nitric oxide: Implications for the perivascular dynamics of NO and O_2. *Proc. Natl. Acad. Sci. USA* **2001**, *98*, 355–360. [CrossRef] [PubMed]
7. Kelm, M. Nitric oxide metabolism and breakdown. *Biochim. Biophys. Acta* **1999**, *1411*, 273–289. [CrossRef] [PubMed]
8. Palmer, R.M.; Ferrige, A.G.; Moncada, S. Nitric oxide release accounts for the biological activity of endothelium-derived relaxing factor. *Nature* **1987**, *327*, 524–526. [CrossRef] [PubMed]
9. Moncada, S.; Radomski, M.W.; Palmer, R.M. Endothelium-derived relaxing factor. Identification as nitric oxide and role in the control of vascular tone and platelet function. *Biochem. Pharmacol.* **1988**, *37*, 2495–2501. [CrossRef] [PubMed]
10. Džoljić, E.; Grbatinić, I.; Kostić, V. Why is nitric oxide important for our brain? *Funct. Neurol.* **2015**, *30*, 159–163. [CrossRef]
11. Joca, S.R.L.; Sartim, A.G.; Roncalho, A.L.; Diniz, C.F.A.; Wegener, G. Nitric oxide signalling and antidepressant action revisited. *Cell Tissue Res.* **2019**, *377*, 45–58. [CrossRef]
12. Toda, N.; Ayajiki, K.; Okamura, T. Control of systemic and pulmonary blood pressure by nitric oxide formed through neuronal nitric oxide synthase. *J. Hypertens.* **2009**, *27*, 1929–1940. [CrossRef] [PubMed]
13. Vidanapathirana, A.K.; Goyne, J.M.; Williamson, A.E.; Pullen, B.J.; Chhay, P.; Sandeman, L.; Bensalem, J.; Sargeant, T.J.; Grose, R.; Crabtree, M.J.; et al. Biological Sensing of Nitric Oxide in Macrophages and Atherosclerosis Using a Ruthenium-Based Sensor. *Biomedicines* **2022**, *10*, 1807. [CrossRef]
14. Di Fenza, R.; Shetty, N.S.; Gianni, S.; Parcha, V.; Giammatteo, V.; Fakhr, B.S.; Tornberg, D.; Wall, O.; Harbut, P.; Lai, P.S.; et al. High-Dose Inhaled Nitric Oxide in Acute Hypoxemic Respiratory Failure Due to COVID-19: A Multicenter Phase II Trial. *Am. J. Respir. Crit. Care Med.* **2023**, *208*, 1293–1304. [CrossRef]
15. Ichinose, F.; Roberts, J.D., Jr.; Zapol, W.M. Inhaled nitric oxide: A selective pulmonary vasodilator: Current uses and therapeutic potential. *Circulation* **2004**, *109*, 3106–3111. [CrossRef]
16. Kamenshchikov, N.O.; Berra, L.; Carroll, R.W. Therapeutic Effects of Inhaled Nitric Oxide Therapy in COVID-19 Patients. *Biomedicines* **2022**, *10*, 369. [CrossRef] [PubMed]
17. Stamler, J.S.; Loh, E.; Roddy, M.A.; Currie, K.E.; Creager, M.A. Nitric oxide regulates basal systemic and pulmonary vascular resistance in healthy humans. *Circulation* **1994**, *89*, 2035–2040. [CrossRef]
18. Persson, M.G.; Gustafsson, L.E.; Wiklund, N.P.; Moncada, S.; Hedqvist, P. Endogenous nitric oxide as a probable modulator of pulmonary circulation and hypoxic pressor response in vivo. *Acta Physiol. Scand.* **1990**, *140*, 449–457. [CrossRef] [PubMed]

19. Singh, J.; Lee, Y.; Kellum, J.A. A new perspective on NO pathway in sepsis and ADMA lowering as a potential therapeutic approach. *Crit. Care* **2022**, *26*, 246. [CrossRef]
20. Ballarin, R.S.; Lazzarin, T.; Zornoff, L.; Azevedo, P.S.; Pereira, F.W.L.; Tanni, S.E.; Minicucci, M.F. Methylene blue in sepsis and septic shock: A systematic review and meta-analysis. *Front. Med.* **2024**, *11*, 1366062. [CrossRef]
21. Sari-Yavuz, S.; Heck-Swain, K.L.; Keller, M.; Magunia, H.; Feng, Y.-S.; Haeberle, H.A.; Wied, P.; Schlensak, C.; Rosenberger, P.; Koeppen, M. Methylene blue dosing strategies in critically ill adults with shock—A retrospective cohort study. *Front. Med.* **2022**, *9*, 1014276. [CrossRef]
22. Ascenzi, P.; di Masi, A.; Sciorati, C.; Clementi, E. Peroxynitrite-An ugly biofactor? *Biofactors* **2010**, *36*, 264–273. [CrossRef] [PubMed]
23. Liew, F.Y. Nitric oxide in infectious and autoimmune diseases. *Ciba Found. Symp.* **1995**, *195*, 234–239; discussion 239–244. [PubMed]

Disclaimer/Publisher's Note: The statements, opinions and data contained in all publications are solely those of the individual author(s) and contributor(s) and not of MDPI and/or the editor(s). MDPI and/or the editor(s) disclaim responsibility for any injury to people or property resulting from any ideas, methods, instructions or products referred to in the content.

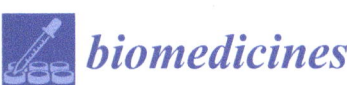

Communication

Total Nitrite and Nitrate Concentration in Human Milk and Saliva during the First 60 Days Postpartum—A Pilot Study

Jenny Ericson [1,2,3,*], Michelle K. McGuire [4], Anna Svärd [2] and Maria Hårdstedt [2]

1 School of Education, Health and Social Studies, Dalarna University, 791 88 Falun, Sweden
2 Center for Clinical Research Dalarna, Uppsala University, 753 10 Uppsala, Sweden; anna.svard@regiondalarna.se (A.S.); maria.hardstedt@regiondalarna.se (M.H.)
3 Department of Pediatrics, Falu Hospital, 791 82 Falun, Sweden
4 Margaret Ritchie School of Family and Consumer Sciences, University of Idaho, Moscow, ID 83844, USA; smcguire@uidaho.edu
* Correspondence: jeer@du.se

Abstract: Nitric oxide (NO) in human milk may have important functions in lactation and infant health. This longitudinal pilot cohort study investigated the total nitrite and nitrate (NOx) concentration in human milk and maternal saliva during the first 60 days postpartum. Additionally, we explored the association between selected breastfeeding variables and milk and saliva NOx concentration. Human milk and maternal saliva samples were collected on days 2, 5, 14, 30, and 60 postpartum and analyzed for NOx concentration. Breastfeeding data were collected through self-assessed questions. Data analyses were performed using mixed models. The concentration of NOx in milk was significantly higher during the first 30 days compared to day 60, and there was a positive association between milk and saliva NOx concentrations throughout the entire study period. In absolute numbers, partially breastfeeding mothers had a lower concentration of NOx in milk on day 2 compared to exclusively breastfeeding mothers (8 vs. 15.1 µM, respectively). Partially breastfeeding mothers reported a later start of secretory activation and fewer mothers in this group started breastfeeding within the first hour after birth. Due to the small numbers, these differences could not be statistically evaluated. Further research is warranted to elucidate the role of NO in lactation success and breastfeeding outcomes.

Keywords: breastfeeding; human milk; nitrate; nitric oxide; nitrite; saliva

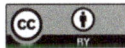

1. Introduction

Breastfeeding provides health benefits for both mothers and infants and reduces healthcare costs even in high-income countries [1]. Human milk fulfills the nutritional needs of the infant, regulates the immune system, protects against pathogens, and promotes neurological and metabolic development. Breastfeeding also offers long-term health advantages for the mother [1–4]. The World Health Organization recommends initiating breastfeeding within the first hour after birth and exclusively breastfeeding for the first six months, followed by continued partial breastfeeding for up to two years or more [5]. However, many mothers cease breastfeeding during the first months, often earlier than intended [6,7], and the underlying causes for this are inadequately understood. Previous studies have shown that the most common reasons for breastfeeding cessation are breastfeeding difficulties, including perceived low milk production [7,8]. As 70% of mothers experience breastfeeding difficulties, a statistic that is associated with higher rates of non-exclusive breastfeeding and subsequent increased risk of breastfeeding cessation, this is an important issue to address [7,8].

Nitric oxide (NO) and its metabolites serve as essential mediators in various physiological processes in the human body including neurotransmission, the regulation of vascular tone, host defense, and cellular respiration [9]. Nitrite and nitrate (referred to collectively, herein, as NOx), which are both relatively high in concentration in human milk [10], are believed to be involved in the physiological adaptation of infants to extrauterine life and may be involved in the process of lactation [11]. During the neonatal period, the infant has an immature immune system, less acidic gastric juices, and reduced bacterial communities in the mouth, which are all associated with increased susceptibility to infections. It is plausible that human milk-borne nitrite may contribute to antimicrobial activity in the infant's gastrointestinal tract [11]. In addition, several studies have indicated that NO may be involved in milk production and/or letdown [11–13].

In adults, the entero-salivary nitrate–nitrite–nitric oxide pathway contributes to a stable nitrite pool in the blood by ensuring an active uptake of dietary nitrate from the circulation by salivary glands and, subsequently, an incorporation of nitrate into saliva [11]. Bacteria in the mouth reduce salivary nitrate to nitrite, which is further reduced to NO and other nitrogen-containing metabolites in the stomach. Nitrite in human milk may compensate for the immature entero-salivary nitrate–nitrite–nitric oxide pathway of the infant. Human milk is an important source of nitrite, which may be relevant for both the formation of NO metabolites in the stomach of the infant as well as NO bioavailability in the systemic circulation [10,14].

The source of NOx in human milk remains unclear, but concentrations in milk appear to be independent of maternal nitrate intake [11]. Previous data suggest that higher nitrite concentrations in milk during the first days after birth are associated with an earlier lactation onset and greater milk output [15,16]. However, associations between concentration of NOx in milk and saliva and breastfeeding outcomes have been underexplored, and very little research has documented NOx concentration in human milk over time. Understanding the NO system and its regulation in breastfeeding women might be a key to understand both breastfeeding success as well as difficulties.

Hence, the primary aim of this pilot study was to document the total NOx concentration in human milk and maternal saliva collected over the first 60 days postpartum. In addition, we explored associations between NOx concentrations in milk and breastfeeding characteristics/outcomes such as exclusive versus partial breastfeeding.

2. Materials and Methods

2.1. Study Design and Participants

Data presented here were collected as part of a longitudinal cohort pilot study designed to understand factors related to lactation success in Swedish women. From 2021 to 2022, pregnant women in the county of Dalarna, Sweden were recruited through social media, leaflets, and/or midwives. Using a consecutive recruitment method, pregnant women ($\geq$18 years) who could answer questionnaires in Swedish and who consented to participate were included in the study.

2.2. Milk, Saliva, and Data Collection

Breastfeeding registration and self-report questionnaires regarding breastfeeding were collected through a mobile application on days 2, 5, 14, 30, and 60 postpartum or until breastfeeding cessation. Exclusive breastfeeding was defined as providing only human milk to the infant whereas partial breastfeeding involved providing a combination of human milk and infant formula.

The mothers provided five 3 mL samples of milk from one breast (not specified which) and three 2 mL samples of saliva on days 2, 5, 14, 30, and 60 postpartum or until breastfeeding cessation. Milk was collected by the mothers in their homes, in the morning, using a conventional manual breast pump provided by the research project. Women were not required to provide complete breast expressions, so milk was generally foremilk. Saliva samples were collected via passive drooling, where mothers allowed saliva to drip naturally into the tubes. Polypropene cryotubes (Sarstedt AG & Co. KG, Nümbrecht, Germany) were used for the saliva, and polystyrene tubes (Sarstedt AG & Co. KG, Nümbrecht, Germany) were used for the milk. Milk and saliva were frozen immediately at home and kept in home freezers (−20 °C) for up to 60 days, when they were transferred to a −80 °C freezer at the hospital.

2.3. Analysis

After thawing, milk was centrifuged three times to separate the aqueous phase from the lipid layer and cells (pellet): twice at 680× g (10 min, 4 °C) and once at 10,000× g (30 min, 4 °C) [17]. Saliva was thawed and centrifuged at 10,000× g for 10 min to separate solid particles (pellet) from the liquid portion (supernatant). Following centrifugation, supernatants from milk and saliva preparations were transferred to 96-well plates and frozen at −80 °C until further analysis. Total concentrations of NOx were measured using the Cayman's nitrite/nitrate colorimetric assay kit (no 780001) according to the manufacturer's instructions [18]. The Cayman colorimetric kit has previously been used for human milk [12]. The intra-assay % coefficients of variability (% CV) were 4.1 (SD 5.1) for breastmilk and 8.8 (SD 12.0) for saliva. Inter-assay % CV based on breastmilk analysis was 13.9 (SD 2.0).

Analyses of somatic cell count (SCC) and levels of sodium (Na) and potassium (K) were performed on whole milk according to the manufacturer's instructions. Somatic cell count was analyzed with DeLaval cell counter (DeLaval International AB, Tumba, Sweden). Sodium and potassium levels were determined using ion selective electrodes (sodium: LAQUAtwin Na-11; potassium: LAQUAtwin K-11; Horiba, Japan). The ratio between sodium and potassium was calculated; a ratio above 0.8 indicated mastitis.

2.4. Statistical Analyses

Data analyses were conducted using IBM SPSS Statistics for Windows (version 28.0). Descriptive statistics are presented here as medians and interquartile ranges (IQRs) or numbers and percentages. Total NOx concentrations in milk and saliva, together with breastfeeding characteristics, have been presented in total (all women) and subdivided by breastfeeding status, and exclusive versus partial breastfeeding, at day 60 postpartum. No analyses of comparative statistics were performed between mothers who exclusively versus partially breastfeed due to few cases in the latter group.

All statistics were performed on log-transformed data due to a right-skewed data distribution. Linear mixed-effect models were used to analyze the trajectory (i.e., days 2, 5, 14, 30, 60 postpartum) of NOx concentrations in milk and saliva. A linear mixed-effect model was also used to evaluate associations between NOx concentrations in milk and saliva. The linear mixed-effects modeling included repeated measurements with fixed effects of time. We used the covariance structure AR1, and model assumptions were checked. Reference levels (coded as 1) were taken at day 60 postpartum. If the value for the estimate was positive, the NOx concentration was lower in the reference group. If the value for the estimate was negative, NOx concentration was higher in the reference group. The linear mixed-effects model offers an advantage in dealing with missing outcome values as it allows for the inclusion of individuals in the analysis even when some outcome values are not available. Furthermore, it is a valuable statistical tool for analyzing longitudinal data due to its ability to accommodate the dependence among repeated measurements from the same individual over time. The results from the linear mixed-effects model analyses are presented here with estimates, which should be interpreted as the mean differences in total NOx concentration, 95% confidence intervals (95% CI), and p-values. Differences were considered significant if $p < 0.05$.

3. Results

Altogether, 25 mothers provided milk and saliva samples. Background characteristics and demographics of the participating mothers and their infants are presented in Table 1. Not all mothers could provide samples at all time points, and the total numbers of samples collected are presented in Table 2.

Table 1. Background demographics of participating mothers and infants ($n = 25$) and data related to pregnancy, delivery, and breastfeeding. Data are presented as medians and interquartile ranges [IQRs] or numbers and percentages (%).

	Total
Maternal demographics and health	
Age at time of birth, y [IQR]	32 [32–35.5]
Completed university education, n (%)	20 (80)
Cohabiting at time of birth, n (%)	21 (88)
Body mass index, kg/m² [IQR]	24.2 [21.5–26.9]
Maternal chronic disease *, n (%)	3 (12)
Mental illness #, n (%)	7 (29)
Diabetes (type 1, type 2, or gestational diabetes), n (%)	3 (13)
Pregnancy, delivery, and breastfeeding characteristics	
Primiparous, n (%)	7 (30)
Pregnancy complication, n (%)	2 (7)
Cesarean section, n (%)	2 (8)
Earlier breastfeeding experience, n (%)	15 (60)
Exclusive breastfeeding at discharge from maternity unit, n (%)	24 (100)
Infant characteristics	
Gestational age at birth, wk [IQR]	39 [39,40]
Male, n (%)	15 (63)
Birth weight, g [IQR]	3599 [3296–3974]

* Two mothers had asthma, one had a non-specified endocrine decease, and one had psoriasis arthritis. # The kind of mental illness was not specified.

Table 2. Total nitrate and nitrite (NOx) concentrations (µM) in milk and saliva and data related to breastfeeding in the 25 participating mothers up to 60 days postpartum. Data are presented as medians and intra-quartile ranges [IQR] or numbers and percentages (%), respectively. Data are given for all women as well as subdivided by breastfeeding status at day 60 postpartum.

	All Women		Exclusive Breastfeeding on Day 60 Postpartum		Partial Breastfeeding on Day 60 Postpartum	
	N	median [IQR] or number (%)	n	median [IQR] or number (%)	n	median [IQR] or number (%)
NOx (µM) in milk						
day 2	17	14.0 [3.2–54.4]	14	15.1 [3.8–54.4]	3	8.0 [3.2–22.2]
day 5	20	12.7 [3.8–28.5]	18	12.7 [3.8–28.5]	2	11.3 [7.5–15.1]
day 14	18	14.4 [5.3–41.3]	15	14.0 [5.3–38.0]	3	23.2 [13.3–41.3]
day 30	22	12 [4.0–48.5]	18	12.6 [4.0–48.5]	4	9.3 [5.7–17.1]
day 60	22	7.7 [3.0–23.8]	18	7.7 [3.0–23.8]	4	8.1 [3.4–13.8]
NOx (µM) in saliva						
day 2	12	28.6 [1.0–113.5]	11	17.5 [1.0–113.5]	1	59.3 [59.3]
day 5	16	59.1 [0.2–327.4]	13	51.4 [0.2–313.1]	3	104.8 [78.3–327.4]
day 14	16	87.6 [1.0–350]	13	82.6 [1.0–171.9]	3	257.4 [84.6–350.0]
day 30	18	63.7 [28.3–350]	15	59.3 [28.3–350.0]	3	87.5 [47.4–350.0]
day 60	17	49.2 [5.9–354.3]	13	43.0 [5.9–354.3]	4	103.7 [28.2–336.3]
Breastfeeding characteristics						
Breastfed during the first hour after birth	23	17 (74)	20	16 (80)	3	1 (33)
Reported secretory activation hours after birth	21	72 [24–120]	19	72 [48–120]	2	84 [72–96]
Exclusive breastfeeding						
day 2	24	22 (92)	21	21 (100)	3	1 (33)
day 5	23	20 (87)	20	19 (95)	3	1 (33)
day 14	23	21 (88)	19	18 (95)	4	1 (25)
day 30	23	19 (86)	19	18 (95)	3	1 (33)
day 60	23	21 (84)	21	21 (100)		
Number of breastfeeding sessions per day						
day 2	14	11 [7]	12	10.5 [5.8]	2	15
day 5	15	11 [7]	13	11 [7.5]	2	10
day 14	15	10 [3]	14	8 [2.8]	1	7 [0]
day 30	14	10 [5]	12	10.5 [5.5]	2	9
day 60	15	9 [6]	13	11 [4]	2	13

NOx Concentration in Milk and Saliva

The median total NOx concentration in milk collected on days 2, 5, 14, 30, and 60 postpartum was 12.3 µM (range 3.0–54.4 µM), and in saliva, it was 53.6 µM (range 0.2–354.3 µM) (Table 2 and Figure 1). The NOx concentration in milk was higher on days 2, 5, 14, and 30 postpartum compared to day 60 (estimate 0.88 (95% CI 0.76–1.00), $p < 0.001$) (Table 3). In saliva, total NOx concentration was lower on day 2 compared to days 5, 14, 30, 60 (estimate 1.72 (95% CI 1.42–2.01), $p < 0.001$) (Table 3). Based on the mixed model analysis, there was an association between NOx concentrations in milk and saliva (estimate 0.16 (95% CI 0.06–0.27), $p = 0.020$, result not shown in the table).

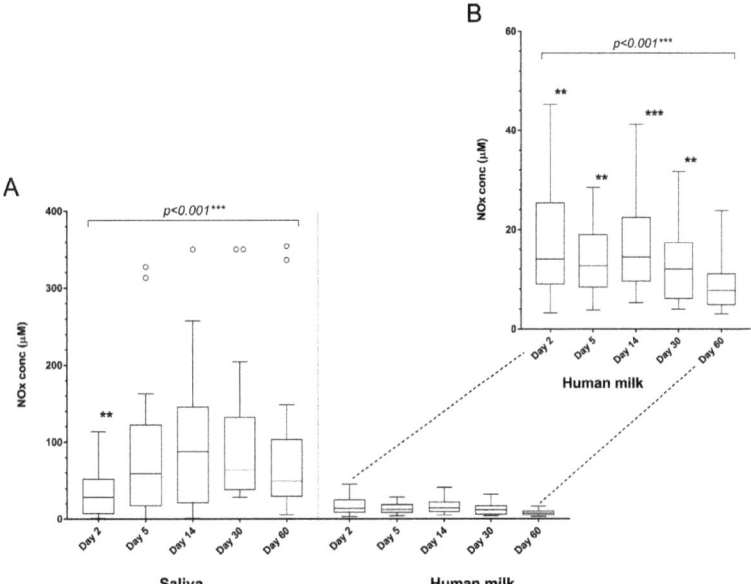

Figure 1. (**A**). Total nitrate and nitrite (NOx) concentration (µM) in milk and saliva on days 2, 5, 14, 30, and 60 postpartum. (**B**). Graph adjusted to better visualize NOx concentration in milk. Data are presented as Tukey boxplots; the box extends from the 25th to the 75th percentile with a horizontal line for the median; whiskers show maximum and minimum values, and outliers (>1.5* interquartile range) are plotted as individual dots. Presented in the figure are significant levels for the overall mixed model analysis and estimated marginal means compared to the concentration at day 60 (** $p < 0.01$, *** $p < 0.001$).

Table 3. Results of mixed model analysis comparing total concentrations of nitrite/nitrate (NOx, µM) in milk and saliva on days 2, 5, 14, 30, and 60 postpartum. Data are presented with estimates, 95% confidence intervals (95% CI), and *p*-values.

	Human Milk			Saliva		
	n	Estimate (95% CI)	*p*-Value	n	Estimate (95% CI)	*p*-Value
Model	25	0.88 (0.76–1.00)	<0.001	20	1.72 (1.42–2.01)	<0.001
day 2		0.27 (0.10–0.44)	0.002		−0.52 (−0.96–0.09)	0.019
day 5		0.22 (0.60–0.38)	0.008		−0.16 (−0.52–0.23)	0.42
day 14		0.29 (0.14–0.44)	<0.001		−0.005 (−0.37–0.36)	0.98
day 30		0.18 (0.05–0.30)	0.005		0.16 (−0.13–0.46)	0.28
day 60		ref			ref	

NOx concentration in milk during the first days postpartum was lower in partially breastfeeding mothers compared to exclusively breastfeeding mothers: 8 µM (range 3.2–22.2) vs. 15.1 µM (range 3.8–54.4), respectively. Partially breastfeeding mothers also reported a longer period of time until secretory activation (also referred to as secretory activation or "milk coming in"): 84 vs. 72 h compared to mothers still exclusively breastfeeding on day 60 postpartum. Furthermore, fewer of the partially breastfeeding mothers had initiated breastfeeding during the first hour after birth compared to mothers still exclusively breastfeeding on day 60 postpartum [1 (33%) vs. 16 (80%)]. However, these differences could not be statistically evaluated due to a small sample size. (Table 2). For two mothers, one at day 14 and one at day 30, self-reported symptoms, a high somatic cell count (1709 and 352 cells/µL) and Na/K ratio (1.04 and 1.24), suggested mastitis at the time of sampling. The total NOx concentrations in milk for these two mothers (16.9 and 15.2 µM) were slightly higher than the median concentrations of 14.4 µM on day 14 and 12 µM on day 30 based on all mothers.

4. Discussion

In summary, we have presented the natural time course of the total NOx concentration in human milk and maternal saliva during the first 60 days postpartum. The NOx concentration was higher on day 2 than on day 60, which was in line with the few previous studies published [14,15]. The NOx concentration remained relatively high until day 30, which means that not only colostrum, but also transitional and mature milk during the first month have high concentrations of NOx.

The concentration of NOx was higher in saliva than in milk, as previously shown [19]. A recent study examining NOx in plasma, saliva, and milk at one time point, at least 120 days after birth, found no association between nitrite concentrations in plasma and nitrite concentrations in milk. The authors suggested that complex mechanisms regulate concentrations of nitrite and nitrate in milk, probably reflecting the fact that NO is synthesized by the L-arginine–NO-synthase pathway locally in the mammary gland [19]. This was supported by data from Iizuka et al. [15] who did not find associations between NOx in plasma and milk. Interestingly, we found an association between NOx concentration in milk and saliva, based on repeated samples over a period of 60 days postpartum. Due to our small sample size, however, these results need to be further evaluated. In this study, we did not collect plasma samples, which was a limitation. Larger studies analyzing NOx, or nitrate and nitrite, simultaneously in milk, saliva, and plasma are needed to explore the association between concentrations in different body fluids in breastfeeding mothers.

Previous studies have suggested that NO may trigger lactation in humans with NOx concentration in milk peaking just before the initial increase in milk volume [16]. Furthermore, the NOx concentration was overall higher in milk produced by mothers characterized as high-milk-secreting compared to those producing lesser amounts of milk during the first days after birth [16]. In the present study, almost all women breastfed exclusively. Thus, we could not fully evaluate the potential association between NOx concentration in milk and breastfeeding exclusivity. However, we noted that mothers who would be only breastfeeding on day 60 postpartum (compared to those who would be exclusively breastfeeding on day 60 postpartum) tended to produce milk with lower NOx concentration at day 2 postpartum. These women also experienced delayed secretory activation, and fewer of them initiated breastfeeding during the first hour after birth compared to exclusively breastfeeding mothers. These differences could, however, not be statistically evaluated due to a small sample size. Only two mothers reported to have experienced mastitis during the study period; hence, our sample size was too small to assess any potential association between mastitis and NOx concentration. Interestingly, in cows and goats, mastitis is linked to increased concentrations of nitric oxide, nitrite, and nitrate [20,21]. Nitric oxide is believed to play a crucial role in the immune system, including antimicrobial effects [22]. Nevertheless, future studies should explore the relationship between mastitis and NO levels in humans as it appears to vary across different species [20].

There were several limitations to this study. First, the sample size was small, and the results should be interpreted with this in mind. Moreover, the duration of the study was only 60 days, and a longer follow-up could possibly allow more insight as to whether early NOx concentrations in milk might predict more long-term breastfeeding outcomes. Not all mothers provided samples at all occasions. However, the statistical mixed model method has the advantage of handling missing data. Another limitation was that the mothers represented a quite homogenous population, having high education levels, being multiparous, and showing a high percentage of exclusive breastfeeding. Previous studies have shown that highly educated women tend to breastfeed more exclusively and for a longer time [1]. For future research, the ability to recruit a broader population is important.

Nonetheless, no studies have documented NOx in milk and maternal saliva as extensively and longitudinally as the current study. Moreover, few studies have explored the physiological mechanisms of breastfeeding success and difficulties, and even fewer have focused on nitrite and nitrate concentration. This pilot study is part of a comprehensive research study with the goal of exploring the physiological causes of breastfeeding difficulties.

5. Conclusions

Based on the presented pilot study, the total concentration of NOx in human milk was higher during the first 30 days compared to day 60 postpartum. An association between NOx concentration in milk and saliva was found over the study period of 60 days postpartum. Since NO and its metabolites are believed to be essential for lactation, besides the suggested importance for the infant, studying NOx can provide clues both to the physiology of successful breastfeeding as well as to breastfeeding difficulties. Further larger longitudinal studies are needed.

Author Contributions: Conceptualization, J.E., M.H., M.K.M. and A.S.; methodology, J.E., M.H. and A.S.; software, J.E.; validation, J.E., M.H. and A.S.; formal analysis, J.E.; investigation, J.E.; data curation, J.E.; writing—original draft preparation, J.E.; writing—review and editing, J.E., M.H., M.K.M. and A.S.; visualization, M.H.; project administration, J.E.; funding acquisition, J.E. All authors have read and agreed to the published version of the manuscript.

Funding: This research was funded by Dalarna University, the Center for Clinical Research Dalarna, under grant number CKFUU-974923, CKFUU-936195, CKFUU-987306 and the Swedish Research Council for Health, Working Life and Welfare under grant number 2019-00634.

Institutional Review Board Statement: The study was conducted in accordance with the Declaration of Helsinki and approved by the Swedish Ethical Review Authority, Dnr 2020/02152. All methods in the study were conducted in accordance with relevant guidelines and regulations.

Informed Consent Statement: Informed consent was obtained from all subjects involved in the study after receiving both verbal and written information.

Data Availability Statement: The dataset generated in the current study is not publicly available due to ethical and legal reasons but is available from the corresponding author on reasonable request.

Acknowledgments: The authors would like to express their deepest gratitude to the women who participated in the study. We also thank Anders Larsson for the analysis of total NOx concentration in his laboratory at Uppsala University.

Conflicts of Interest: The authors declare no conflicts of interest in this research. The funders had no role in the design of the study; in the collection, analyses, or interpretation of data; in the writing of the manuscript; or in the decision to publish the results.

References

1. Victora, C.G.; Bahl, R.; Barros, A.J.D.; Franca, G.V.A.; Horton, S.; Krasevec, J.; Murch, S.; Sankar, M.J.; Walker, N.; Rollins, N.C.; et al. Breastfeeding in the 21st century: Epidemiology, mechanisms, and lifelong effect. *Lancet* **2016**, *387*, 475–490. [CrossRef]
2. Gila-Diaz, A.; Arribas, S.M.; Algara, A.; Martín-Cabrejas, M.A.; López de Pablo, Á.L.; Sáenz de Pipaón, M.; Ramiro-Cortijo, D. A Review of Bioactive Factors in Human Breastmilk: A Focus on Prematurity. *Nutrients* **2019**, *11*, 1307. [CrossRef]

3. Perez-Escamilla, R.; Tomori, C.; Hernandez-Cordero, S.; Baker, P.; Barros, A.J.D.; Begin, F.; Chapman, D.J.; Grummer-Strawn, L.M.; McCoy, D.; Menon, P.; et al. Breastfeeding: Crucially important, but increasingly challenged in a market-driven world. *Lancet* **2023**, *401*, 472–485. [CrossRef] [PubMed]
4. Bode, L.; Raman, A.S.; Murch, S.H.; Rollins, N.C.; Gordon, J.I. Understanding the mother-breastmilk-infant "triad". *Science* **2020**, *367*, 1070–1072. [CrossRef] [PubMed]
5. World Health Organization (WHO). Breastfeeding. Available online: https://www.who.int/health-topics/breastfeeding#tab=tab_2 (accessed on 18 February 2024).
6. The National Board of Health and Welfare in Sweden. Breastfeeding Statistics. Available online: http://www.socialstyrelsen.se/statistik/statistikdatabas/amning (accessed on 19 January 2020).
7. Gianni, M.L.; Bettinelli, M.E.; Manfra, P.; Sorrentino, G.; Bezze, E.; Plevani, L.; Cavallaro, G.; Raffaeli, G.; Crippa, B.L.; Colombo, L.; et al. Breastfeeding Difficulties and Risk for Early Breastfeeding Cessation. *Nutrients* **2019**, *11*, 2266. [CrossRef] [PubMed]
8. Karall, D.; Ndayisaba, J.P.; Heichlinger, A.; Kiechl-Kohlendorfer, U.; Stojakovic, S.; Leitner, H.; Scholl-Bürgi, S. Breast-feeding Duration: Early Weaning-Do We Sufficiently Consider the Risk Factors? *J. Pediatr. Gastroenterol. Nutr.* **2015**, *61*, 577–582. [CrossRef] [PubMed]
9. Moncada, S.; Higgs, A. The L-Arginine-Nitric Oxide Pathway. *NEJM* **1993**, *329*, 2002–2012. [PubMed]
10. Hord, N.G.; Ghannam, J.S.; Garg, H.K.; Berens, P.D.; Bryan, N.S. Nitrate and nitrite content of human, formula, bovine, and soy milks: Implications for dietary nitrite and nitrate recommendations. *Breastfeed. Med.* **2011**, *6*, 393–399. [CrossRef] [PubMed]
11. Kobayashi, J. Nitrite in breast milk: Roles in neonatal pathophysiology. *Pediatr. Res.* **2021**, *90*, 30–36. [CrossRef] [PubMed]
12. Ohta, N.; Tsukahara, H.; Ohshima, Y.; Nishii, M.; Ogawa, Y.; Sekine, K.; Kasuga, K.; Mayumi, M. Nitric oxide metabolites and adrenomedullin in human breast milk. *Early Hum. Dev.* **2004**, *78*, 61–65. [CrossRef] [PubMed]
13. Tezer, M.; Ozluk, Y.; Sanli, O.; Asoglu, O.; Kadioglu, A. Nitric oxide may mediate nipple erection. *J. Androl.* **2012**, *33*, 805–810. [CrossRef] [PubMed]
14. Jones, J.A.; Ninnis, J.R.; Hopper, A.O.; Ibrahim, Y.; Merritt, T.A.; Wan, K.; Power, G.G.; Blood, A.B. Nitrite and nitrate concentrations and metabolism in breast milk, infant formula, and parenteral nutrition. *J. Parenter. Enteral Nutr.* **2014**, *38*, 856–866. [CrossRef] [PubMed]
15. Iizuka, T.; Sasaki, M.; Oishi, K.; Uemura, S.; Koike, M.; Minatogawa, Y. Nitric oxide may trigger lactation in humans. *J. Pediatrics* **1997**, *131*, 839–843. [CrossRef] [PubMed]
16. Akçay, F.; Aksoy, H.; Memisogullari, R. Effect of breast-feeding on concentration of nitric oxide in breast milk. *Ann. Clin. Biochem.* **2002**, *39*, 68–69. [CrossRef] [PubMed]
17. Kverka, M.; Burianova, J.; Lodinova-Zadnikova, R.; Kocourkova, I.; Cinova, J.; Tuckova, L.; Tlaskalova-Hogenova, H. Cytokine profiling in human colostrum and milk by protein array. *Clin. Chem.* **2007**, *53*, 955–962. [CrossRef] [PubMed]
18. Green, L.C.; Wagner, D.A.; Glogowski, J.; Skipper, P.L.; Wishnok, J.S.; Tannenbaum, S.R. Analysis of nitrate, nitrite, and [15N] nitrate in biological fluids. *Anal. Biochem.* **1982**, *126*, 131–138. [CrossRef] [PubMed]
19. Fernandes, J.O.; Tella, S.O.C.; Ferraz, I.S.; Ciampo, L.A.D.; Tanus-Santos, J.E. Assessment of nitric oxide metabolites concentrations in plasma, saliva, and breast milk and their relationship in lactating women. *Mol. Cell Biochem.* **2021**, *476*, 1293–1302. [CrossRef] [PubMed]
20. Novac, C.S.; Andrei, S. The Impact of Mastitis on the Biochemical Parameters, Oxidative and Nitrosative Stress Markers in Goat's Milk: A Review. *Pathogens* **2020**, *9*, 882. [CrossRef]
21. Atakisi, O.; Oral, H.; Atakisi, E.; Merhan, O.; Pancarci, S.M.; Ozcan, A.; Marasli, S.; Polat, B.; Colak, A.; Kaya, S. Subclinical mastitis causes alterations in nitric oxide, total oxidant and antioxidant capacity in cow milk. *Res. Vet. Sci.* **2010**, *89*, 10–13. [CrossRef] [PubMed]
22. Bogdan, C. Nitric oxide and the immune response. *Nat. Immunol.* **2001**, *2*, 907–916. [CrossRef] [PubMed]

Disclaimer/Publisher's Note: The statements, opinions and data contained in all publications are solely those of the individual author(s) and contributor(s) and not of MDPI and/or the editor(s). MDPI and/or the editor(s) disclaim responsibility for any injury to people or property resulting from any ideas, methods, instructions or products referred to in the content.

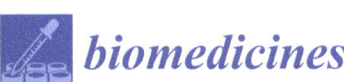

Article

Exhaled Nitric Oxide Reflects the Immune Reactions of the Airways in Early Rheumatoid Arthritis

Tomas Weitoft [1,2,*], Johan Rönnelid [3], Anders Lind [1], Charlotte de Vries [4], Anders Larsson [5], Barbara Potempa [6], Jan Potempa [6,7], Alf Kastbom [8], Klara Martinsson [8], Karin Lundberg [4] and Marieann Högman [9]

1. Centre for Research and Development, Uppsala University, Region Gävleborg, 801 88 Gävle, Sweden; anders.lind@regiongavleborg.se
2. Rheumatology, Department of Medical Science, Uppsala University, 751 85 Uppsala, Sweden
3. Department of Immunology, Genetics and Pathology, Uppsala University, 751 85 Uppsala, Sweden; johan.ronnelid@igp.uu.se
4. Rheumatology Unit, Department of Medicine, Karolinska University Hospital, 171 76 Solna, Sweden; charlotte.de.vries@ki.se (C.d.V.); karin.lundberg@ki.se (K.L.)
5. Clinical Chemistry, Department of Medical Science, Uppsala University, 751 85 Uppsala, Sweden; anders.larsson@akademiska.se
6. Department of Oral Immunity and Infectious Diseases, School of Dentistry, University of Louisville, 501 S. Preston St., Louisville, KY 40202, USA; barbara.potempa@louisville.edu (B.P.); jan.potempa@icloud.com (J.P.)
7. Faculty of Biochemistry, Biophysics and Biotechnology, Jagiellonian University, Gronostajowa St. 7, 31-387 Krakow, Poland
8. Department of Biomedical and Clinical Sciences, Linköping University, 581 83 Linköping, Sweden; alf.kastbom@liu.se (A.K.); klara.martinsson@liu.se (K.M.)
9. Department of Medical Science, Respiratory, Allergy and Sleep Research, Uppsala University, 751 85 Uppsala, Sweden; marieann.hogman@uu.se
* Correspondence: thomas.weitoft@regiongavleborg.se

Abstract: Patients with rheumatoid arthritis (RA) have altered levels of exhaled nitric oxide (NO) compared with healthy controls. Here, we investigated whether the clinical features of and immunological factors in RA pathogenesis could be linked to the NO lung dynamics in early disease. A total of 44 patients with early RA and anti-citrullinated peptide antibodies (ACPAs), specified as cyclic citrullinated peptide 2 (CCP2), were included. Their exhaled NO levels were measured, and the alveolar concentration, the airway compartment diffusing capacity and the airway wall concentration of NO were estimated using the Högman–Meriläinen algorithm. The disease activity was measured using the Disease Activity Score for 28 joints. Serum samples were analysed for anti-CCP2, rheumatoid factor, free secretory component, secretory component containing ACPAs, antibodies against *Porphyromonas gingivalis* (Rgp) and total levels of IgA, IgA1 and IgA2. Significant negative correlations were found between the airway wall concentration of NO and the number of swollen joints (Rho -0.48, $p = 0.004$), between the airway wall concentration of NO and IgA rheumatoid factor (Rho -0.41, $p = 0.017$), between the alveolar concentration and free secretory component (Rho -0.35, $p = 0.023$) and between the alveolar concentration and C-reactive protein (Rho -0.36, $p = 0.016$), but none were found for anti-CCP2, IgM rheumatoid factor or the anti-Rgp levels. In conclusion, altered NO levels, particularly its production in the airway walls, may have a role in the pathogenesis of ACPA-positive RA.

Keywords: rheumatoid arthritis; free secretory component; ACPA; exhaled nitric oxide; lung; pathogenesis; rheumatoid factor

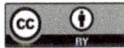

1. Introduction

Rheumatoid arthritis (RA) is a systemic inflammatory disease mainly affecting the joints and may lead to joint destruction and disability. In 50–80% of cases, autoantibodies against citrullinated proteins (ACPAs) or the Fc part of immunoglobulin G (IgG), rheumatoid factor (RF), are found [1]. ACPAs probably have an essential role in the disease, as they are also associated with a more severe disease course [2,3]. Consequently, RA with ACPAs and without ACPAs are often regarded as two different disease entities and may have different aetiologies [4].

Theories on the aetiology of RA involve a genetic predisposition and triggering exogenous factors, such as smoking [5], which may lead to a posttranslational shift in the amino acid arginine to citrulline in specific proteins, induced by the enzyme peptidyl arginine deaminase (PAD) [6]. This immune reaction may be triggered by inhaled agents and start in the mucosa of the gums, airways or lungs. The locally produced secretory antibodies (IgA and IgM) are transported through the mucosa by the polymeric immunoglobulin (poly Ig) receptor [7]. A shredded part of this receptor, free secretory component (free SC), is elevated in the serum of patients with ACPA-positive RA already before arthritis onset [8].

Another theory includes the bacterium *Porphyromonas gingivalis*, involved in periodontitis disease, which also expresses a PAD enzyme which may induce protein citrullination [9]. In accordance, RA patients have increased anti-*P. gingivalis* antibody levels, even before arthritis onset [10], and RA is four times more frequent in patients with periodontitis compared to the general population [11].

Nitric oxide (NO) is an important molecule in the inflammation process, inducing vascular dilatation and permeability [12], and is relevant in the cellular reactions of oxidative stress [13]. Elevated levels are found in the serum and synovial fluid of patients with RA [14]. In exhaled gas, the measured NO is produced by the cells of the airways and alveoli but is also influenced by the capillary diffusion of NO in the airways. In an extended NO analysis, using multiple NO measurements at different exhaled flows, it is possible to determine in which part of the lungs NO is produced. The Högman–Meriläinen algorithm (HMA) [15] gives estimates of the alveolar concentration (CA_{NO}), the airway compartment diffusing capacity (Daw_{NO}) and the airway wall concentration of NO (Caw_{NO}). Altered levels are found in disorders with inflammatory changes in the lungs and airways, such as asthma and chronic obstructive pulmonary disease [14], but also in rheumatic diseases, such as Sjögren's disease [16] and systemic sclerosis [17].

In a previous cross-sectional study on patients with chronic RA, we found not only lower NO levels in terms of CA_{NO} and Caw_{NO} but also a higher Daw_{NO} when compared with matched healthy controls [18]. Similar results were found in ACPA-positive RA patients with early disease investigated before any treatments were initiated, suggesting that these changes may reflect pulmonary involvement in its pathogenesis [19]. These subjects, representing a homogenous autoimmune disease entity, all with ACPAs, were re-analysed in the present study, where the objectives were to elucidate whether their exhaled NO levels were associated with characteristic RA autoantibodies and other markers of the autoimmune process.

2. Materials and Methods

2.1. Study Population

Patients (n = 51) with recent-onset ACPA-positive RA according to the 2010 classification criteria [20] were recruited at diagnosis on their first visit to the rheumatology department at Gävle Hospital, Sweden. After their informed consent and physical examination by a rheumatologist, the patients were included in the study. Patients with a symptom duration of more than two years at diagnosis, those treated with >10 mg prednisolone and those with difficulties understanding the study information were excluded (n = 7). The disease activity was measured using the Disease Activity Score for 28 joints (DAS28) [21], and disability was assessed according to the Health Assessment Questionnaire (HAQ) [22].

2.2. NO Analysis

The NO measurements were performed in accordance with the 2005 American Thoracic Society [23] and the European Respiratory Society [24]. The exhaled NO was analysed at an exhalation flow of 50 mL/s ($FE_{NO,50}$) using an EcoMedics DLC 88 (Eco Medics AG, Dürnten, Switzerland). The NO parameters were calculated using the nonlinear HMA method with exhalation target flows of 20, 100 and 300 mL/s or using the Tsoukias and George method with flows of 100, 200 and 300 mL/s [24] when the participants could not perform the lowest flow of 20 mL/s. A constant exhaled flow was facilitated using flow resistors, and a visual feedback system guided the patients in maintaining the targeted flow throughout the exhalation. The exact flow was measured. A calculated $FE_{NO,50}$ value for the HMA was derived for each subject and compared with the measured value as quality control [24]. The HMA method estimates the NO parameters CA_{NO}, Caw_{NO} and Daw_{NO}.

Serum nitrate/nitrite (NOx) was analysed using a Cayman nitrate/nitrite colorimetric assay kit (Ann Arbor, MI, USA). The total coefficient of variation for the NOx assay was 3.4%, and the detection limit was 1 µM/L.

2.3. Spirometry

Pre-bronchodilator spirometry was performed after the NO analysis using a Welch Allyn Spiro Perfect II (Welch Allyn, Skaneateles Falls, NY, USA). The reference values are presented as the percentages predicted using the Swedish reference values [25,26].

2.4. Blood Analyses

Samples were collected for analysis of their inflammatory markers, such as the erythrocyte sedimentation rate (ESR), C-reactive protein (CRP) and autoantibodies, including RF (IgA and IgM) and ACPAs (anti-CCP2 IgA and IgG), as well as free secretory component (SC), secretory component containing ACPAs (SC ACPAs) and antibodies against the *P. gingivalis* virulence factor arginine gingipain (Rgp) as a marker for periodontal infection/periodontitis.

2.5. Analyses of ACPA and RF

IgG and IgA anti-CCP2 and IgA and IgM RF were analysed using a fluorescence enzyme immunoassay (Elia, Thermo Fischer Scientific, Uppsala, Sweden) and using a Phadia 250 instrument (Thermo Fisher Scientific) according to the manufacturer's instructions. The cut-off levels for anti-CCP2 IgG and IgA were 7 arbitrary units (AU). For RF IgM, the cut-off was 5 AU, and for RF IgA, it was 20 AU, as suggested by the manufacturer.

2.6. Analyses of Free SC, SC ACPAs, Anti-Rgp IgG and Total IgA, IgA1 and IgA2

Free SC was analysed using an in-house sandwich ELISA [8,27]. Briefly, the serum samples were diluted 1:25, added to microtiter plates pre-coated overnight with 10 µg/mL of anti-free SC 6B3 monoclonal antibody (mAb) and incubated at 37 °C for 90 min for the serum and 60 min for the detection antibody. Following washing, an HRP-conjugated anti-SC mAb 5D8, diluted 1:100, was added and incubated at 37 °C for 60 min. TMB (Merck, Darmstadt, Germany) was added as substrate, and the reaction was stopped with 1 M sulfuric acid and the plates read at an optical density (OD) of 450 nm (SpectraMax ABS Plus, Molecular Devices, San Jose, CA, USA). We used a 7-step serially diluted SC-positive serum pool as the standard curve to recalculate the OD values into concentrations. All the samples were analysed in duplicate and reanalysed if the coefficient of variation (CV) between the duplicates was >20%. The inter-assay CV was 9%, and the intra-assay CV was 2%, respectively.

The serum SC ACPAs were measured by modifying anti-CCP2 ELISA kits (CCPlus® Immunoscan; Svar Life Science, Malmö, Sweden). In brief, the serum samples were diluted 1:25 in kit buffer, and the secondary antibody, detecting human secretory component, was diluted 1:2000 (polyclonal goat antibody conjugated to horseradish peroxidase, GAHu/SC/PO; Nordic Biosite, Täby, Sweden). Incubation and washing were performed according to the manufacturer's instructions. The reaction was stopped and the plates read at OD_{450nm} (SpectraMax ABS Plus). A 7-step standard curve based on a serum sample with known high levels of SC ACPAs was used to recalculate the OD values into arbitrary units. All the samples were analysed in duplicate and reanalysed if the CV between the duplicates was >20%. The inter-assay CV was 10%, and the intra-assay CV was 5%.

The presence of antibodies (IgG) against the oral pathogen *P. gingivalis* virulence factor arginine gingipains (Rgp) was assessed using an in-house ELISA, using the RgpB protein, purified from *P. gingivalis* cultures, as the coating antigen, as previously described [9]. The samples were analysed in duplicate, and a standard curve (pool of Rgp IgG-positive sera) was used to present the antibody levels in arbitrary units (AU).

The total levels of IgA, IgA1 and IgA2 were measured using in-house ELISAs. The total IgA ELISA utilised F(ab′)2 fragment goat anti-alpha chain antibodies for capture and detection (Jackson ImmunoResearch, West Grove, PA, USA), and the subclass-specific ELISAs both used the same capture antibody as for total IgA and the detection antibodies ABIN135642 for IgA1 and ABIN135646 for IgA 2, respectively (www.antibodies-online.com, accessed on 19 February 2024). The same normal serum was used as the standard curve for all the analyses; the levels of total IgA, IgA1 and IgA2 were determined at the Uppsala University laboratory.

2.7. Statistical Analysis

All the statistical analyses were performed using SPSS v. 28 for Windows (SPSS Inc., Chicago, IL, USA). The data tested for normality using the Shapiro–Wilk test are expressed as means ± SD and the skew-distributed data as medians and lower and upper quartiles. An independent t-test and the Mann–Whitney U test were used to compare current smokers and non-smokers. For the frequency distribution, Pearson's χ^2-test was used. Correlations were tested using Spearman's rank order correlation. A *p*-value of <0.05 was considered significant. The significance levels are presented both without and with Bonferroni correction for the number of NO variables investigated.

3. Results

3.1. Baseline Characteristics of the Study Population

As smoking affects pulmonary NO [28], the study participants (n = 44), 26 females and 18 males, were divided into subgroups depending on their current smoking status. The smoking subjects had significantly lower $FE_{NO,50}$ and CA_{NO} values but higher free SC levels in their serum (Table 1). A total of 10 subjects could not perform the lowest exhalation flow, and the results for Caw_{NO} and Daw_{NO} are given for 34 subjects in Table 1.

Table 1. Characteristics of participants with recent-onset ACPA-positive RA.

	All (n = 44)	Non-Smokers (n = 32)	Current Smokers (n = 12)	*p*-Value
Age (years)	60 ± 14	59 ± 16	62 ± 9	0.521
Sex (% female)	59%	66%	42%	0.150
BMI	28 ± 5	28 ± 5	28 ± 4	0.665
Symptom duration (months)	4 (2, 8)	5 (3, 8)	3 (2,11)	0.195
DAS28	4.47 ± 1.06	4.40 ± 1.19	4.65 ± 0.59	0.495
- Swollen joints	4 (2, 6)	3 (2, 5)	5 (3, 8)	0.153
- Tender joints	4 (2, 5)	4 (2, 6)	4 (1, 5)	0.866
- Global health	45 ± 24	42 ± 25	50 ± 21	0.478
- ESR	24 (12, 42)	20 (12, 40)	30 (13, 42)	0.679
CRP	7.9 (3.2, 20)	8.1 (2.6, 23)	7.1 (3.3, 14)	0.576
NOx	2.3 (1.8, 3.1)	2.4 (1.6, 3.1)	2.1 (1.3, 3.0)	0.243
HAQ	0.92 ± 0.46	0.89 ± 0.47	0.98 ± 0.45	0.591
Immunological markers				
IgA anti-CCP2 AU/mL	10.5 (3.1, 23)	6.8 (3.6, 21)	15.5 (2.4, 28)	0.668
IgG anti-CCP2 AU/mL	299 (93, 600)	288 (122, 600)	527 (56, 600)	0.706
IgA RF AU/mL	26 (12, 94)	25 (10, 56)	56 (25, 136)	0.059
IgM RF IU/mL	62 (20, 179)	49 (18, 131)	165 (34, 250)	0.100
Anti-Rgp AU/mL	361 (174, 727)	348 (168, 766)	369 (175, 563)	0.969
SC	0 (0, 30)	0 (0, 13)	24 (0, 47)	0.035
SC ACPAs	29 (12, 130)	24 (11, 62)	119 (16, 217)	0.082
Total IgA g/L	4.72 (3.77, 6.07)	4.76 (3.78, 6.31)	4.72 (3.85, 6.07)	0.645
Total IgA1, g/L	4.15 (2.74, 7.18)	4.15 (2.75, 7.18)	4.32 (2.56, 9.25)	1.000
Total IgA2, g/L	0.81 (0.48, 1.25)	0.78 (0.45, 1.23)	0.90 (0.54, 1.66)	0.377

Table 1. Cont.

	All (n = 44)	Non-Smokers (n = 32)	Current Smokers (n = 12)	p-Value
NO analysis				
$FE_{NO,50}$ ppb	16 (10, 24)	19 (13, 25)	10 (5, 16)	**0.002**
CA_{NO} ppb	1.6 (1.0, 2.2)	1.9 (1.2, 2.3)	1.0 (0.4, 1.3)	**0.004**
Caw_{NO} ppb (n = 34)	55 (24, 106)	64 (33, 115)	24 (20, 75)	0.086
Daw_{NO} mL/s (n = 34)	17 (8, 30)	16 (9, 31)	19 (7, 29)	0.809
Lung function				
FEV_1 % predicted	84 ± 15	87 ± 15	78 ± 15	0.446
FVC % predicted	86 ± 11	87 ± 11	84 ± 13	0.071

Data presented as means ± SD, and for skewed data, as medians (25–75-percentile); *p*-value of <0.05 was considered significant (highlighted in bold). BMI, body mass index; DAS28, Disease Activity Score for 28 joints; ESR, erythrocyte sedimentation rate; CRP, C-reactive protein; NOx, serum nitrate/nitrite; HAQ, the Swedish version of the Stanford Health Assessment Questionnaire; RF, rheumatoid factor; ACPA, anti-citrullinated protein antibody; anti-CCP2, antibody against cyclic citrullinated peptide, second generation; anti-Rgp; antibody against *P. gingivalis* arginine gingipains; IgA/IgG/IgM, immunoglobulin isotypes A, G and M; SC, secretory component; SC ACPAs, SC ACPA immune complex; $FE_{NO,50}$, fraction of exhaled nitric oxide at a flow of 50 mL/s; CA_{NO}, alveolar nitric oxide; Caw_{NO}, nitric oxide content in the airway wall; Daw_{NO}, nitric oxide diffusion capacity over airway wall; FEV_1, forced expiratory volume at 1 s; FVC, forced vital capacity.

3.2. NO in Relation to Clinical and Inflammation Markers

The serum levels of NO were correlated weakly with $FE_{NO,50}$ (Rho 0.304, $p = 0.048$). As in our previous study, we found no association with DAS28, but when splitting DAS28 into separate components (swollen joints, tender joints, general health and ESR), we found a negative correlation between the number of swollen joints and $FE_{NO,50}$ and especially Caw_{NO} (Table 2 and Figure 1A,B). For Daw_{NO}, this correlation was positive (Table 2). CA_{NO} was correlated with both CRP and SC (Table 2).

Table 2. Correlation of $FE_{NO,50}$ and NO parameters representing the airways and lungs in all participants.

	$FE_{NO,50}$ (n = 44)		Caw_{NO} (n = 34)		Daw_{NO} (n = 34)		CA_{NO} (n = 44)	
	Rho	p-Value	Rho	p-Value	Rho	p-Value	Rho	p-Value
DAS28								
Total score	−0.248	0.109	−0.327	0.063	0.150	0.406	0.169	0.279
Number of swollen joints	−0.336	**0.026**	−0.479	**0.004 ***	0.385	**0.025**	0.023	0.882
Number of tender joints	−0.171	0.268	−0.140	0.430	−0.076	0.669	−0.025	0.870
Global Health	−0.130	0.406	−0.023	0.901	−0.129	0.473	−0.068	0.666
ESR	−0.001	0.995	−0.111	0.532	0.167	0.346	0.285	0.064
CRP	0.030	0.848	−0.136	0.442	0.172	0.332	0.362	**0.016**
Immunological markers								
IgA anti-CCP2	−0.113	0.465	−0.180	0.309	0.138	0.435	0.063	0.686
IgG anti-CCP2	−0.148	0.311	−0.181	0.305	0.107	0.547	−0.027	0.860
IgA RF	−0.171	**0.036**	−0.406	**0.017**	0.357	**0.037**	−0.001	0.994
IgM RF	−0.173	0.262	−0.151	0.394	0.001	0.994	0.039	0.804
IgG anti-Rgp	−0.063	0.683	−0.044	0.803	0.027	0.878	0.015	0.922
SC	−0.173	0.266	−0.007	0.971	−0.160	0.366	−0.345	**0.023**
SC ACPA	−0.255	0.103	−0.050	0.783	−0.093	0.608	−0.131	0.408
Total IgA	0.184	0.231	0.087	0.624	0.141	0.427	0.071	0.646
Total IgA1	0.270	0.076	−0.035	0.844	0.242	0.168	0.128	0.406
Total IgA2	0.062	0.689	−0.169	0.339	0.130	0.462	−0.047	0.759

* = remains significant ($p = 0.020$) after Bonferroni correction. *p*-value of <0.05 was considered significant (highlighted in bold). DAS28, Disease Activity Score for 28 joints; ESR, erythrocyte sedimentation rate; CRP, C-reactive protein; RF, rheumatoid factor; ACPA, anti-citrullinated protein antibody; anti-CCP2, antibody against cyclic citrullinated peptide, second generation; anti-Rgp, antibody against *P. gingivalis* arginine gingipains; IgA/IgG/IgM, immunoglobulin isotypes A, G and M; SC, secretory component; SC ACPAs, SC ACPA immune complex; $FE_{NO,50}$, fraction of exhaled nitric oxide at a flow of 50 mL/s; CA_{NO}, alveolar nitric oxide; Caw_{NO}, nitric oxide content in the airway wall; Daw_{NO}, nitric oxide diffusion capacity over airway wall.

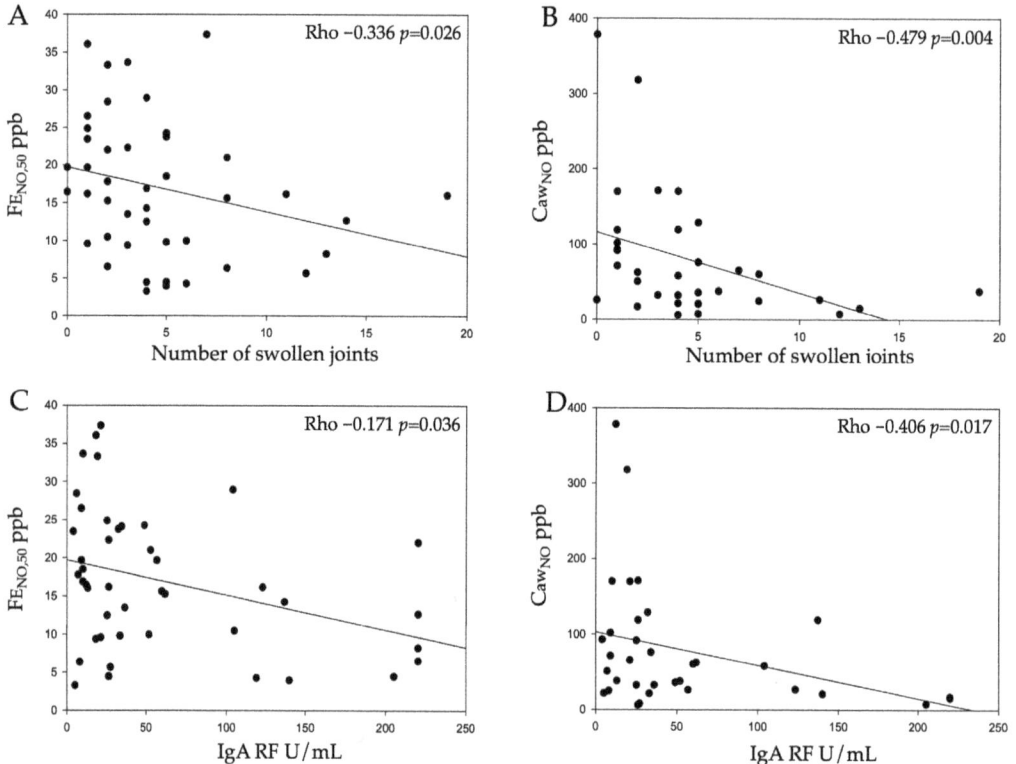

Figure 1. Correlation plots for $FE_{NO,50}$ and Caw_{NO} for the number of swollen joints (**A,B**), and for IgA RF (**C,D**).

3.3. NO in Relation to Antibodies

In this material, of the anti-CCP-IgG-positive RA participants, 52% also had anti-CCP2 IgA, 93% had IgM RF and 64% had IgA RF. The levels of anti-CCP2 (IgA and IgG) and IgM RF did not correlate with the exhaled NO parameters (Table 2). IgA RF was correlated negatively with Caw_{NO} and $FE_{NO,50}$, while Daw_{NO} showed a positive correlation (Table 2 and Figure 1C,D). Among the smokers, the proportion of IgA-RF-positive parties was 83% compared with 67% in the non-smokers (n.s.). When comparing the non-smoking patients with the current smokers, there were no statistical differences in any antibody level.

Free SC in the serum was found in 44% of patients (67% current smokers, 36% non-smokers, $p = 0.065$), and its levels were negatively correlated with CA_{NO}. The SC ACPAs, anti-Rgp IgG and the total levels of the IgA and IgA subclasses did not correlate with the exhaled NO parameters (Table 2).

4. Discussion

The main findings in the present study were negative correlations between the exhaled NO levels, especially the airway wall concentration of NO (Caw_{NO}), and the number of swollen joints and IgA RF levels, respectively, in ACPA-positive RA. In addition, the lack of an association with the anti-CCP2 antibody levels or the SC ACPAs suggests that altered NO dynamics in the lungs reflect another biological process in early RA.

We have previously found that patients with recent-onset RA have significantly lower exhaled NO parameters than matched healthy control subjects [18]. It is known that smoking decreases these levels in healthy individuals. Our studies confirm that this is true for patients with early and chronic RA as well [18,19]. However, the levels were also low in the non-smoking patients, especially Caw$_{NO}$, suggesting that smoking reduces the already low NO levels in the airways of ACPA-positive RA patients. It is not known whether other inhaled agents associated with RA pathogenesis, such as silica and textile dust, may also reduce the exhaled NO levels in non-smoking RA patients.

As smoking is a known triggering factor in the pathogenesis of seropositive RA [29], we looked for an association between RA-specific autoantibodies and the exhaled NO levels. We found a significant negative correlation between IgA RF and the NO levels in the airway wall compartment but not for the NO levels in the alveoli, suggesting an immune-mediated process localised to the airways. The link between airway diseases and ACPA-positive RA is excellently described by Matson et al. [30]. The authors also present theories on the immune reactions of the airways and their relevance to RA's pathogenesis.

Generally, IgA is a secretory antibody dominating the mucosal tissue. Smoking in healthy individuals may increase serum IgA levels [31], including IgA RF, as shown in a non-arthritic population from Iceland, where the presence of IgA RF was more frequent in smokers than in non-smokers [32]. Also, among RA patients, smokers also have elevated IgA RF levels compared to non-smokers [31], and we saw the same trend in our early RA cohort. Additionally, smoking has been linked to increased RA disease activity [33] and a reduced RA treatment response to anti-rheumatic therapies, such as anti-TNF treatment [34].

In patients with RA, serum IgA RF levels correlate with saliva and tear fluid levels, which may support local mucosal IgA RF production [35]. In our study, IgA RF was correlated negatively with Caw$_{NO}$ and FE$_{NO,50}$, and since IgA antibodies are present mainly in the mucosa, our data support the hypothesis that immune reactions in the airway mucosa are essential in early seropositive RA.

RA patients have elevated levels of total IgA [36,37], and serum levels of IgA and IgG can predict future RA development [38], while serum levels of IgA, but not IgG or IgM, have been associated with the degree of cartilage erosions in patients with established RA for $\geq$1 year [39]. Due to the unique association between IgA RF and the NO parameters in our study, pointing towards primarily airway involvement, we also analysed the total levels of IgA as well as the IgA subclasses in relation to the NO parameters (Table 2) and smoking (Table 1), but we did not find any associations.

In line with previous findings [8], the free SC in the serum was increased among the currently or previously smoking RA patients. Therefore, the negative correlation between CA$_{NO}$ and free SC in the serum is difficult to disentangle since smoking is associated with reduced NO levels. Nevertheless, the poly Ig receptor is readily expressed in small airways [40], and RA-related pro-inflammatory cytokines such as interferon gamma and TNF are known to upregulate poly Ig receptor expression [41]. Thus, a potential link between local NO production, inflammation and free SC release may exist but needs further characterisation [41].

We found no correlation between the exhaled NO parameters and the ACPA levels, measured as IgG and IgA anti-CCP2 or SC ACPAs. We deliberately focused this investigation on ACPA-positive RA, as this is the subgroup of patients with the most severe prognosis and most probably represents a disease entity on its own [42]. Therefore, we do not know how these analyses would have looked if we had included both (IgG) ACPA-positive and ACPA-negative patients, nor did we find any associations between the NO levels and antibodies against the *P. gingivalis* antigen Rgp. The low NO levels in the exhaled gas may reflect NO-consuming processes in RA pathogenesis, such as oxidative stress during inflammation and the production of reactive oxygen species [43]. Alternatively, this may depend on arginine depletion because of the increased arginase activity seen in RA and the subsequent substrate competition with inducible nitric oxide synthase (iNOS) [44]. Both enzymes use arginine as a substrate for their activity.

One or more swollen joints are required for RA diagnosis [20], and this clinical finding is essential to and the basis for all arthritis diagnoses. The strong correlation observed between the number of swollen joints and decreasing exhaled NO parameters in early ACPA-positive RA, which remained after Bonferroni correction for multiple testing, supports the need for future studies on exhaled NO as a predictor of arthritis onset in ACPA-positive at-risk individuals. This is further corroborated by our own recent findings, showing that in early RA, ACPAs but not RF are specifically associated with a lower number of inflamed joints as compared to ACPA-negative patients [45]. Together, these findings implicate that in early ACPA-positive RA, a low number of swollen joints is strongly associated with a higher airway NO concentration (but still lower than that of healthy controls) [18] and that this local change in NO in the airway walls might be specifically associated with ACPA-positive RA. Further studies regarding exhaled NO in ACPA-positive individuals who subsequently develop RA are therefore needed. What impacts the size of the swollen joints and the NO levels in synovial fluid may have has not been investigated either. The exhaled NO levels in other arthritis diseases have also been incompletely studied. Several questions remain to be answered on this topic.

Our findings of reduced exhaled NO parameters in association with IgA RF levels—but not IgM RF or ACPA levels—may indicate that several different inflammatory and immunological reactions are present in the airway mucosa of patients with early RA. The lack of an association with ACPA levels may suggest that our findings reflect another parallel and independent smoking-related immunological process. Moreover, the lack of an association between NO and anti-Rgp IgG levels (reflecting periodontitis) suggests that periodontal inflammation, which is linked to ACPA-positive RA, does not influence the exhaled NO levels.

A limitation of this study is the small number of participating subjects, and a larger study is needed to confirm the results. In addition, parallel examinations of ACPA-positive and ACPA-negative RA patients, and high-resolution computed tomography of the lungs to detect parenchymal changes, would be desired. As interstitial lung disease is common but present only in a minority of patients with early RA [46], a future investigation correcting for these limitations should be a larger multicentre study.

In conclusion, the altered NO dynamics of the lungs in patients with early ACPA-positive RA were correlated with IgA RF levels and the number of swollen joints, suggesting that NO, especially a reduced NO concentration in the airway walls, may be relevant to RA pathogenesis.

Author Contributions: T.W., M.H. and J.R. designed the study. T.W. and A.L. (Anders Lind) recruited the patients. J.R. and A.L. (Anders Larsson) performed the chemical and immunological analysis. A.K. and K.M. analysed the free SC and SC ACPAs. K.L. and C.d.V. were responsible for performing the anti-Rgp IgG ELISA and the related analyses. B.P. and J.P. purified and supplied the RgpB protein. T.W., M.H. and J.R. were responsible for the acquisition and statistical analysis of the data. All authors have read and agreed to the published version of the manuscript.

Funding: Local funding was sourced from the Centre for Research and Development, Uppsala University/Region Gävleborg. The NO analyser was paid for with funds from Gävle Cancer Foundation. The Rgp IgG analyses performed at Karolinska Institutet were funded by research grants from King Gustaf V's 80-year Foundation (FAI-2021-0771) and the Swedish Rheumatism Foundation (R-969194). B.P. and J.P. are supported by grants from US NIH/NIDCR (DE 022597) and the National Science Center (UMO-2018/30/A/NZ5/00650, NCN, Krakow, Poland).

Institutional Review Board Statement: The Regional Review Board in Uppsala, Sweden, approved the study on 7 October 2015 (Dnr 2015/370-1). The study was performed in accordance with the Declaration of Helsinki.

Informed Consent Statement: Written informed consent was obtained from all subjects involved in the study.

Data Availability Statement: Data are available upon reasonable request by contacting the corresponding author.

Acknowledgments: The authors wish to thank the participating patients and Liselotte Sundgren, the research nurse at the Centre for Research and Development, Uppsala University/Region Gävleborg.

We also thank Irina Griazeva and Marina Samoylovich at Granov Russian Research Center of Radiology and Surgical Technologies, Sankt-Petersburg, Russia, for the collaboration on the free SC. We are grateful to Kyra Gerderman at Sanquin Diagnostics, Amsterdam, the Netherlands, and to Anna Svanqvist and Christine Möller Westerberg, who assisted in and performed the analyses of the total levels of IgA, IgA1 and IgA2 in the samples.

Conflicts of Interest: The authors declare no conflicts of interest.

Abbreviations

ACPA	anti-citrullinated protein/peptide antibody
AU	arbitrary unit
Anti-CCP2	anti-cyclic citrullinated peptide version 2
BMI	body mass index
CA_{NO}	alveolar NO
Caw_{NO}	NO content in the airway walls
CV	coefficient of variation
DAS28	Disease Activity Score for 28 joints
Daw_{NO}	NO diffusion capacity over the airway wall
ESR	erythrocyte sedimentation rate
$FE_{NO,50}$	fraction of exhaled nitric oxide at a flow of 50 mL/s
FEV_1	forced expiratory volume at 1 s
FVC	forced vital capacity
HAQ	Health Assessment Questionnaire
HMA	Högman–Meriläinen algorithm
Ig	immunoglobulin
mAb	monoclonal antibody
NO	nitric oxide
iNOS	nitric oxide synthase
NOx	nitrate/nitrite in serum
OD	optical density
PAD	peptidyl arginine deaminase
Poly Ig	polymeric immunoglobulin
ppb	parts per billion
RF	rheumatoid factor
Rgp	arginine gingipain
SC	secretory component
CRP	C-reactive protein
TNF	tumour necrosis factor

References

1. Scott, D.L.; Wolfe, F.; Huizinga, T.W. Rheumatoid arthritis. *Lancet* **2010**, *376*, 1094–1108. [CrossRef]
2. Rönnelid, J.; Wick, M.C.; Lampa, J.; Lindblad, S.; Nordmark, B.; Klareskog, L.; van Vollenhoven, R. Longitudinal analysis of anti-citrullinated protein/peptide antibodies (anti-CP) during 5 year follow-up in early rheumatoid arthritis: Anti-CP status is a stable phenotype that predicts worse disease activity and greater radiological progression. *Ann. Rheum. Dis.* **2005**, *64*, 1744–1749. [CrossRef] [PubMed]
3. Kastbom, A.; Strandberg, G.; Lindroos, A.; Skogh, T. Anti-CCP antibody test predicts the disease course during 3 years in early rheumatoid arthritis (the Swedish TIRA project). *Ann. Rheum. Dis.* **2004**, *63*, 1085–1089. [CrossRef]
4. Malmström, V.; Catrina, A.I.; Klareskog, L. The immunopathogenesis of seropositive rheumatoid arthritis: From triggering to targeting. *Nat. Rev. Immunol.* **2017**, *17*, 60–75. [CrossRef] [PubMed]
5. Catrina, A.I.; Ytterberg, A.J.; Reynisdottir, G.; Malmstrom, V.; Klareskog, L. Lungs, joints and immunity against citrullinated proteins in rheumatoid arthritis. *Nat. Rev. Rheumatol.* **2014**, *10*, 645–653. [CrossRef]
6. Curran, A.M.; Naik, P.; Giles, J.T.; Darrah, E. PAD enzymes in rheumatoid arthritis: Pathogenic effectors and autoimmune targets. *Nat. Rev. Rheumatol.* **2020**, *16*, 301–315. [CrossRef]
7. Brandtzaeg, P. Mucosal immunity: Induction, dissemination, and effector functions. *Scand. J. Immunol.* **2009**, *70*, 505–515. [CrossRef] [PubMed]
8. Martinsson, K.; Ljungberg, K.R.; Ziegelasch, M.; Cedergren, J.; Eriksson, P.; Klimovich, V.; Reckner, Å.; Griazeva, I.; Sjöwall, C.; Samoylovich, M.; et al. Elevated free secretory component in early rheumatoid arthritis and prior to arthritis development in patients at increased risk. *Rheumatology* **2020**, *59*, 979–987. [CrossRef]

9. de Molon, R.S.; Rossa, C., Jr.; Thurlings, R.M.; Cirelli, J.A.; Koenders, M.I. Linkage of Periodontitis and Rheumatoid Arthritis: Current Evidence and Potential Biological Interactions. *Int. J. Mol. Sci.* **2019**, *20*, 4541. [CrossRef]
10. Kharlamova, N.; Jiang, X.; Sherina, N.; Potempa, B.; Israelsson, L.; Quirke, A.M.; Eriksson, K.; Yucel-Lindberg, T.; Venables, P.J.; Potempa, J.; et al. Antibodies to *Porphyromonas gingivalis* Indicate Interaction Between Oral Infection, Smoking, and Risk Genes in Rheumatoid Arthritis Etiology. *Arthritis Rheumatol.* **2016**, *68*, 604–613. [CrossRef]
11. Mercado, F.; Marshall, R.I.; Klestov, A.C.; Bartold, P.M. Is there a relationship between rheumatoid arthritis and periodontal disease? *J. Clin. Periodontol.* **2000**, *27*, 267–272. [CrossRef] [PubMed]
12. Ricciardolo, F.L.; Sterk, P.J.; Gaston, B.; Folkerts, G. Nitric oxide in health and disease of the respiratory system. *Physiol. Rev.* **2004**, *84*, 731–765. [CrossRef] [PubMed]
13. Ricciardolo, F.L.; Di Stefano, A.; Sabatini, F.; Folkerts, G. Reactive nitrogen species in the respiratory tract. *Eur. J. Pharmacol.* **2006**, *533*, 240–252. [CrossRef] [PubMed]
14. Farrell, A.J.; Blake, D.R.; Palmer, R.M.; Moncada, S. Increased concentrations of nitrite in synovial fluid and serum samples suggest increased nitric oxide synthesis in rheumatic diseases. *Ann. Rheum. Dis.* **1992**, *51*, 1219–1222. [CrossRef] [PubMed]
15. Högman, M.; Holmkvist, T.; Wegener, T.; Emtner, M.; Andersson, M.; Hedenström, H.; Meriläinen, P. Extended NO analysis applied to patients with COPD, allergic asthma and allergic rhinitis. *Respir. Med.* **2002**, *96*, 24–30. [CrossRef] [PubMed]
16. Högman, M. Extended NO analysis applied to patients with known altered values of exhaled NO. In *Disease Markers in Exhaled Breath Basic Mechanism and Clinical Application*; Marczin, N., Yacoub, M.H., Eds.; NATO Science Series: Series I: Life Behavioural Sciences 346; IOS Press: Amsterdam, The Netherlands, 2002; pp. 187–190.
17. Tiev, K.P.; Le-Dong, N.N.; Duong-Quy, S.; Hua-Huy, T.; Cabane, J.; Dinh-Xuan, A.T. Exhaled nitric oxide, but not serum nitrite and nitrate, is a marker of interstitial lung disease in systemic sclerosis. *Nitric Oxide* **2009**, *20*, 200–206. [CrossRef] [PubMed]
18. Thornadtsson, A.; Lind, A.; Weitoft, T.; Högman, M. Altered levels of exhaled nitric oxide in rheumatoid arthritis. *Nitric Oxide* **2018**, *76*, 1–5. [CrossRef] [PubMed]
19. Weitoft, T.; Lind, A.; Larsson, A.; Rönnelid, J.; Högman, M. Exhaled nitric oxide in early rheumatoid arthritis and effects of methotrexate treatment. *Sci. Rep.* **2022**, *12*, 6489. [CrossRef] [PubMed]
20. Aletaha, D.; Neogi, T.; Silman, A.J.; Funovits, J.; Felson, D.T.; Bingham, C.O., 3rd; Birnbaum, N.S.; Burmester, G.R.; Bykerk, V.P.; Cohen, M.D.; et al. 2010 Rheumatoid arthritis classification criteria: An American College of Rheumatology/European League Against Rheumatism collaborative initiative. *Ann. Rheum. Dis.* **2010**, *69*, 1580–1588. [CrossRef] [PubMed]
21. Prevoo, M.L.; van t'Hof, M.A.; Kuper, H.H.; van Leeuwen, M.A.; van de Putte, L.B.; van Riel, P.L. Modified disease activity scores that include twenty-eight-joint counts. Development and validation in a prospective longitudinal study of patients with rheumatoid arthritis. *Arthritis Rheum.* **1995**, *38*, 44–48. [CrossRef]
22. Ekdahl, C.; Eberhardt, K.; Andersson, S.I.; Svensson, B. Assessing disability in patients with rheumatoid arthritis. *Scand. J. Rheumatol.* **1988**, *17*, 263–271. [CrossRef] [PubMed]
23. The American Thoracic Society (ATS); The European Respiratory Society (ERS). ATS/ERS recommendations for standardized procedures for the online and offline measurement of exhaled lower respiratory nitric oxide and nasal nitric oxide, 2005. *Am. J. Respir. Crit. Care Med.* **2005**, *171*, 912–930. [CrossRef] [PubMed]
24. Horváth, I.; Barnes, P.J.; Loukides, S.; Sterk, P.J.; Högman, M.; Olin, A.-C.; Amann, A.; Antus, B.; Baraldi, E.; Bikov, A.; et al. A European Respiratory Society technical standard: Exhaled biomarkers in lung disease. *Eur. Respir. J.* **2017**, *49*, 1600965. [CrossRef]
25. Hedenström, H.; Malmberg, P.; Agarwal, K. Reference values for lung function tests in female. Regression equations with smoking variables. *Bull. Eur. Physiopathol. Respir.* **1985**, *21*, 551–557. [PubMed]
26. Hedenström, H.; Malmberg, P.; Fridriksson, H.V. Reference values for pulmonary function test in men: Regression equations which include tobacco smoking variables. *Upsala J. Med. Sci.* **1986**, *91*, 299–310. [CrossRef] [PubMed]
27. Griazeva, I.V.; Samoĭlovich, M.P.; Klimovich, B.V.; Pavlova, M.S.; Vartanian, N.L.; Kirienko, A.N.; Klimovich, V.B. Monoclonal antibodies against human secretory component: Epitope specificity and utility for immunoanalysis. *Zhurnal Mikrobiol. Epidemiol. Immunobiol.* **2010**, *4*, 54–59.
28. Malinovschi, A.; Janson, C.; Holmkvist, T.; Norbäck, D.; Meriläinen, P.; Högman, M. Effect of smoking on exhaled nitric oxide and flow-independent nitric oxide exchange parameters. *Eur. Respir. J.* **2006**, *28*, 339–345. [CrossRef] [PubMed]
29. Tarbiah, N.; Todd, I.; Tighe, P.J.; Fairclough, L.C. Cigarette smoking differentially affects immunoglobulin class levels in serum and saliva: An investigation and review. *Basic Clin. Pharmacol. Toxicol.* **2019**, *125*, 474–483. [CrossRef] [PubMed]
30. Matson, S.M.; Demoruelle, M.K.; Castro, M. Airway Disease in Rheumatoid Arthritis. *Ann. Am. Thorac. Soc.* **2022**, *19*, 343–352. [CrossRef]
31. Jonsson, T.; Thorsteinsson, J.; Valdimarsson, H. Does smoking stimulate rheumatoid factor production in non-rheumatic individuals? *APMIS* **1998**, *106*, 970–974. [CrossRef]
32. Manfredsdottir, V.F.; Vikingsdottir, T.; Jonsson, T.; Geirsson, A.J.; Kjartansson, O.; Heimisdottir, M.; Sigurdardottir, S.L.; Valdimarsson, H.; Vikingsson, A. The effects of tobacco smoking and rheumatoid factor seropositivity on disease activity and joint damage in early rheumatoid arthritis. *Rheumatology* **2006**, *45*, 734–740. [CrossRef] [PubMed]
33. Abhishek, A.; Butt, S.; Gadsby, K.; Zhang, W.; Deighton, C.M. Anti-TNF-alpha agents are less effective for the treatment of rheumatoid arthritis in current smokers. *J. Clin. Rheumatol.* **2010**, *16*, 15–18. [CrossRef]

34. Bobbio-Pallavicini, F.; Caporali, R.; Alpini, C.; Avalle, S.; Epis, O.M.; Klersy, C.; Montecucco, C. High IgA rheumatoid factor levels are associated with poor clinical response to tumour necrosis factor alpha inhibitors in rheumatoid arthritis. *Ann. Rheum. Dis.* **2007**, *66*, 302–307. [CrossRef] [PubMed]
35. Otten, H.G.; Daha, M.R.; Maarl, M.G.J.; Hoogendoorn, L.I.; Beem, E.M.; Rooy, H.H.; Breedveld, F.C. IgA rheumatoid factor in mucosal fluids and serum of patients with rheumatoid arthritis: Immunological aspects and clinical significance. *Clin. Exp. Immunol.* **1992**, *90*, 256–259. [CrossRef] [PubMed]
36. Marcolongo, R., Jr.; Carcassi, A.; Frullini, F.; Bianco, G.; Bravi, A. Levels of serum immunoglobulins in patients with rheumatoid arthritis. *Ann. Rheum. Dis.* **1967**, *26*, 412–418. [CrossRef] [PubMed]
37. Veys, E.M.; Claessens, H.E. Serum levels of IgG, IgM, and IgA in rheumatoid arthritis. *Ann. Rheum. Dis.* **1968**, *27*, 431–440. [CrossRef] [PubMed]
38. Aho, K.; Heliovaara, M.; Knekt, P.; Reunanen, A.; Aromaa, A.; Leino, A.; Kurki, P.; Heikkila, R.; Palosuo, T. Serum immunoglobulins and the risk of rheumatoid arthritis. *Ann. Rheum. Dis.* **1997**, *56*, 351–356. [CrossRef] [PubMed]
39. He, Y.; Zha, Q.; Liu, D.; Lu, A. Relations between serum IgA level and cartilage erosion in 436 cases of rheumatoid arthritis. *Immunol. Invest.* **2007**, *36*, 285–291. [CrossRef] [PubMed]
40. Blackburn, J.B.; Schaff, J.A.; Gutor, S.; Du, R.-H.; Nichols, D.; Sherrill, T.; Gutierrez, A.J.; Xin, M.K.; Wickersham, N.; Zhang, Y.; et al. Secretory cells are the primary source of pIgR in small airways. *Am. J. Respir. Cell Mol. Biol.* **2022**, *67*, 334–345. [CrossRef]
41. Pilette, C.; Ouadrhiri, Y.; Godding, V.; Vaerman, J.P.; Sibille, Y. Lung mucosal immunity: Immunoglobulin-A revisited. *Eur. Respir. J.* **2001**, *18*, 571–588. [CrossRef]
42. Klareskog, L.; Stolt, P.; Lundberg, K.; Kallberg, H.; Silva, C.; Grunewald, J.; Ronnelid, J.; Harris, H.E.; Ulfgren, A.; Dahlqvist, S.R.; et al. A new model for an etiology of RA; Smoking may trigger HLA-DR (SE)—Restricted immune reactions to autoantigens modified by citrullination. *Arthritis Rheum.* **2006**, *54*, 38–46. [CrossRef] [PubMed]
43. Herlitz-Cifuentes, H.; Vejar, C.; Flores, A.; Jara, P.; Bustos, P.; Castro, I.; Poblete, E.; Saez, K.; Opazo, M.; Gajardo, J.; et al. Plasma from patients with rheumatoid arthritis reduces nitric oxide synthesis and induces reactive oxygen species in a cell-based biosensor. *Biosensors* **2019**, *9*, 32. [CrossRef]
44. Chandrasekharan, U.M.; Wang, Z.; Wu, Y.; Tang, W.H.W.; Hazen, S.L.; Wang, S.; Husni, M.E. Elevated levels of plasma symmetric dimethylarginine and increased arginase activity as potential indicators of cardiovascular comorbidity in rheumatoid arthritis. *Arthritis Res. Ther.* **2018**, *20*, 123. [CrossRef] [PubMed]
45. Pertsinidou, E.; Manivel, V.A.; Klareskog, L.; Alfredsson, L.; Mathsson, L.; Hansson, M.; Cornillet, M.; Serre, G.; Holmdahl, R.; Skriner, K.; et al. In early rheumatoid arthritis anti-citrullinated peptide antibodies associate with lower number of affected joints, and Rheumatoid factor associates with systemic inflammation. *Ann. Rheum. Dis.* **2024**, *83*, 277–287. [CrossRef] [PubMed]
46. Koduri, G.; Solomon, J.J. Identification, Monitoring, and Management of Rheumatoid Arthritis-Associated Interstitial Lung Disease. *Arthritis Rheumatol.* **2023**, *75*, 2067–2077. [CrossRef]

Disclaimer/Publisher's Note: The statements, opinions and data contained in all publications are solely those of the individual author(s) and contributor(s) and not of MDPI and/or the editor(s). MDPI and/or the editor(s) disclaim responsibility for any injury to people or property resulting from any ideas, methods, instructions or products referred to in the content.

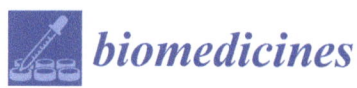

Article

New Nitric Oxide-Releasing Compounds as Promising Anti-Bladder Cancer Drugs

María Varela [1,2], Miriam López [1,2], Mariana Ingold [2], Diego Alem [1], Valentina Perini [1], Karen Perelmuter [3], Mariela Bollati-Fogolín [3], Gloria V. López [2,4,*] and Paola Hernández [1,*]

1. Departamento de Genética, Instituto de Investigaciones Biológicas Clemente Estable, Avenida Italia 3318, Montevideo 11600, Uruguay
2. Laboratorio de Biología Vascular y Desarrollo de Fármacos, Institut Pasteur Montevideo, Mataojo 2020, Montevideo 11400, Uruguay
3. Cell Biology Unit, Institut Pasteur Montevideo, Mataojo 2020, Montevideo 11400, Uruguay
4. Departamento de Química Orgánica, Facultad de Química, Universidad de la República, Avenida General Flores 2124, Montevideo 11800, Uruguay
* Correspondence: vlopez@fq.edu.uy (G.V.L.); phernandez@iibce.edu.uy (P.H.); Tel.: +598-2-4871616 (ext. 232) (P.H.); Fax: +598-2-4875461 (P.H.)

Abstract: Bladder cancer is a worldwide problem and improved therapies are urgently needed. In the search for newer strong antitumor compounds, herein, we present the study of three nitric oxide-releasing compounds and evaluate them as possible therapies for this malignancy. Bladder cancer cell lines T24 and 253J were used to evaluate the antiproliferative, antimigratory, and genotoxic effects of compounds. Moreover, we determined the NF-κB pathway inhibition, and finally, the survivin downregulation exerted by our molecules. The results revealed that compounds **1** and **3** exerted a high antiproliferative activity against bladder cancer cells through DNA damage and survivin downregulation. In addition, compound **3** reduced bladder cancer cell migration. We found that nitric oxide donors are promising molecules for the development of a new therapeutic targeting the underlying mechanisms of tumorigenesis and progression of bladder cancer.

Keywords: bladder cancer; furoxans; nitric oxide donors; NF-κB; survivin

Citation: Varela, M.; López, M.; Ingold, M.; Alem, D.; Perini, V.; Perelmuter, K.; Bollati-Fogolín, M.; López, G.V.; Hernández, P. New Nitric Oxide-Releasing Compounds as Promising Anti-Bladder Cancer Drugs. *Biomedicines* **2023**, *11*, 199. https://doi.org/10.3390/biomedicines11010199

Academic Editor: Amirata Saei Dibavar

Received: 22 December 2022
Revised: 5 January 2023
Accepted: 10 January 2023
Published: 12 January 2023

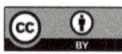

Copyright: © 2023 by the authors. Licensee MDPI, Basel, Switzerland. This article is an open access article distributed under the terms and conditions of the Creative Commons Attribution (CC BY) license (https://creativecommons.org/licenses/by/4.0/).

1. Introduction

Bladder cancer (BC) is one of the most common genitourinary malignancies and represents a serious health problem worldwide. Its incidence rises with age and it is three times more common in men than in women [1]. BC risk factors include genetic and molecular abnormalities, chemical or environmental exposures, and chronic irritation [2].

Cisplatin-based combination chemotherapy has been the first-line treatment for metastatic BC, providing an overall survival of 14–15 months and 5-year survival of 13–15% [3]. Yet, two-thirds of patients are ineligible due to impaired performance status or comorbidities [4] while 30% of patients do not respond to initial chemotherapy or have recurrence within the first year of treatment [5]. Over this past decade, the emergence of contemporary immunotherapy, targeted inhibitors, and antibody–drug conjugates has significantly changed the long-standing, predominantly chemotherapy-based option, giving a second wave of hope and prolonging overall survival [6]. Still, low objective response rates and poor survival demand further investigation of new and more effective therapeutic strategies for BC.

The selective inhibition of cell proliferation and the induction of apoptosis are crucial aspects of anticancer therapies. Nitric oxide (·NO)-releasing compounds alone or in combination with traditional chemo- or radiotherapy are promising agents for the treatment of BC [7]. ·NO can induce a multitude of antitumor effects such as the inhibition of cell proliferation; apoptosis stimulation; sensitization to chemo-, radio-, or immunotherapy; and the impairment of angiogenesis, invasion, and metastasis [8]. High local ·NO concentrations increase the intracellular content of nitrogen and oxygen-reactive species generating nitrosative and oxidative stress inducing cytotoxic effects in cancer cells [9]. Under this oxidative state, nitrous anhydride and peroxynitrite generated by ·NO are the major inductors of genotoxicity leading to the deamination of DNA bases, the oxidation of bases and deoxyribose, strand breaks, and multiple types of cross-linking events [10]. Moreover, ·NO can inhibit the nuclear factor kappa-B (NF-κB) by S-nitrosylation modulating its gene products [11]. Dysregulation of the NF-κB pathway plays an important role in cancer progression and metastasis by inducing gene transcription of growth-promoting, anti-apoptotic, and epithelial mesenchymal transition factors (EMT) [12,13]. In BC cells, it has been demonstrated that NF-κB activation enhances survivin expression which in turn promotes apoptosis resistance and cancer cell proliferation [14]. Elevated expression of survivin has been associated with an advanced cancer stage, poor prognosis, and decreased response to therapy [15,16]. In addition, survivin is an independent predictor of recurrence and cancer-specific survival [17]. Thus, therapies based on ·NO-releasing compounds represent an attractive approach for BC treatment.

In previous works, we showed the promising potential application of ·NO-releasing compounds for the treatment of BC [18]. Herein, continuing with our efforts to explore the anticancer action of arylsulfonylfuroxan derivatives, we performed the chemical synthesis of three new ·NO-releasing compounds (Figure 1) and evaluated their potential use as drug candidates in BC.

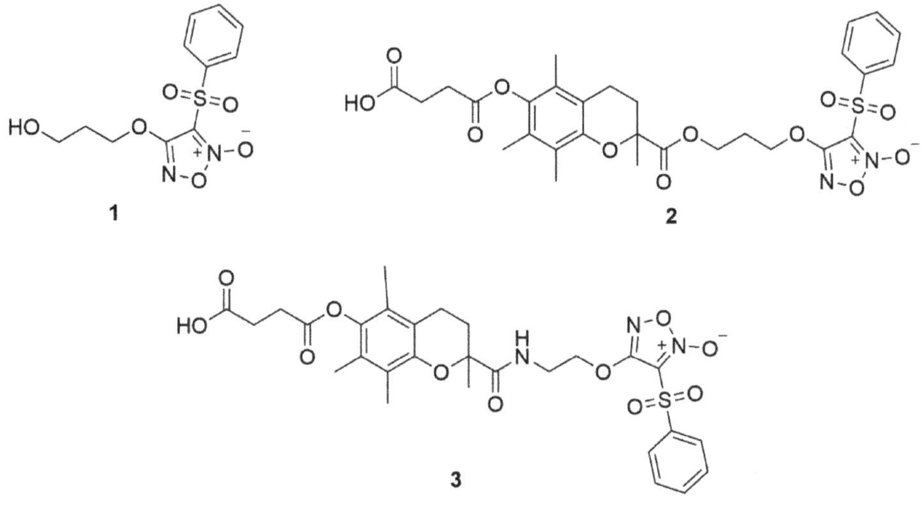

Figure 1. Structures of compounds **1**, **2**, and **3**.

To assess these objectives, we employed two BC cell lines: T24 cells derived from a primary grade 3 transitional cell carcinoma [19] and 253J cells derived from a metastatic transitional cell tumor of the urinary tract [20]. We found that compounds **1** and **3** were excellent antiproliferative agents toward BC cells by inducing DNA damage and survivin downregulation. Both molecules showed an improved selectivity toward cancer cells compared to the drug cisplatin indicating the therapeutic potential of these compounds. The ·NO release exerted by these molecules was involved in the antiproliferative activity against cancer cells. However, compounds showed differences in their mode of action. Compound **1** showed an important inhibition of the NF-κB pathway and a moderate ability to downregulate the survivin level, while compound **3** behaved as a strong antiproliferative agent in both 2D and 3D cancer cell cultures, a cell migration inhibitor, and a potent survivin downregulator. Thus, compound **3** emerges as a promising molecule for BC treatment. Moreover, since the overexpression of survivin confers chemo- and radioresistance in a variety of human cancers [21,22], we highlight the use of ·NO-releasing compounds as a promising hit and scaffold for future drug design for cancer treatments in which survivin is upregulated. In this sense, this study opens the possibility for further approaches combining these ·NO donors with classical therapies, with the aim to sensitize tumor cells and enhance the efficacy of the drugs in clinical use.

2. Materials and Methods

2.1. General Experimental Information

Chemical supplies were from Sigma-Aldrich (Saint Louis, MO, USA). Compounds **1** [23], **4** [24], and **5** [24] were prepared as reported. Electron impact mass spectra (MS) were performed on a Shimadzu GC–MS QP 1100 EX instrument and high-resolution mass analysis was performed on a Thermo Scientific Q Exactive Hybrid Quadrupole-Orbitrap Mass Spectrometer using MeOH as a solvent. ^{1}H NMR and ^{13}C NMR spectra were obtained on a Bruker Avance DPX-400 spectrometer, using TMS as internal reference. The chemical shifts (δ) are reported in parts per million (ppm) relative to the center line of the corresponding solvent. The reaction progress was analyzed by TLC (silica gel 60F-254 plates visualized with UV light (254 nm)). Column chromatography was carried out using silica gel (230–400 mesh).

Cell culture supplies were from Biological Industries (Beit Haemek, Israel) and Capricorn Scientific (Ebsdorfergrund, Germany). Sulforhodamine B, cisplatin, and propidium iodide were from Sigma-Aldrich (St. Louis, MO, USA). SAHA was from Acade (Hong Kong, China). Protease inhibitors were purchased from Roche. Antibodies against survivin (ab76424) and alpha-tubulin (ab15246) and the ECL chemiluminescence kit were from Abcam (Cambridge, MA, USA). The secondary antibody goat-anti-rabbit HRP (G21234) was from Invitrogen (Rockford, IL, USA) and the PVDF membrane (RPN303F) was from GE Healthcare Life Sciences (Little Chalfont, Buckinghamshire, UK). The bladder cancer cell line T24 (ATCC HBT-4) was purchased from the Cell Repository ABAC (Asociación Banco Argentino de Células). The bladder cancer cell line 253J and immortalized human keratinocyte cell line HaCaT (BCRJ batch number 001071) were kindly provided by Dr. Wilner Martínez-López and Dr. Jimena Hochmann, respectively.

2.2. Experimental Procedures and Characterization Data for the Compounds

3-(3-Phenylsulfonyl-N^2-oxide-1,2,5-oxadiazole-4-oxy)propyl 6-((3-carboxypropanoyl)oxy)-2,5,7,8-tetramethylchroman-2-carboxylate (**2**). A solution of 3-(3-phenylsulfonyl-N^2-oxide-1,2,5-oxadiazole-4-yl)oxypropyl 6-hydroxy-2,5,7,8-tetramethylchroman-2-carboxylate (**4**, 0.090 mmol), succinic anhydride (0.135 mmol), and cesium carbonate (0.180 mmol) in 1.5 mL acetonitrile was stirred at room temperature for 24 h and the completion of the reaction was monitored by TLC. The solvent was evaporated under reduced pressure and the reaction crude was diluted with a 10% HCl solution and extracted with EtOAc. The combined organic layers were dried with Na_2SO_4 and filtered, and the solvent was evaporated under reduced pressure. The residue was purified by flash column chromatography (SiO_2, Hexane/EtOAc, 7/3) to render the desired product as a colorless oil that crystallized at 4 °C, yield 59%. ^{1}H and ^{13}C NMR spectra are provided in the Supplementary Material. ^{1}H NMR (400 MHz, CDCl$_3$) δ 8.04 (d, J = 7.4 Hz, 2H), 7.75 (t, J = 7.5 Hz, 1H), 7.61 (t, J = 7.9 Hz, 2H), 4.40–4.35 (m, 1H), 4.16–4.02 (m, 3H), 2.91 (bs, 2H), 2.82 (bs, 2H), 2.65–2.60 (m, 1H), 2.51–2.45 (m, 2H), 2.16 (s, 3H), 2.09–2.04 (m, 2H), 2.01 (s, 3H), 1.95–1.92 (m, 1H), 1.89 (s, 3H), 1.65 (s, 3H). ^{13}C NMR (101 MHz, CDCl$_3$) δ 173.9, 173.7, 171.5, 156.7, 149.5, 138.1, 135.6, 129.7, 128.5, 127.4, 125.3, 122.9, 117.1, 110.5, 77.5, 67.3, 60.4, 30.9, 30.5, 28.5, 20.9, 12.9, 12.0, 11.8. MS (IE, 70 eV) m/z (%): 532 (M^+-Succ.Ac., 12), 516 (17), 391 (M^+-Fx, 10), 333 (2), 232 (7), 217 (6), 205 (91), 142 (28), 77 (100). HRMS (ESI+): m/z calculated for $C_{29}H_{32}N_2O_{12}SNa$: 655.1574 $[M + Na]^+$; found 655.1608.

6-((3-carboxypropanoyl)oxy)-2,5,7,8-tetramethyl-N-[2-(3-phenylsulfonyl-N^2-oxide-1,2,5-oxadiazole-4-yl)oxyethyl]chroman-2-carboxamide (**3**). The title compound was prepared from 6-hydroxy-2,5,7,8-tetramethyl-N-[2-(3-phenylsulfonyl-N^2-oxide-1,2,5-oxadiazole-4-

yl)oxyethyl]chroman-2-carboxamide (**5**, 0.200 mmol), succinic anhydride (0.400 mmol), and cesium carbonate (0.3 mmol) in 3 mL of DMF with stirring at room temperature for 3 h; the completion of the reaction was monitored by TLC. Subsequently, the reaction mixture was diluted with a 10% HCl solution and extracted with ethyl ether. The combined organic layers were dried with Na_2SO_4, filtered, and the solvent evaporated under reduced pressure. The residue was purified by flash column chromatography (SiO_2, Hexane/EtOAc, 4/6) to render the desired product as a white solid, m.p. 79-81 °C, yield 30%. ^{1}H and ^{13}C NMR spectra are provided in the Supplementary Material. ^{1}H NMR (400 MHz, acetone-d_6) δ 8.10 (d, J = 7.4 Hz, 2H), 7.88–7.84 (m, 1H), 7.72–7.69 (m, 2H), 4.54 (bs, 2H), 3.80–3.70 (m, 2H), 2.97–2.93 (m, 2H), 2.77–2.74 (m, 2H), 2.66–2.54 (m, 2H), 2.36–2.28 (m, 1H), 2.17 (s, 3H), 2.02 (s, 3H), 1.98 (s, 3H), 1.92—1.85 (m, 1H), 1.52 (s, 3H). ^{13}C NMR (101 MHz, acetone-d_6) δ 174.0, 172.6, 170.7, 159.3, 148.1, 141.7, 138.1, 135.8, 129.8, 128.6, 127.3, 125.6, 122.5, 118.1, 110.7, 78.5, 70.0, 38.6, 28.4, 28.2, 23.1, 20.0, 12.2, 11.3. MS (IE, 70eV) *m/z* (%): 375 (M$^+$-Fx, 4), 275 (16), 203 (2), 141 (27), 101 (2), 77 (100). HRMS (ESI+): *m/z* calculated for $C_{28}H_{31}N_3O_{11}SNa$: 640.1577 [M + Na]$^+$; found 640.1592.

2.3. Cell Cultures

Human bladder cancer cells T24 (derived from transitional cell carcinoma) and 253J (developed from a retroperitoneal metastasis) were grown in McCoy's 5A medium (Biological Industries) supplemented with 10% FBS (Capricorn Scientific). The non-cancer keratinocyte cell line HaCaT was grown in DMEM (Biological Industries) and the reporter cell line HT-29-NF-κB-hrGFP was grown in RPMI supplemented with 10% FBS (Capricorn Scientific). The cells were passaged twice per week, and the culture medium was changed with the same frequency. Cell cultures were maintained under humidified 5% CO_2 atmosphere at 37 °C.

2.4. Antiproliferative Activity

The antiproliferative effect of compounds in BC cells and in the non-cancer cells HaCaT was evaluated as follows. T24 and 253J cells (8×10^3 cells per well) and HaCaT keratinocytes (10×10^3 cells per well) were seeded in a 96-well plate and allowed to attach for 24 h. Afterward, the culture media was removed and the solubilized compounds in DMSO were added at increasing concentrations (0.1–50 µM) diluted in fresh culture medium in triplicate. The reference anticancer compounds cisplatin and suberoylanilide hydroxamic acid (SAHA) were included in each experiment. The cells were further incubated at 37 °C and 5% CO_2 for 24 h. Then, the antiproliferative activity of the compounds was determined using the sulforhodamine B method [25]. Absorbance was measured at 510 nm and background at 620 nm using a microplate spectrophotometer (Varioskan Flash Microplate spectrophotometer, Thermo Fisher, Waltham, MA, USA). The IC_{50} was determined as the concentration that reduces absorbance by 50% compared with the control 0.5% DMSO and was determined by linear regression analysis. Each assay was repeated at least three times.

2.5. NO Release in Cell Culture Media

T24 and 253J cells (8×10^3 cells per well) were seeded in a 96-well plate and allowed to attach for 24 h. Culture media were removed and the solubilized compounds in DMSO were added at 50 µM diluted in fresh culture medium in sextuplicate. The control with 0.5% DMSO was included in the experiments. After that, cells were incubated at 37 °C and 5% CO_2 for 3 h. Then, the ·NO production as the nitrate/nitrite content was measured by the Griess reaction assay [26]. Briefly, 50 µL of culture medium was transferred to a new 96-well plate. Subsequently, 50 µL of 1% sulfanilamide solution was added to each well and incubated for 10 min protected from light. Finally, 50 µL of 0.1% N-1-naphtilethylenrdiamine dihydrochloride solution was added and incubated for an additional 10 min. A reference curve with $NaNO_2$ was performed at serial dilutions between 0 and 100 µM in 50 µL of culture medium. Absorbance was measured at 540 nm using a microplate spectrophotometer.

2.6. NO Release in Physiological Solution

NO released by the compounds during incubation in a physiological solution in the presence of L-cysteine was determined [27]. The compounds were solubilized in DMSO and then diluted at 50 µM in a mixture of 50 mM pH 7.4 PBS solution/MeOH (1% DMSO) 50/50 v/v. Afterward, they were incubated in the presence of L-cysteine at a 0.25 mM concentration (a 5-fold excess compared to the ·NO-donor derivative) for 1, 3, and 6 h at 37 °C. The presence of nitrite in the sample was determined using the Griess reaction assay. At the same time, a standard curve with $NaNO_2$ was performed at serial dilutions between 0 and 100 µM in 50 µL of the PBS/MeOH mixture. The absorbance was measured at 540 nm using a microplate spectrophotometer.

2.7. Antiproliferative Activity with Hemoglobin

To investigate the contribution of antiproliferative–proliferative activity of the studied compounds, we evaluated their effect on T24 and 253J bladder cancer cell culture's growth in the absence and presence of Hb. Cells were seeded into a 96-well plate at 8×10^3 cells per well and were allowed to attach for 24 h. The cultures were pretreated with hemoglobin (Hb) at 0 µM or 50 µM for 1 h and then treated with 50 µM of the selected compounds for 24 h. Then, the antiproliferative activity was assessed by the sulforhodamine B assay [18]. Statistical analysis was carried out using a two-way ANOVA analysis test followed by Bonferroni's multiple comparison test.

2.8. Clonogenic Assay

Compounds were tested for their ability to inhibit T24 and 253J bladder cancer cell colonies. Cells were seeded (500 cells per well) in 60 mm plates and allowed to attach for 5 h after seeding. Then, compounds were added at a final concentration of 10 µM. The control with 0.5% DMSO was included in the experiments After 6 days, the clones were fixed with a solution of acetic acid in methanol 1%, stained with crystal violet 0.5%, and counted. The colonies formed (CF) were counted and then the plating efficiency (PE) and the survival fraction (SF) were calculated for each compound. The PE was calculated by dividing the CF by the number of cells plated. The SF was determined by dividing the PE of the treated cells by the PE of the control cells and then multiplying by 100 [28].

2.9. Spheroids

To evaluate the effects of our compounds in 3D spheroids, 96-well plates were pretreated with 1.5% agarose in PBS. Then, cells were seeded (3×10^4 cells per well) in 200 µL of cell culture media. The culture was placed in culture conditions for 3 days to allow spheroid production. At day 3, 100 µL of the media was removed carefully and replaced with 100 µL 2X of the final concentration of our compounds. DMSO was used as a control. Finally, at 24, 48, and 72 h, the culture media were replaced by resazurin 2× in PBS and fluorescence at 530 nm (ex) and 590 nm (em) was measured in a microplate reader [29].

2.10. Scratch Assay

The ability to inhibit the cancer cell migration was evaluated using a scratch assay. T24 and 253J cells were seeded at 5×10^5 cells per well in six-well plates and incubated for 24 h. Cell culture media were removed and washed with PBS. Cultures were incubated with mitomycin-c at 5 µg/mL in a culture medium supplemented with 1% SFB for 2 h. Then, cells were washed with PBS and wounds were created by scratching cell monolayers with a sterile 200 µL plastic pipette tip. Compounds were added at 5 and 10 µM in fresh culture media supplemented with 1% SFB for 17 h. Six images per well were taken in a phase contrast microscopy Olympus IX-81 with a 10× objective at 0 and 17 h and quantified using the ImageJ program [30]. Statistical analysis was performed using a one-way ANOVA test followed by Dunnett's test.

2.11. Comet Assay

The genotoxic damage induced in T24 and 253J cells after 3 h of treatment with compounds was evaluated by alkaline single-cell gel electrophoresis (comet assay). Cells were seeded in 35 mm plates at 2×10^5 cells per well and allowed to attach for 24 h in a humidified 5% CO_2 atmosphere at 37 °C. Afterward, the culture media were removed and compounds were added at 50 μM in a fresh culture medium. Hydrogen peroxide at 100 μM was included a positive control. The cells were further incubated for 3 h at 37 °C and 5% CO_2. After the incubation step, cells were detached and centrifuged for 10 min at 1200 rpm and the cell pellet was resuspended in PBS. Cell suspensions were mixed with 1.5% low-melting-point agarose and immediately placed on slides pre-coated with normal-melting-point agarose. The agarose was allowed to set for 15 min at 4 °C and cells were lysed through the immersion of slides in a cold solution of lysis buffer (2.5 M NaCl, 100 mM Na_2EDTA, 10 mM Trizma-HCl, NaOH to pH 10 and 1% Triton X-100) for 12 h at 4 °C. Slides were incubated in a cold alkaline electrophoresis solution (300 mM NaOH and 1 mM Na_2EDTA, pH 13) for 20 min to DNA unwinding and expression of alkali labile sites were allowed. Electrophoresis was performed at 25 V (300 mA) for 20 min in a cold unit at 4 °C. Samples were washed three times with neutralization buffer pH 7.5 (0.4 M Tris–HCl). Finally, slides were stained with bromodeoxyuridine (10 μg/mL) [31]. Images were taken using an epifluorescence microscopy Olympus IX-81 with a 20× objective. A total of 100 comets on each comet slide were visually scored and classified as belonging to one of the five classes according to the tail length and given a value from 0 (undamaged) to 4 (maximum damage). The DNA damage score in the range of 0 to 400 was calculated using the equation: $\Sigma(n.\alpha)$, where n is the percentage of cells in a class of tail length and α is the class of tail length [32,33].

2.12. NF-κB Pathway Inhibition

To determine if these ·NO-releasing compounds inhibit the NF-κB pathway, we used the reporter cell line HT-29-NF-κB-hrGFP as we previously described [34].

A—HT-29-NF-κB-hrGFP cells cytotoxicity assay: 4×10^4 cells per well were seeded in a 96-well plate in RPMI and incubated for 24 h at 37 °C and 5% CO_2. The culture media were removed and the compounds, dissolved in DMSO (lower than 0.5%, v/v, in the final volume of RPMI), were added at the desired final concentrations diluted in fresh RPMI (0.19–50 μM) and the cells were further incubated for 24 h at 37 C, 5% CO_2. Afterward, the culture supernatant was removed and cell viability was determined by the MTT assay. Absorbance measurements were performed at 570 nm in a spectrophotometer plate reader.

B—NF-κB pathway inhibition assay: Cells were seeded in a 96-well plate (4×10^4 cells per well) in a fresh RPMI culture media and incubated for 24 h. Cell cultures were pretreated with compounds at 5 and 10 μM for 1 h prior to pro-inflammatory stimuli with TNF-α (1 ng/mL) and cultures were further incubated for 24 h. Three controls were included: cells treated only with TNF-α, cells treated only with compounds, and cells treated with BAY 11-7082 at 10 μM and TNF-α (1 ng/mL). Cells were detached and resuspended to perform flow cytometry analysis. Cells were analyzed using a BD Accuri™ C6 (Biosciences, BD, USA) flow cytometer equipped with 488 and 640 nm lasers. Data acquisition and analysis was achieved using BD Accuri C6 Software V1.0.264.21. The GFP and propidium iodide fluorescence emissions were detected using band-pass filters 533/30 and 585/40, respectively. For each sample, 5000 counts gated on an FSC versus SSC dot plot (excluding doublets) were recorded. For analysis, only single living cells (those that excluded propidium iodide) were considered. The percentage of GFP positive was normalized against the percentage of GFP cells obtained with the TNF-α control. Statistical analysis was carried out using a one-way ANOVA test and Dunnett's test.

2.13. Western Blotting

The capability of compounds to reduce survivin levels in BC cells was determined through a Western blot. T24 or 253J cells (5×10^5 cells) were seeded in 10 cm Petri dishes in a complete medium and allowed to attach for 24 h. Cells were treated with compounds **1** and **3** at 10 µM or 0.5% DMSO for 24 h. At the end of the incubation period, cells were washed twice with PBS 1X and harvested. Proteins were solubilized in Laemmli buffer plus protease inhibitors (NaF, PMSF and protease inhibitor mixture) followed by denaturation at 95 °C for 5 min and resolved on a 15% SDS-PAGE. For immunoblotting, proteins were electro-transferred onto a PVDF membrane and blocked with 5% nonfat milk in TBS-0.10% Tween 20 (TBST) at room temperature for 1 h. Then, the membrane was incubated with the primary antibodies rabbit anti-survivin (1/5000) and rabbit tubulin (1/200) at 4 °C overnight. After washing (TBST) and subsequent blocking, the blot was incubated with the secondary antibody goat-anti-rabbit HRP (1/5000) for 1 h at room temperature. The blots were developed using an enhanced chemiluminescence ECL detection reagent. Quantification was performed with ImageJ software. Statistical analysis was carried out using two-way ANOVA followed by a Bonferroni multiple comparison test.

3. Results

3.1. Chemistry

Chemical Synthesis

Furoxan **1** was synthesized as previously [23] and furoxan derivatives **2** and **3** were synthesized from **4** and **5** [24] by treatment with succinic anhydride in the presence of cesium carbonate as illustrated in Scheme 1.

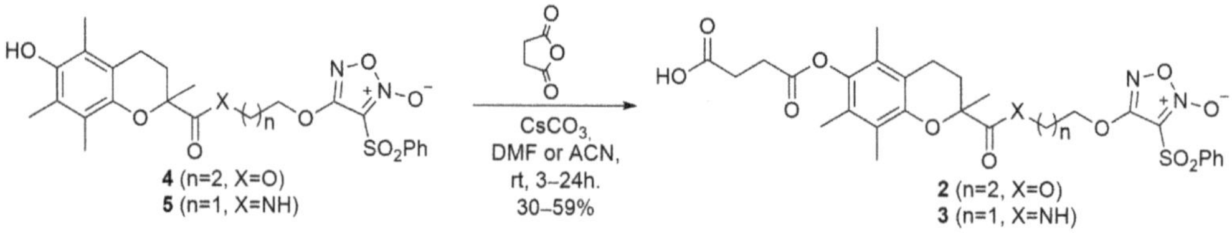

Scheme 1. Synthesis of furoxan derivatives **2** and **3**.

3.2. Biology

3.2.1. Antiproliferative Activity

The in vitro antiproliferative activity of the compounds was determined in bladder-cancer-derived cell lines T24 and 253J and in the non-cancer HaCaT cells to determine the cytotoxic selectivity index against cancer cells. The cells were incubated in the presence of the compounds for 24 h. The antiproliferative activity was determined using the sulforhodamine B assay. The results presented in Table 1 are expressed as IC_{50} in µM, which is the drug concentration resulting in a 50% reduction in cellular net growth when compared with the negative control DMSO 0.5%. The standard anticancer drug cisplatin and SAHA were used as positive controls.

Table 1. Antiproliferative activity in T24 and 253J cancer cells along with selectivity index and the antiproliferative activity in the non-cancer cell line HaCaT.

Compound	T24		253J		HaCaT
	IC_{50} (µM)	SI	IC_{50} (µM)	SI	IC_{50} (µM)
1	2.48 ± 1.15	8.04	3.59 ± 1.11	5.55	19.93 ± 1.12
2	4.97 ± 1.08	0.90	2.27 ± 1.08	1.86	4.49 ± 1.11
3	2.57 ± 1.10	6.48	2.01 ± 1.13	8.28	16.65 ± 1.12
SAHA	14.65 ± 1.25	0.37	11.83 ± 1.20	0.46	5.39 ± 1.10
Cisplatin	12.38 ± 1.11	2.11	63.84 ± 1.09	0.41	26.18 ± 1.17

IC_{50} values are expressed as mean ± standard deviation. Selectivity index (SI) determined by the IC_{50} HaCaT/IC_{50} cancer cell lines.

Compounds **1**, **2**, and **3** showed an important antiproliferative activity in T24 and 253J cancer cell lines. As an attempt to approximate the safety profile and selectivity toward cancer cells, we further studied the antiproliferative activity in non-cancerous HaCaT cells. The selectivity index (SI) was calculated as the ratio between the IC_{50} for HaCaT cells and the IC_{50} for BC cells. The results show that compounds **1** and **3** provided a higher selectivity for cancer cells than the chemotherapeutic drug cisplatin. It is worth mentioning that compound **3** exhibited the highest antiproliferative effect on the cisplatin-resistant cell line 253J and a 20-fold higher SI value 20 than cisplatin. Thus, this study suggests that compounds **1** and **3** presented the best profile for further studies in BC cells.

3.2.2. Nitric-Oxide-Releasing Activity

Furoxan heterocycles are antitumor pharmacophores that are capable of releasing ·NO via a thiol-dependent mechanism [35]. In this regard, the ·NO-releasing activity of compounds was determined at 50 µM incubated for 3 h in T24 and 253J cell cultures was determined by the Griess assay. The strong nitric-oxide-releasing compound SNAP was used as a control.

The results indicate that the compounds were able to release nitric oxide in cell culture media after 3 h of incubation (Figure 2). Compound **3** produced higher ·NO levels in T24 cell culture, while compound **2** produced higher ·NO levels in 253J cell culture. Compound **1** induced the lowest nitrate/nitrite levels.

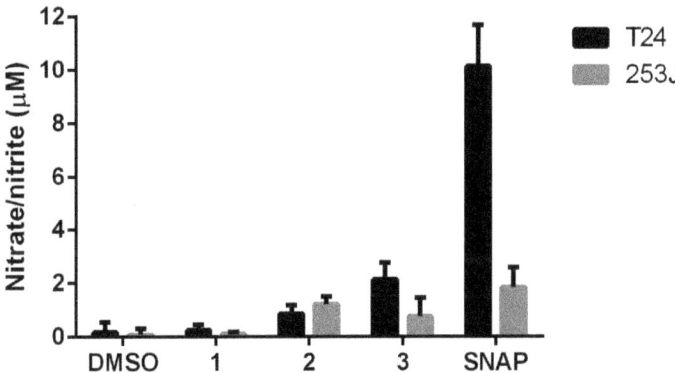

Figure 2. Levels of ·NO produced by furoxans derivatives in T24 and 253J bladder cancer cell cultures. The results are the means ± standard deviation of three independent experiments. SNAP is the ·NO-releasing positive control compound.

The ·NO production by furoxans at 50 µM was also measured in physiological solution in the presence of L-cysteine (5-fold molar excess) after incubation for 1, 3, and 6 h at 37 °C.

The results indicated that in the physiological solution, the compounds **1**, **2**, and **3** and SNAP released higher ·NO levels at 3 h as we indicated previously [18] (Figure 3). Moreover, the results showed that the ·NO-releasing capacity of the products in the cell milieu differed from that under physiological conditions, suggesting that they exhibited different physicochemical properties and reactivity towards thiols.

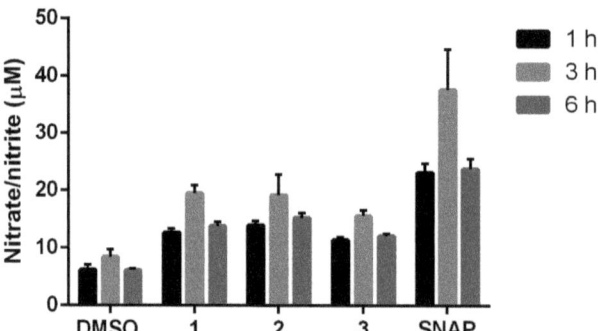

Figure 3. Levels of ·NO produced by furoxans derivatives in physiological solution at pH 7.4 and 37 °C. The results are the means ± standard deviation of three independent experiments. SNAP is the ·NO-releasing positive control compound.

3.2.3. Antiproliferative Activity with Hemoglobin

The contribution of ·NO to the antiproliferative activity of the studied compounds was evaluated on BC cells grown in the absence and presence of hemoglobin. Cultures were pretreated with or without hemoglobin (50 μM) for 1 h and then treated with compounds (10 μM) for 24 h until the sulforhodamine B assay. The results indicated that the antiproliferative activity of the compounds decreased in the presence of an ·NO scavenger (hemoglobin), suggesting that the ·NO release was involved in their anticancer mechanism (Figure 4).

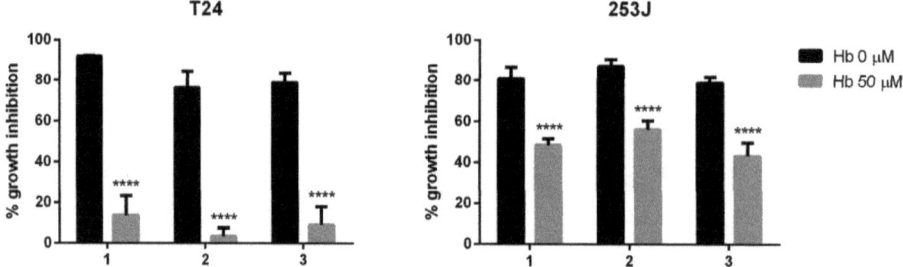

Figure 4. Effects of hemoglobin (Hb) on the antiproliferative effect of ·NO-donor compounds. The results are expressed as the percentage of cell growth inhibition relative to the control cells. The data are the means ± standard deviation obtained from three determinations. Statistical analysis: a two-way ANOVA followed by a Bonferroni multiple comparison test: **** $p < 0.0001$.

We observed that the antiproliferative activity of the compounds **1**, **2**, and **3** in T24 cells was mainly due to ·NO-releasing activity. On the other hand, in 253J cells, the ·NO-releasing activity was partially involved in the antiproliferative effect. Therefore, these results suggest that the invasive BC cell line T24 is highly sensitive to ·NO while the cisplatin-resistant cell line 253J is moderately sensitive to ·NO.

3.2.4. Clonogenic Assay

A clonogenic assay was performed in T24 and 253J cells. The results are shown in Figure 5 and the SFs determined by the ratio between the PE of the treated and control cells are presented in Table 2. Compounds **1** and **3** were able to inhibit the clonogenic ability of both cancer cell lines. Compound **2** only inhibited the clonogenic survival in 253J cells. According to these results and the antiproliferative activity, we selected compounds **1** and **3** for further studies.

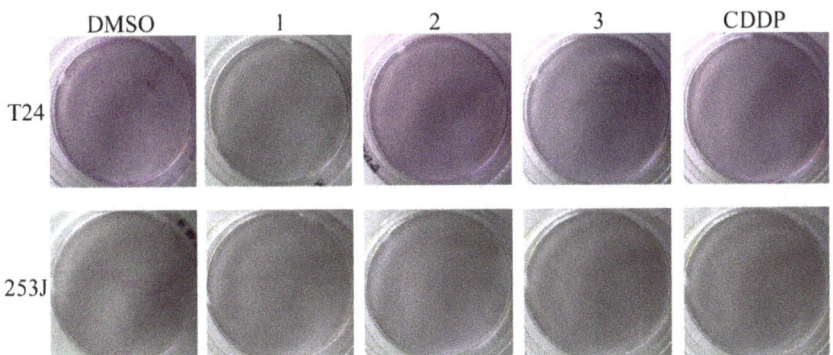

Figure 5. Clonogenic assay performed in T24 and 253J cells. Cultures were exposed to compounds **1**, **2**, and **3** or cisplatin (CDDP) at 10 µM.

Table 2. Clonogenic assay of T24 and 253J cells treated with compounds at 10 µM.

Cell Line	Clonogenic Score	DMSO	1	2	3	Cisplatin
	CF	221	0	56	0	0
T24	PE (%)	44	0	11	0	0
	SF	100	0	25	0	0
	CF	271	0	0	0	0
253J	PE (%)	54	0	0	0	0
	SF	1	0	0	0	0

CF: colonies formed, PE: plating efficiency, SF: survival fraction.

3.2.5. Spheroids

The capacity of the compounds to inhibit cell growth in 3D cultures was determined in T24 cancer cell spheroids. In this assay, spheroids of T24 cells were incubated with compounds **1** or **3** or cisplatin for 24, 48, and 72 h. Cell viability was then determined using the resazurin method. The results indicate that compound **3** had a strong inhibitor effect on 3D cell growth (Figure 6). Even at 24, 48, and 72 h, this compound exerted a higher antiproliferative activity than the reference compound cisplatin.

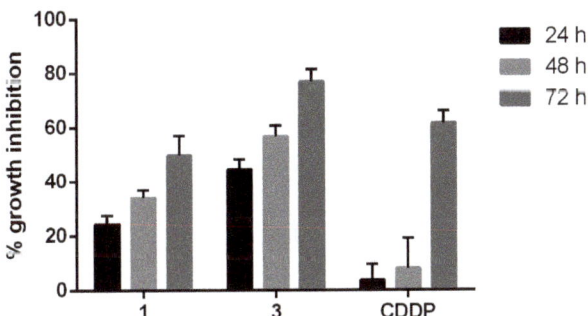

Figure 6. Growth inhibition percentage in T24 spheroids by compounds **1**, **3** or cisplatin (CDDP) at IC_{50} during 24, 48 and 72 h. The data are the means ± standard deviation obtained from three determinations.

The fact that the potent antiproliferative activity of compound **3** increased over the time suggests that BC cells are unable to avoid its anticancer effect.

3.2.6. Migration Assay

The ability to inhibit cell migration was determined using a scratch assay. Considering the above results, **1** and **3** were selected to perform this study. To suppress cell proliferation, cells were incubated with mitomycin-c for 2 h and then removed by washing before making the scratch. Images were immediately taken (0 h). Cells were incubated for 17 h in the presence of compounds **1** and **3** at 5 and 10 µM. SAHA at 10 µM, a pan-HDAC inhibitor, was included as a control. After this period, images were captured to measure gaps. results indicate (Figure 7) that in T24 cells, compound **3** was the most potent compound able to reduce cell migration (57%), even better than SAHA (47%). On the other hand, in 253J cells, SAHA reduced cell migration by 60%, whereas compound **3** reduced cell migration by 30%.

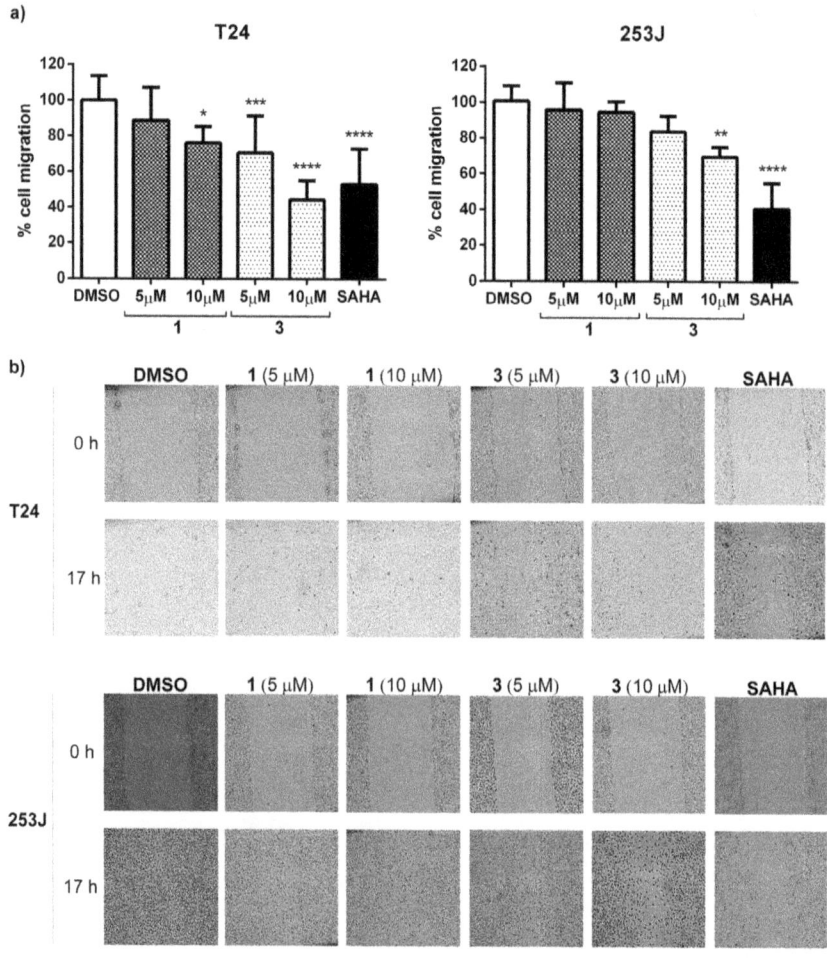

Figure 7. Effect of compounds on T24 and 253J cell migration. (**a**) Percentage of cell migration in the presence of compounds **1** and **3** at 5 and 10 µM during a 17 h period. SAHA at 10 µM was included as a positive control. The graph represents the mean ± standard deviation obtained from six measurements per well in three independent experiments. Statistical analysis was performed using one-way ANOVA test followed by Dunnett's test with * $p \leq 0.05$, ** $p \leq 0.01$, *** $p \leq 0.001$ and **** $p \leq 0.0001$. (**b**) Representative images of the scratch assay from each experimental condition are shown in (**a**) graphical view at 0 and 17 h for both cell lines.

3.2.7. Comet Assay

The induction of genotoxic effect by ·NO-releasing compounds was assessed by measuring DNA migration caused by strand breaks in the alkaline single-cell electrophoresis assay. BC cells were incubated in the presence of compounds **1** and **3** at 50 µM or H_2O_2 at 100 µM for 3 h. The results indicate that ·NO-releasing molecules induced DNA strand breaks in cancer cells (Figure 8). Compound **1** induced mainly class 3 DNA damage in both cell lines. Compound **3** also induced strand breaks, although the effect in T24 cells was lower than 253J cells. While in T24 this compound induced different degrees of DNA damage, in 253J cells, we identified comets that corresponded mainly to class 3. The positive control H_2O_2 induced a higher genotoxic effect with a high prevalence of class 4 DNA damage score.

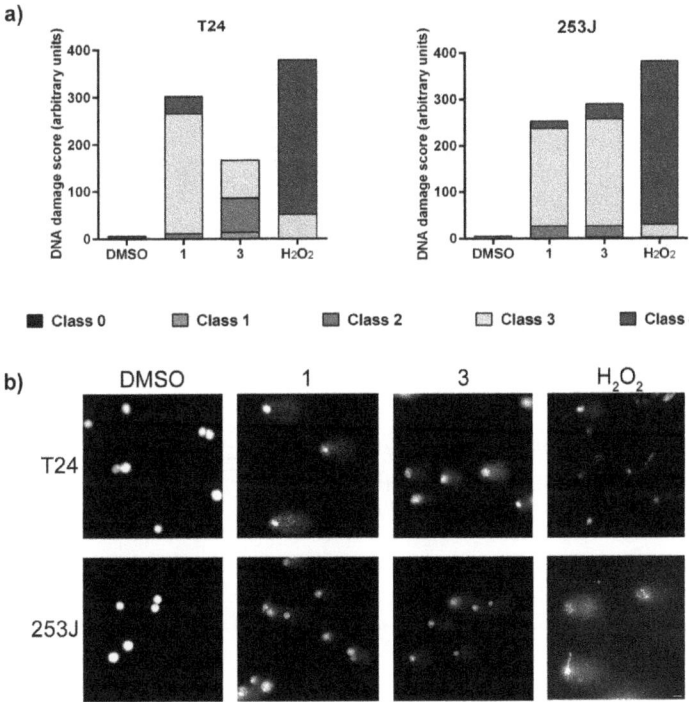

Figure 8. Alkaline comet assay in T24 and 253J cells incubated with compounds **1** and **3** for 3 h. (**a**) DNA damage score was calculated from each comet classified into five classes corresponding to the amount of DNA in the tail from 0 to 4. (**b**) Representative single-cell electrophoresis images of each experimental condition are shown in a) graphical view. Bar: 20 µM.

3.2.8. NF-κB Pathway Inhibition

Using a human pathway-specific reporter cell system (HT-29-NF-κB-hrGFP), the in vitro capability to decrease the activation of NF κB level was determined. Human intestinal cells HT-29 stably transfected with the pNF-κB-hrGFP plasmid were stimulated with the pro-inflammatory cytokine TNF-α. NF-κB activation was estimated by measuring the percentage of GFP-expressing cells. Determinations were performed in the absence and presence of compounds **1** and **3** at the non-cytotoxic doses of 5 and 10 µM (100% of cell survival on HT-29-NF-κB-hrGFP cells). BAY-117082 at 10 µM was used as a reference compound. Controls without TNF-α stimulation were also included to evaluate the compounds' intrinsic pro-inflammatory properties, finding that compounds were not pro-inflammatory per se.

The results shown in Figure 9 demonstrated that compound **1** at 10 µM inhibited NF-κB activation almost as well as the positive control BAY-117082. On the other hand, compound **3** was found to be inactive at the evaluated doses. Thus, compound **1** may suppress cancer cell proliferation by modulating the NF-κB pathway.

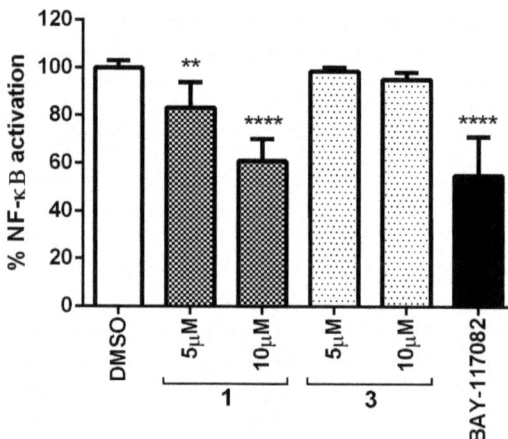

Figure 9. Percentage of NF-κB activation in the presence of compounds **1** and **3** at 5 and 10 µM. BAY-117082 at 10 µM was included as a positive control. The graph represents the mean ± standard deviation of three independent experiments. Statistical analysis was performed using one-way ANOVA test and Dunnett's test with ** $p \leq 0.01$ and **** $p \leq 0.0001$.

3.2.9. Survivin Expression Inhibition

Survivin is known to be involved in cancer cell proliferation and apoptosis inhibition. Thus, inhibition of survivin expression holds promise for BC therapies. T24 and 253J cells were exposed to compounds **1** and **3** at 10 µM for 24 h and a Western blot assay was performed. Our results suggest that compound **1** is a moderate inhibitor of survivin expression in both cell lines (Figure 10). Taking into consideration the above results, compound **1** could induce the antiproliferative activity by modulating the NF-κB and reducing the survivin expression. On the other hand, compound **3** showed a strong downregulation of survivin level in both BC cell lines. Therefore, compound **3** emerges as a promising survivin inhibitor for cancer treatment.

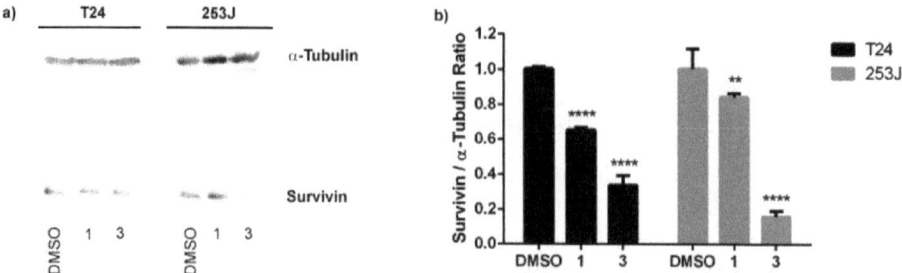

Figure 10. Expression profile of survivin in T24 and 253 J cells treated with compounds **1** and **3**. (**a**) Protein expression of survivin from Western blot analysis. α-Tubulin was used as an internal control for total protein measurement. (**b**) Survivin/α-Tubulin ratio of the Western blot analysis. The graph represents the mean ± standard deviation of three independent experiments. Statistical analysis was carried out using two-way ANOVA followed by a Bonferroni multiple comparison test with ** $p < 0.01$ and **** $p < 0.0001$.

4. Discussion

BC is one of the most frequent cancers and a worldwide health problem. There is an urgent need to develop new therapeutic agents targeting the underlying mechanisms that trigger the tumorigenesis and progression of BC. The main antitumor effects of ·NO include apoptosis, necrosis, and cytotoxicity stimulation; the inhibition of tumor cell proliferation; DNA fragmentation; the inhibition of NF-κB and the modulation of its gene products; and the impairment of angiogenesis and metastasis [8]. Continuing our efforts in the search for new arylsulfonylfuroxans with potent anticancer activity, herein, we describe the study of three ·NO-donor compounds as potential therapeutic agents for BC. Our results indicate that compounds **1**, **2**, and **3** exert a high antiproliferative activity against BC cells.

In previous studies, in the BC cell lines described here, compounds analogs to **2** and **3**, including **4** and **5**, and the furoxan precursor of the latter were tested [18]. From these studies, compound **4** was found to have the highest antiproliferative activity and selectivity towards tumor cells in the 253J cell line (Table 3), while for the T24 cell line, compound **5** stands out, with an acceptable IC_{50} but with a relatively low selectivity index (Table 3). In the search to improve these results and to further study the underlying mechanisms of action, we started to work on the synthesis of hydroxamic acid derivatives of these compounds. However, the synthesis was very challenging and it was not possible to obtain these derivatives, but it was possible to obtain the synthetic intermediates described here, **2** and **3**, which we studied as shown, and achieved comparable-to-better activities than their precursors **4** and **5**.

Table 3. Antiproliferative activity (IC_{50} values in µM ± standard deviation) and selectivity index (SI) of arylsulfonylfuroxan derivatives in 253J and T24 cancer cells.

	253J			T24		
Compound	IC_{50}	SI	Compound		IC_{50}	SI
1	3.59 ± 1.11	5.55			12.26 ± 1.26 *	2.81 *
4	4.94 ± 1.22 *	5.09 *	5		3.69 ± 1.12 *	1.31 *
2	2.27 ± 1.08	1.86	3		2.57 ± 1.10	6.48

* Data from [18].

In this line of thought, if we compare the results of antiproliferative activity in the 253J cell line for compounds **1**, **4**, and **2**, going from a simple to a more complex arylsulfonylfuroxan, incorporating a tocopherol-mimetic pharmacophore with known antitumor activity [36,37], it was observed that compound **1** stood out for its antiproliferative activity and selectivity and was therefore selected for further studies. The proposed structural changes did not significantly improve its activity or its selectivity. In contrast, when we performed the same analysis on the T24 cell line for compound **3** and its precursors, it was observed that the structural changes introduced improved both its antiproliferative activity and selectivity (Table 3). Moreover, compound **3** also stood out for its antiproliferative activity in the 253J cell line, and was therefore selected for further studies.

Compounds **1** and **3** proved to have a higher selectivity for T24 and 253J cancer cells than for non-cancer cells HaCaT, surpassing the chemotherapeutic drug cisplatin. Compound **2** showed a high inhibition of cell growth in 253J cells and a moderate effect in T24 cells; however, its selectivity toward BC cells was low, indicating possible side effects. In addition, we observed that the ·NO-releasing activity of compounds was primarily responsible for the anticancer effect in T24 cells, whereas in 253J cells, the ·NO-releasing capacity was partially involved. These observations confirm previously reported studies that emphasise the importance of ·NO donors for BC [7,18]. A clonogenic assay showed similar anticancer behavior of compounds as was observed in the sulforhodamine B assay, indicating that compounds **1** and **3** are suitable for further studies in BC cells. In this sense, we performed a three-dimensional antiproliferative assay as an approach to determine the antitumor effect of compounds in a small tumor. As we have shown above (Figure 6), compound **3** exhibited higher toxicity towards cancer cells, increasing its antiproliferative effect between 24 and 72 h of treatment. Thus, compound **3** appears to be a promising molecule to perform future in vivo studies for BC. With the aim to identify possible mechanisms of action exerted by compounds **1** and **3**, additional studies were performed. It is well-known that ·NO can react with molecular oxygen to generate secondary species which induce DNA damage. Via an alkaline comet assay, we observed the induction of DNA strand breaks in the BC nucleus after incubation with **1** and **3** (Figure 8). However, this assay did not discriminate between alkali-labile sites and single- or double-strand breaks. Further studies will be performed to elucidate precisely the DNA damage induced by these ·NO donors. As we pointed out before, the NF-κB pathway has been described as an EMT and metastasis positive regulator [13]. Moreover, NF-κB activation upregulates survivin expression enhancing the proliferation and resistance to the apoptosis of BC cells [14]. In this regard, inhibition of the NF-κB pathway and downregulation of the growth-promoting and anti-apoptotic protein survivin is suitable for cancer therapy. Our results suggest that compound **1** inhibited the NF-κB pathway, slightly reduced cell migration, and moderately reduced survivin expression in BC cell lines. On the other hand, compound **3** significantly decreased cell migration and strongly downregulated survivin in BC cells, although it did not seem to affect the NF-κB pathway. Therefore, this molecule could impair the initial stage of the EMT process and reduce the survivin intracellular level through a different mechanism than compound **1**. Survivin plays an important role in DNA double-strand-break repair regulation through its interaction with proteins involved in double-strand-break repair machinery [38]. In this way, our results indicate that the synthetized ·NO-releasing compounds **1** and **3** induce DNA strand breaks and avoid DNA repair through survivin downregulation. Hence, in this work, we evidenced that the ·NO donors **1** and **3** inhibit BC cell proliferation with high selectivity and induce DNA damage through a mechanism that involves ·NO-releasing capacity and survivin downregulation. A general scheme of the identified mechanisms of action exerted by ·NO donors **1** and **3** in this work can be seen below (Figure 11). We highlight compound **3** as a promising therapy for BC. In the future, further studies of this ·NO donor will be performed.

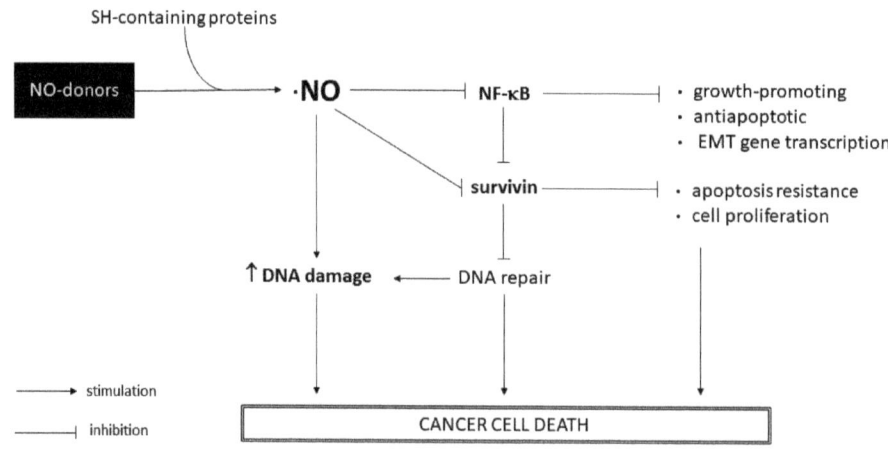

Figure 11. Schematic overview of the main pathways involved in the mode of action of ·NO-releasing compounds **1** and **3**.

Finally, herein, we confirmed that the generation of arylsulfonylfuroxans and their hybridization with tocopherol-mimetic pharmacophores is a promising strategy for BC treatment. The combined administration of these ·NO-releasing compounds and traditional cancer therapies must be considered to enhance its efficacy. To the best of our knowledge, this is the first report of ·NO-releasing compounds with survivin-downregulating activity proposed for BC treatment. Future approaches of ·NO donors in other cancer types in which survivin is upregulated will be performed.

5. Conclusions

In conclusion, we report three ·NO-releasing compounds as promising anti-bladder-cancer drugs. We demonstrate that compound **3** is a potent inhibitor of cell proliferation and a strong downregulator of survivin levels in BC cells. Therefore, we believe that the development of ·NO donors is a promising therapeutic directed against the underlying mechanism of BC development.

Supplementary Materials: The following supporting information can be downloaded at: https://www.mdpi.com/article/10.3390/biomedicines11010199/s1, Figure S1: 1H and 13C-NMR spectra of synthesized compounds **2** and **3**.

Author Contributions: Conceptualization, G.V.L. and P.H.; methodology, M.V., M.L., M.I., D.A., V.P., and K.P.; validation, M.V., M.L., M.I., D.A., K.P., M.B.-F., G.V.L. and P.H.; formal analysis, M.V., M.L., M.I., D.A., K.P., G.V.L. and P.H.; investigation, M.V., M.L., M.I., D.A., V.P., K.P. and P.H.; resources, M.V., M.L., M.I., D.A., V.P. and K.P.; data curation, M.V., M.L., M.I., D.A., K.P. and P.H.; writing—original draft preparation, M.V., G.V.L. and P.H.; writing—review and editing, M.V., G.V.L. and P.H.; visualization, P.H.; supervision, M.B.-F., G.V.L. and P.H.; project administration, G.V.L.; funding acquisition, G.V.L. All authors have read and agreed to the published version of the manuscript.

Funding: This research was funded by CSIC, Udelar, and PEDECIBA-Química, Uruguay (2018 - FID 37 - Grupo ID 882469). The research that gave rise to the results presented in this article received funding from the Agencia Nacional de Investigación e Innovación (ANII) under the code POS_NAC_2021_1_169813.

Institutional Review Board Statement: Not applicable.

Informed Consent Statement: Not applicable.

Data Availability Statement: Not applicable.

Acknowledgments: The authors are thankful for the technical support provided by Horacio Pezaroglo from Universidad de la República, and Alejandro Leyva from Institut Pasteur de Montevideo.

Conflicts of Interest: The authors declare no conflict of interest.

Sample Availability: Samples of the compounds are available from the authors.

References

1. Siegel, R.L.; Miller, K.D.; Fuchs, H.E.; Jemal, A. Cancer Statistics, 2022. *CA Cancer J. Clin.* **2022**, *72*, 7–33. [CrossRef] [PubMed]
2. Kaufman, D.S.; Shipley, W.U.; Feldman, A.S. Bladder Cancer. *Lancet* **2009**, *374*, 239–249. [CrossRef] [PubMed]
3. Ghatalia, P.; Zibelman, M.; Geynisman, D.M.; Plimack, E. Approved Checkpoint Inhibitors in Bladder Cancer: Which Drug Should Be Used When? *Ther. Adv. Med. Oncol.* **2018**, *10*, 1–10. [CrossRef] [PubMed]
4. Witjes, J.A.; Bruins, H.M.; Cathomas, R.; Compérat, E.M.; Cowan, N.C.; Gakis, G.; Hernández, V.; Linares Espinós, E.; Lorch, A.; Neuzillet, Y., et al. European Association of Urology Guidelines on Muscle-Invasive and Metastatic Bladder Cancer: Summary of the 2020 Guidelines. *Eur. Urol.* **2021**, *79*, 82–104. [CrossRef] [PubMed]
5. Yoon, C.Y.; Park, M.J.; Lee, J.S.; Lee, S.C.; Oh, J.J.; Park, H.; Chung, C.W.; Abdullajanov, M.M.; Jeong, S.J.; Hong, S.K.; et al. The Histone Deacetylase Inhibitor Trichostatin a Synergistically Resensitizes a Cisplatin Resistant Human Bladder Cancer Cell Line. *J. Urol.* **2011**, *185*, 1102–1111. [CrossRef]
6. Knowles, M.; Dyrskjøt, L.; Heath, E.I.; Bellmunt, J.; Siefker-Radtke, A.O. Metastatic Urothelial Carcinoma. *Cancer Cell* **2021**, *39*, 583–585. [CrossRef]
7. Seabra, A.B.; Durán, N. Nitric Oxide Donors for Prostate and Bladder Cancers: Current State and Challenges. *Eur. J. Pharmacol.* **2018**, *826*, 158–168. [CrossRef]

8. Huang, Z.; Fu, J.; Zhang, Y. Nitric Oxide Donor-Based Cancer Therapy: Advances and Prospects. *J. Med. Chem.* **2017**, *60*, 7617–7635. [CrossRef]
9. Korde Choudhari, S.; Chaudhary, M.; Bagde, S.; Gadbail, A.R.; Joshi, V. Nitric Oxide and Cancer: A Review. *World J. Surg. Oncol.* **2013**, *11*, 1–11. [CrossRef]
10. Thomas, S.; Lowe, J.E.; Knowles, R.G.; Green, I.C.; Green, M.H.L. Factors Affecting the DNA Damaging Activity of Superoxide and Nitric Oxide. *Mutat. Res.-Fundam. Mol. Mech. Mutagen.* **1998**, *402*, 77–84. [CrossRef]
11. Marshall, H.E.; Stamler, J.S. Inhibition of NF-Kappa B by S-Nitrosylation. *Biochemistry* **2001**, *40*, 1688–1693. [CrossRef]
12. Plenchette, S.; Romagny, S.; Laurens, V.; Bettaieb, A. S-Nitrosylation in TNF Superfamily Signaling Pathway: Implication in Cancer. *Redox Biol.* **2015**, *6*, 507–515. [CrossRef]
13. Huber, M.A.; Azoitei, N.; Baumann, B.; Grünert, S.; Sommer, A.; Pehamberger, H.; Kraut, N.; Beug, H.; Wirth, T. NF-κB Is Essential for Epithelial-Mesenchymal Transition and Metastasis in a Model of Breast Cancer Progression. *J. Clin. Investig.* **2004**, *114*, 569–581. [CrossRef]
14. Cui, X.; Shen, D.; Kong, C.; Zhang, Z.; Zeng, Y.; Lin, X.; Liu, X. NF-κB Suppresses Apoptosis and Promotes Bladder Cancer Cell Proliferation by Upregulating Survivin Expression in Vitro and in Vivo. *Sci. Rep.* **2017**, *7*, 1–13. [CrossRef]
15. Shariat, S.F.; Ashfaq, R.; Karakiewicz, P.I.; Saeedi, O.; Sagalowsky, A.I.; Lotan, Y. Survivin Expression Is Associated with Bladder Cancer Presence, Stage, Progression, and Mortality. *Cancer* **2007**, *109*, 1106–1113. [CrossRef]
16. Altieri, D.C. Survivin, Versatile Modulation of Cell Division and Apoptosis in Cancer. *Oncogene* **2003**, *22*, 8581–8589. [CrossRef]
17. Shariat, S.F.; Karakiewicz, P.I.; Godoy, G.; Karam, J.A.; Ashfaq, R.; Fradet, Y.; Isbarn, H.; Montorsi, F.; Jeldres, C.; Bastian, P.J.; et al. Survivin as a Prognostic Marker for Urothelial Carcinoma of the Bladder: A Multicenter External Validation Study. *Clin. Cancer Res.* **2009**, *15*, 7012–7019. [CrossRef]
18. Pérez, F.; Varela, M.; Canclini, L.; Acosta, S.; Martínez-López, W.; López, G.V.; Hernández, P. Furoxans and Tocopherol Analogs-Furoxan Hybrids as Anticancer Agents. *Anticancer. Drugs* **2019**, *30*, 330–338. [CrossRef]
19. Bubeník, J.; Barešová, M.; Viklický, V.; Jakoubková, J.; Sainerová, H.; Donner, J. Established Cell Line of Urinary Bladder Carcinoma (T24) Containing Tumour-specific Antigen. *Int. J. Cancer* **1973**, *11*, 765–773. [CrossRef] [PubMed]
20. Elliott, A.Y.; Cleveland, P.; Cervenka, J.; Castro, A.E.; Stein, N.; Hakala, T.R.; Fraley, E.E. Characterization of a Cell Line from Human Transitional Cell Cancer of the Urinary Tract. *J. Natl. Cancer Inst.* **1974**, *53*, 1341–1349. [CrossRef]
21. Singh, N.; Krishnakumar, S.; Kanwar, R.K.; Cheung, C.H.A.; Kanwar, J.R. Clinical Aspects for Survivin: A Crucial Molecule for Targeting Drug-Resistant Cancers. *Drug Discov. Today* **2015**, *20*, 578–587. [CrossRef] [PubMed]
22. Rödel, F.; Hoffmann, J.; Distel, L.; Herrmann, M.; Noisternig, T.; Papadopoulos, T.; Sauer, R.; Rödel, C. Survivin as a Radioresistance Factor, and Prognostic and Therapeutic Target for Radiotherapy in Rectal Cancer. *Cancer Res.* **2005**, *65*, 4881–4887. [CrossRef] [PubMed]
23. Lolli, M.L.; Cena, C.; Medana, C.; Lazzarato, L.; Morini, G.; Coruzzi, G.; Manarini, S.; Fruttero, R.; Gasco, A. A New Class of Ibuprofen Derivatives with Reduced Gastrotoxicity. *J. Med. Chem.* **2001**, *44*, 3463–3468. [CrossRef] [PubMed]
24. López, G.V.; Blanco, F.; Hernández, P.; Ferreira, A.; Piro, O.E.; Batthyány, C.; González, M.; Rubbo, H.; Cerecetto, H. Second Generation of α-Tocopherol Analogs-Nitric Oxide Donors: Synthesis, Physicochemical, and Biological Characterization. *Bioorganic Med. Chem.* **2007**, *15*, 6262–6272. [CrossRef] [PubMed]
25. Vichai, V.; Kirtikara, K. Sulforhodamine B Colorimetric Assay for Cytotoxicity Screening. *Nat. Protoc.* **2006**, *1*, 1112–1116. [CrossRef]
26. Griess, P. Bemerkungen Zu Der Abhandlung Der HH. Weselsky Und Benedikt „Ueber Einige Azoverbindungen". *Ber. Der Dtsch. Chem. Ges.* **1879**, *12*, 426–428. [CrossRef]
27. Sodano, F.; Gazzano, E.; Rolando, B.; Marini, E.; Lazzarato, L.; Fruttero, R.; Riganti, C.; Gasco, A. Tuning NO Release of Organelle-Targeted Furoxan Derivatives and Their Cytotoxicity against Lung Cancer Cells. *Bioorg. Chem.* **2021**, *111*, 104911. [CrossRef]
28. Franken, N.A.P.; Rodermond, H.M.; Stap, J.; Haveman, J.; van Bree, C. Clonogenic Assay of Cells in Vitro. *Nat. Protoc.* **2006**, *1*, 2315–2319. [CrossRef]
29. Ivanov, D.P.; Parker, T.L.; Walker, D.A.; Alexander, C.; Ashford, M.B.; Gellert, P.R.; Garnett, M.C. Multiplexing Spheroid Volume, Resazurin and Acid Phosphatase Viability Assays for High-Throughput Screening of Tumour Spheroids and Stem Cell Neurospheres. *PLoS ONE* **2014**, *9*, 1–14. [CrossRef]
30. Schneider, C.A.; Rasband, W.S.; Eliceiri, K.W. NIH Image to ImageJ: 25 Years of Image Analysis. *Nat. Methods* **2012**, *9*, 671–675. [CrossRef]
31. Singh, N.P.; McCoy, M.T.; Tice, R.R.; Schneider, E.L. A Simple Technique for Quantitation of Low Levels of DNA Damage in Individual Cells. *Exp. Cell Res.* **1988**, *175*, 184–191. [CrossRef]
32. Anderson, D.; Yu, T.W.; Phillips, B.J.; Schmezer, P. The Effect of Various Antioxidants and Other Modifying Agents on Oxygen-Radical-Generated DNA Damage in Human Lymphocytes in the COMET Assay. *Mutat. Res.-Fundam. Mol. Mech. Mutagen.* **1994**, *307*, 261–271. [CrossRef]
33. Collins, A.R.; Ai-guo, M.; Duthie, S.J. The Kinetics of Repair of Oxidative DNA Damage (Strand Breaks and Oxidised Pyrimidines) in Human Cells. *Mutat. Res. Repair* **1995**, *336*, 69–77. [CrossRef]

34. Hernández, P.; Cabrera, M.; Lavaggi, M.L.; Celano, L.; Tiscornia, I.; Rodrigues Da Costa, T.; Thomson, L.; Bollati-Fogolín, M.; Miranda, A.L.P.; Lima, L.M.; et al. Discovery of New Orally Effective Analgesic and Anti-Inflammatory Hybrid Furoxanyl N-Acylhydrazone Derivatives. *Bioorganic Med. Chem.* **2012**, *20*, 2158–2171. [CrossRef]
35. Burov, O.N.; Kletskii, M.E.; Fedik, N.S.; Lisovin, A.V.; Kurbatov, S.V. Mechanism of Thiol-Induced Nitrogen(II) Oxide Donation by Furoxans: A Quantum-Chemical Study. *Chem. Heterocycl. Compd.* **2015**, *51*, 951–960. [CrossRef]
36. Kanai, K.; Kikuchi, E.; Mikami, S.; Suzuki, E.; Uchida, Y.; Kodaira, K.; Miyajima, A.; Ohigashi, T.; Nakashima, J.; Oya, M. Vitamin E Succinate Induced Apoptosis and Enhanced Chemosensitivity to Paclitaxel in Human Bladder Cancer Cells in Vitro and in Vivo. *Cancer Sci.* **2010**, *101*, 216–223. [CrossRef]
37. Yang, C.S.; Luo, P.; Zeng, Z.; Wang, H.; Malafa, M.; Suh, N. Vitamin E and Cancer Prevention: Studies with Different Forms of Tocopherols and Tocotrienols. *Mol. Carcinog.* **2020**, *59*, 365–389. [CrossRef]
38. Capalbo, G.; Dittmann, K.; Weiss, C.; Reichert, S.; Hausmann, E.; Rödel, C.; Rödel, F. Radiation-Induced Survivin Nuclear Accumulation Is Linked to DNA Damage Repair. *Int. J. Radiat. Oncol. Biol. Phys.* **2010**, *77*, 226–234. [CrossRef]

Disclaimer/Publisher's Note: The statements, opinions and data contained in all publications are solely those of the individual author(s) and contributor(s) and not of MDPI and/or the editor(s). MDPI and/or the editor(s) disclaim responsibility for any injury to people or property resulting from any ideas, methods, instructions or products referred to in the content.

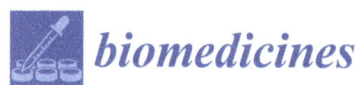

Article

Alveolar Nitric Oxide in Chronic Obstructive Pulmonary Disease—A Two-Year Follow-Up

Marieann Högman [1,*], Andreas Palm [1], Johanna Sulku [2], Björn Ställberg [3], Karin Lisspers [3], Kristina Bröms [3], Christer Janson [1] and Andrei Malinovschi [4]

1 Department of Medical Sciences, Respiratory, Allergy and Sleep Research, Uppsala University, 751 85 Uppsala, Sweden
2 Department of Pharmacy, Uppsala University, 751 23 Uppsala, Sweden
3 Department of Public Health and Caring Sciences, Family Medicine and Preventive Medicine, Uppsala University, 751 22 Uppsala, Sweden
4 Department of Medical Sciences, Clinical Physiology, Uppsala University, 751 85 Uppsala, Sweden
* Correspondence: marieann.hogman@medsci.uu.se

Abstract: Chronic obstructive pulmonary disease (COPD) affects the airways and gas exchange areas. Nitric oxide (NO) production from the airways is presented as F_ENO_{50} and from the gas exchange areas as alveolar NO (C_ANO). We aimed to evaluate, over two years, the consistency of the C_ANO estimations in subjects with COPD. A total of 110 subjects (45 men) who completed the study were included from primary and secondary care settings. C_ANO was estimated using the two-compartment model. C_ANO increased slightly during the two-year follow-up ($p = 0.01$), but F_ENO_{50} remained unchanged ($p = 0.24$). Among the subjects with a low C_ANO (<1 ppb) at inclusion, only 2% remained at a low level. For those at a high level (>2 ppb), 29% remained so. The modified Medical Research Council dyspnoea scale (mMRC) score increased at least one point in 29% of the subjects, and those subjects also increased in C_ANO from 0.9 (0.5, 2.1) ppb to 1.8 (1.1, 2.3) ppb, $p = 0.015$. We conclude that alveolar NO increased slightly over two years, together with a small decline in lung function. The increase in C_ANO was found especially in those whose levels of dyspnoea increased over time.

Keywords: COPD; fraction exhaled nitric oxide and lung function tests; comorbidity; GOLD; mathematical model; gas exchange

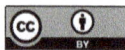

1. Introduction

Chronic obstructive pulmonary disease (COPD) affects the conducting airways and gas exchange areas. Post-bronchodilator spirometry sets a COPD diagnosis in individuals with typical respiratory symptoms such as dyspnoea and chronic cough, often together with a history of relevant exposure to smoke, usually cigarette smoke. Emphysema with the destruction of lung parenchyma can develop after many years of smoking and cannot be reversed.

In a meta-analysis, the fraction of exhaled nitric oxide (F_ENO) was slightly increased in persons with COPD compared to healthy controls [1]. F_ENO is further increased if there is an eosinophilic inflammation, such as type-2 inflammation [2]. Tobacco smoke will interfere with nitric oxide (NO) production in the airway epithelia. Patients with COPD who are currently smoking will therefore have a lower F_ENO than ex-smokers. Additionally, ex-smokers have lower values than never-smokers [3]. Thus, the clinical significance of F_ENO in stable COPD patients is unclear, as was summarised in a recent scoping review [4].

The NO production in the lungs can be traced to the exhalation gas. Fractional exhaled nitric oxide at 50 mL/s (F_ENO_{50}) represents the NO production in the airways, and the alveolar NO (C_ANO) represents production from the gas exchange areas. In COPD, there is an involvement in the lung parenchyma, which can manifest as emphysema. Higher values of C_ANO in COPD patients have been reported [5–8], but also values that did not differ from healthy controls [9]. There are also methodological issues associated with the estimation of C_ANO, which were reviewed in 2017 by a European Respiratory Society task force [10]. The task force recommended two methods to determine estimation: the linear method by Tsoukias & George and the non-linear Högman-Meriläinen algorithm. Both methods refer to Fick's first law of diffusion, where a bolus of gas (alveolar gas) transported up into the conducting airways picks up NO driven by a concentration gradient from the bronchial wall. These methods are explained, and the equations for the calculations can be found together with the usefulness of these methods in respiratory diseases in Högman et al., 2014, 2017 [11,12].

A limited number of studies have followed C_ANO values in patients with COPD over a more extended period. Lehouck et al. followed 22 patients in stable condition for four months. There were no statistically significant differences in the C_ANO values compared to those at inclusion [9]. Lázár et al. investigated patients in a stable disease state and patients experiencing an acute exacerbation, and they found that the C_ANO values were elevated compared to healthy controls [13]. However, no difference was found between the stable and the exacerbated patients. In 26 patients, there was no difference between the C_ANO at the time of the acute exacerbation and discharge from the hospital. Two other studies looked at the effect of corticosteroid treatment after one week [14] and after four weeks [15]. Both studies showed no difference in C_ANO between the visits.

This study aimed to evaluate, over two years, the consistency of the C_ANO estimations in subjects with COPD and the associations of the C_ANO changes to the clinical progression of the disease.

2. Materials and Method

2.1. Study Design and Subjects

The research subjects were recruited from the Swedish multicentre study: Tools Identifying Exacerbations in COPD (TIE-study) [16]. Those included were participants over the age of 40 with a diagnosis of COPD from primary and secondary care settings who came from one of the research centres that could measure C_ANO at inclusion and at the one and two-year follow-ups (Figure 1). The measurements were performed only when the study participants were in a stable disease state, i.e., no exacerbation within the last three weeks. Recruitment to the study occurred from September 2014 until October 2016. The study was completed in October 2018.

2.2. Methods

The COPD diagnosis was set by a physician and confirmed by spirometry. The measurement was obtained using a post-bronchodilator (400 μg salbutamol) forced expiratory volume in one second (FEV_1) divided by the highest value of vital capacity (VC) or forced vital capacity (FVC) with a ratio of <0.70 (SpiroPerfect spirometer, Welch Allyn, Skaneateles Falls, NY, USA). FEV_1 and FVC are presented as per cent predicted using Swedish reference values [17,18].

According to the 2005 standardised measurements recommendation, the measurement of exhaled NO was performed at a flow of 50 mL/s (F_ENO_{50}) [19]. In addition to F_ENO_{50}, exhaled NO at flows of 20, 100, and 300 mL/s were measured in duplicate for the non-linear Högman-Meriläinen algorithm (HMA) modelling of NO exchange. The NO analyser was equipped with the software for the HMA estimation (Eco Medics CLD 88, Eco Medics, Dürnten, Switzerland). HMA estimates the C_ANO, airway wall NO content (C_{aw}NO), the diffusing capacity of NO from the airway wall (D_{aw}NO), and F_ENO_{50}. For quality control, the measured and the estimated F_ENO_{50} were compared for a difference not exceeding 5 ppb [10]. For subjects who could not perform the HMA, the linear modelling method was applied with flows of 100, 200, and 300 mL/s and an r-value > 0.95 [10].

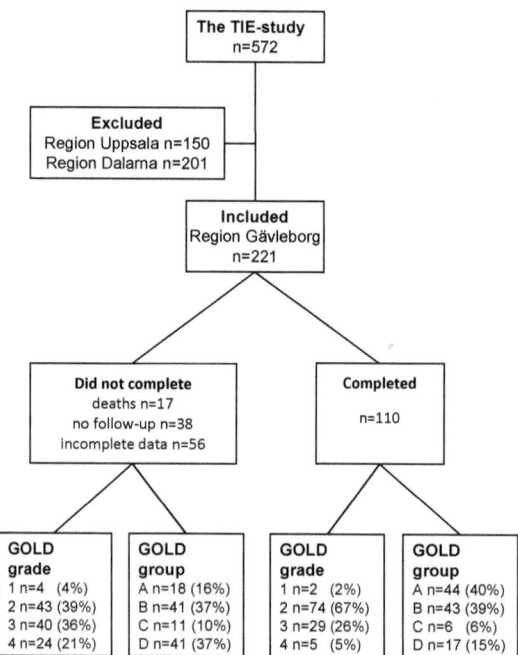

Figure 1. Flow chart of excluded and included COPD subjects. Subjects were grouped according to whether they completed or did not complete the study. Further grouping at inclusion was according to the GOLD 2021 assessment of airflow limitations (GOLD grade) and symptom/risk of exacerbation (GOLD group) (https://goldcopd.org, accessed on 1 March 2022).

Blood cell counts analysing neutrophils (B-Neu) and eosinophils (B-Eos) were performed (Cell-Dyn 4000, Abbott, Abbott Park, IL, USA and Sysmex XN-10, Sysmex America Inc, Lincoinshire, IL, USA). Additionally, questionnaires including the COPD Assessment Test (CAT), the Clinical COPD Questionnaire (CCQ) and the modified Medical Research Council Dyspnoea Scale (mMRC) were used [20]. A clinical difference in CAT was set at ≥2 points [21] and CCQ at ≥0.4 points [22]. For statistical comparisons, mMRC scores were grouped as <2 and ≥2. Questions regarding demographics, smoking habits, comorbidities and inhaled COPD treatment were also assessed. The research nurse reviewed the answers to the questionnaires with the research subjects to assure accuracy.

2.3. Data Analysis

To classify the COPD subjects' disease severity, the GOLD risk assessment version 2021 with assessments of airflow limitations and symptoms/risk of exacerbations (CAT scale) was used together with the history of exacerbations/hospitalisations. An exacerbation was defined as an unscheduled health care visit, and/or a course of oral corticosteroids, and/or a course of antibiotics due to COPD deterioration (questionnaire assessed). Information about hospitalisation admittance was retrieved from hospital records. A questionnaire gathered the exacerbation history for the year prior to each visit.

Binominal test, Pearson χ^2-test, Kolmogorov–Smirnov normality test, and non-parametric tests, i.e., McNemar χ^2-test, Mann–Whitney U test, Friedman's test and Spearman's rho (SPSS, v. 24 for Windows, SPSS Inc., Chicago, IL, USA) were used for the statistical calculations. Descriptive statistics are given as frequencies and percentages, mean ± SD, or median with lower quartile (Q1) and upper quartile (Q3). A p-value of $p < 0.05$ was considered significant.

3. Results

Of the 221 included subjects, 111 did not complete the study. Non-completion was due to death, lack of participation in all follow-up visits, or incomplete data collection (Figure 1). F_ENO_{50} could not be collected from six subjects, and the C_ANO estimations were missing from 51 subjects. More severe disease was found in the subjects who did not complete the study, as validated by lung function, higher B-Neu levels, lower F_ENO_{50} and higher C_ANO values. The symptom burden according to the CAT, CCQ, and mMRC was also higher, and they had a greater number of comorbidities, exacerbations, and treatments with triple therapy (an inhaled corticosteroid in combination with a long-acting beta-2-agonist and a long-acting muscarinic antagonist) than the subjects who completed the study, see Table 1. The C_ANO and F_ENO_{50} were 2.3 (0.6, 3.5) and 12 (5, 15) ppb, respectively in participants who died before completing the study. The 51 subjects whose NO modelling was missing had a $FEV_{1.0}$ of 1.33 (0.94, 1.56) L and a FVC of 2.40 (1.97, 2.96) L.

Table 1. Characteristics of the study subjects at inclusion who completed or did not complete the study.

	Did Not Complete n = 111	Completed n = 110	p-Value
Women n (%)	67 (60%)	65 (59%)	0.847
Age years	69 ± 8	68 ± 8	0.113
Current daily smokers n (%)	25 (23%)	28 (26%)	0.506
BMI	26 (23, 30)	27 (23, 32)	0.185
Comorbidity			
Asthma	45%	33%	0.060
Chronic bronchitis	45%	25%	**0.002**
Heart infarction/angina	11%	12%	0.813
Heart failure	6%	1%	**0.032**
Heart fibrillation	19%	6%	**0.005**
Hypertension	47%	46%	0.836
Diabetes	13%	5%	**0.034**
Anxiety/depression	30%	21%	0.132
Lung function			
$FEV_{1.0}$ L	1.17 (0.79, 1.51)	1.53 (1.24, 1.86)	**<0.001**
$FEV_{1.0}$ % predicted	45 (31, 58)	57 (49, 67)	**<0.001**
FVC L	2.38 (1.89, 3.16)	2.83 (2.47, 3.45)	**<0.001**
FVC % predicted	57 (47, 74)	67 (61, 76)	**<0.001**
Inflammatory markers			
B-Neu 10^9/L	5.4 (4.3, 6.1)	4.3 (3.5, 4.9)	**<0.001**
B-Eos 10^9/L	0.14 (0.08, 0.23)	0.18 (0.10, 0.28)	0.094
Exhaled NO			
F_ENO_{50} ppb	11 (6, 17) [1]	14 (9, 21)	**0.006**
C_ANO ppb	1.5 (0.9, 2.7) [2]	1.3 (0.6, 2.1)	**0.043**
$C_{aw}NO$ ppb	35 (16, 95) [2]	65 (30, 136)	**0.007**
$D_{aw}NO$ mL/s	22 (10, 34) [2]	15 (7, 30)	0.084
Symptom burden			
CAT	14 (9, 22)	11 (6, 16)	**<0.001**
mMRC ≥ 2	65 (59%)	46 (42%)	**0.013**
CCQ	2.0 (1.1, 3.1)	1.3 (0.7, 2.1)	**<0.001**
Exacerbations			
Questionnaire ≥ 1 (%)	67 (61%)	48 (44%)	**<0.001**
Inhaled treatment			
ICS + LABA + LAMA [3]	73 (66%)	46 (42%)	**<0.001**

[1] Missing 6 subjects, [2] missing 51 subjects; [3] regular treatment with inhaled corticosteroids (ICS) in combination with long-acting beta-2-agonist (LABA), and long-acting muscarinic antagonist (LAMA). Body mass index (BMI), forced expiratory volume at 1 s ($FEV_{1.0}$), forced vital capacity (FVC), blood neutrophils (B-Neu), blood eosinophils (B-Eos), fraction of exhaled nitric oxide at 50 mL/s (F_ENO_{50}), alveolar NO (C_ANO), airway wall NO content ($C_{aw}NO$), diffusing capacity of NO from the airway wall ($D_{aw}NO$), COPD Assessment Test (CAT), modified Medical Research Council dyspnoea scale (mMRC), Clinical COPD Questionnaire (CCQ). Data are given in percentage, median (Q1, Q3), or mean ± SD.

A total of 110 subjects completed the two-year follow-up. They were aged 68 ± 8 years and 59% were women. Among the comorbidities reported were: asthma (33%) and chronic bronchitis (25%). However, the distribution of C_ANO was not different from those subjects who did not report asthma or chronic bronchitis, $p = 0.81$ and $p = 0.26$, respectively. Other comorbidities were hypertension (46%), anxiety/depression (21%), heart disease (19%), and diabetes (5%). Additional characteristics of the study participants are presented in Table 2 and Figure 1.

Table 2. Characteristics of the subjects completing the study at inclusion, and their one and two-year follow-ups.

	Inclusion n = 110	1-Year n = 110	2-Year n = 110	*p*-Value
Current daily smokers n (%)	28 (26%)	22 (20%)	27 (24%)	1.0
BMI	27 (23, 32)	27 (23, 31)	27 (24, 31)	0.559
Lung function				
$FEV_{1.0}$ L	1.53 (1.24, 1.86)	1.53 (1.20, 1.94)	1.49 (1.15, 1.89)	**0.024**
$FEV_{1.0}$ % predicted	57 (49, 67)	58 (48, 68)	56 (46, 66)	0.429
FVC L	2.83 (2.47, 3.45)	2.78 (2.27, 3.18)	2.68 (2.23, 3.27)	**<0.001**
FVC % predicted	67 (61, 76)	66 (57, 76)	65 (56, 76)	**0.007**
Inflammatory markers				
B-Neu 10^9/L	4.3 (3.5, 4.9)	4.3 (3.2, 5.3)	4.2 (3.6, 5.4)	0.890
B-Eos 10^9/L	0.18 (0.10, 0.28)	0.17 (0.11, 0.29)	0.16 (0.11, 0.24)	0.072
Exhaled NO				
F_ENO_{50} ppb	14 (9, 21)	14 (9, 23)	13 (8, 19)	0.238
C_ANO ppb	1.3 (0.6, 2.1)	1.5 (1.0, 2.2)	1.7 (1.1, 2.3)	**0.013**
$C_{aw}NO$ ppb	65 (30, 136)	49 (21, 111)	52 (25, 96)	0.089
$D^{aw}NO$ mL/s	15 (7, 30)	18 (9, 36)	16 (6, 33)	0.553
Symptom burden				
CAT	11 (6, 16)	10 (6, 15)	11 (7, 17)	0.523
mMRC n 0/1/2/3/4	17/47/23/14/9	16/48/20/14/12	11/51/16/15/17	
CCQ	1.3 (0.7, 2.1)	1.3 (0.8, 2.1)	1.3 (0.8, 2.4)	0.537
Exacerbations ≥ 1/year	48 (44%)	25 (23%)	29 (27%)	**0.002**
Treatment				
No regular treatment n (%)	21 (19%)	22 (20%)	18 (16%)	0.863
Bronchodilators [1] n (%)	26 (24%)	22 (20%)	27 (25%)	
ICS [2] n (%)	63 (57%)	63 (57%)	64 (58%)	
SABA last week	50 (45%)	48 (44%)	47 (43%)	0.584

[1] Regular treatment with long-acting beta-2-agonist and/or long-acting or short-acting muscarinic antagonist alone or in combination, [2] regular treatment with inhaled corticosteroid alone or in any combination with bronchodilators. Body mass index (BMI), forced expiratory volume at 1 s ($FEV_{1.0}$), forced vital capacity (FVC), blood neutrophils (B-Neu), blood eosinophils (B-Eos), fraction of exhaled nitric oxide at 50 mL/s (F_ENO_{50}), alveolar NO (C_ANO), airway wall NO content ($C_{aw}NO$), diffusing capacity of NO from the airway wall ($D_{aw}NO$), COPD Assessment Test (CAT), modified Medical Research Council dyspnoea scale (mMRC), Clinical COPD Questionnaire (CCQ), inhaled corticosteroids (ICS), short-acting beta-2-agonist (SABA). Data are given in percentage or median (Q1, Q3).

Most of our subjects could perform the multiple flows for the HMA to estimate the C_ANO, but the linear model was used for two subjects at the inclusion, for seven subjects at the one-year visit and for 24 subjects at the two-year visit. There was no statistically significant change in F_ENO_{50} between the visits. F_ENO_{50} was lower in subjects who were currently smoking at inclusion compared to ex-smokers, F_ENO_{50} 9 (6, 16) ppb and 15 (11, 24) ppb respectively, $p = 0.004$. $C_{aw}NO$ was also lower, 34 (21, 94) ppb and 74 (36, 154) ppb respectively, $p = 0.018$, while $D_{aw}NO$ and C_ANO were not affected by smoking status ($p = 0.56$ respectively $p = 0.27$). C_ANO increased during the study period while the other parameters of the HMA did not change (Table 2). C_ANO had no correlation to age. There was no statistically significant difference in C_ANO between females and males, 1.3 (0.7, 2.3) ppb and 1.3 (0.5, 2.0) ppb respectively, $p = 0.38$. C_ANO was 1.3 (0.6, 2.1) ppb in subjects without ICS and 1.3 (0.5, 2.2) ppb in subjects taking ICS, $p = 0.68$. During the two-year follow-up, the FEV$_1$ % predicted was not significantly changed, but the FVC % predicted decreased slightly ($p < 0.001$), see Table 2. There were no correlations between lung function and F$_E$NO$_{50}$ or C$_A$NO at any point in time. Additionally, there was no correlation between the change in F$_E$NO$_{50}$ or C$_A$NO and the change in lung function.

To evaluate the consistency of the C$_A$NO measurements, we divided the participants into three groups: low <1 ppb, medium 1–2 ppb, and high >2 ppb (Figure 2). Only 2% of the subjects who had a low C$_A$NO at inclusion consistently remained at a low level at the last follow-up. In the medium group 18% remained at the same level, and in the high C$_A$NO group 29% remained the same.

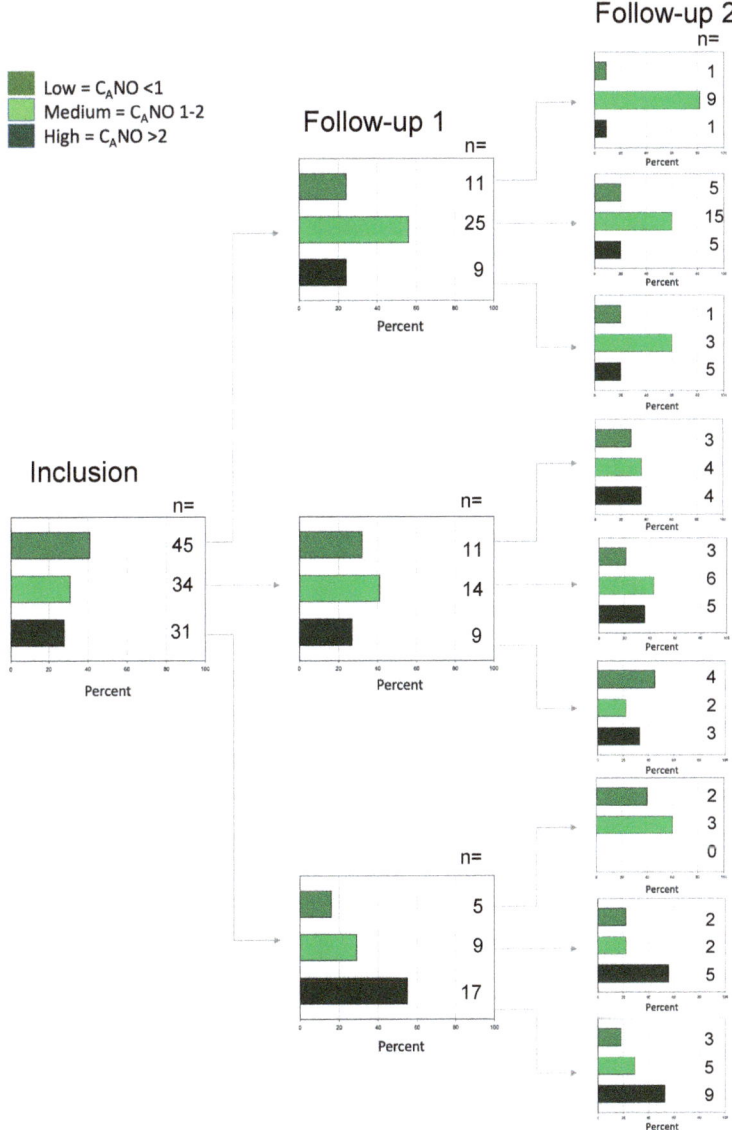

Figure 2. The estimation of C$_A$NO at inclusion and each follow-up during the two-year period. The subjects are grouped in low <1 ppb, medium 1–2 ppb, and high >2 ppb.

The symptom burden assessed by CAT and CCQ did not change during the two-year follow-up period (Table 2). A clinical increase in CAT scores was seen in 44 subjects, but there was no difference in the change in C_ANO in those with and those without an increase ($p = 0.38$). In CCQ scores, a clinical decrease was seen in 36 subjects also without a difference in the change in C_ANO ($p = 0.08$). There were changes in the mMRC dyspnoea scores over the study period, with a shift toward higher values as illustrated in Figure 3 and seen in Table 2. The subjects were divided into two groups, one that increased their mMRC scores by 1–3 points (n = 32) and another that scored minus 1 or had the same value (n = 78) between inclusion and the two-year follow-up. The distribution of C_ANO at inclusion was the same for the two mMRC groups. As seen in Figure 4, the subjects who had an increase in their mMRC, also had an increase in C_ANO.

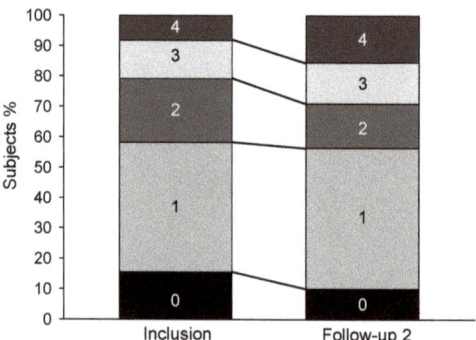

Figure 3. The modified Medical Research Council dyspnoea scale (mMRC) (ordinal scale 0–4) at inclusion and after two years.

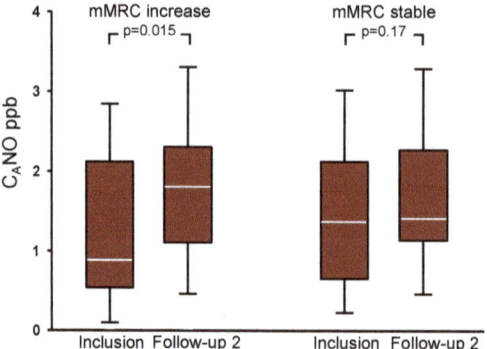

Figure 4. C_ANO values for the subjects that increased their modified Medical Research Council dyspnoea scale (mMRC) by 1–3 points (n = 32, left) and the subjects that had a stable mMRC, minus 1 or the same value (n = 78, right) at inclusion and after two years. The horizontal line in each box corresponds to the median value, the upper and lower margins correspond to Q1 and Q3, and the whiskers correspond to the 10th and 90th percentiles.

The inhaled COPD treatment of our participants that completed the study was similar during the study period (Table 2). The frequency of exacerbations for the subjects with ≥1 exacerbation(s) the year prior to inclusion decreased at the one and two-year follow-ups (Table 2).

4. Discussion

This study showed that over a period of two years, subjects with COPD who had stable treatment had a progression of the disease; as evidenced by slightly lower FVC measurements, higher $C_A NO$ values, and a shift towards higher dyspnoea scores. The subjects who increased their dyspnoea scores had a higher $C_A NO$. Only a third of our subjects with a higher $C_A NO$ value, defined as above 2 ppb, remained at the same level after two years.

When $C_A NO$ values from this study were compared to those from healthy subjects, the values from the COPD subjects were found to be slightly lower. The subjects completing the study aged 47–83 years had a $C_A NO$ of 1.3 that increased to 1.7 ppb, the subjects not completing aged 40–87 years had at inclusion a $C_A NO$ of 1.5 ppb, and the healthy comparison subjects from the literature aged 50–78 years had 2.2 (1.5, 2.9) ppb [11]. $C_A NO$ increases with age in healthy subjects [11], but there was no correlation between age and $C_A NO$ among our COPD subjects.

$C_A NO$ values have been found to be not increased in COPD patients [9], but contradictory results with higher values have also been found [5,6,23]. These divergent results might be related to differences in the populations studied, but also to methodological aspects. For example, the lowest flow to use with the linear method is 100 mL/s [10], and using a flow lower than that will give a falsely high $C_A NO$ level. However, we found higher $C_A NO$ values in a small sample of COPD patients when using the HMA as in the present study [8]. This difference is, therefore, most likely due to the subjects being in different stages of the disease, since $C_A NO$ increased with disease progression. The subjects who did not complete the study and had a higher disease burden had higher $C_A NO$ values than the subjects who completed the study.

Good consistency of $C_A NO$ estimation over the follow-up period was lacking. Only 29% of our subjects with a higher $C_A NO$ value, defined as above 2 ppb, remained at the same level after two years. However, in this study, there was an increase in $C_A NO$ over time. The increase was mainly seen in participants that had increased problems with dyspnoea. In COPD, the alveolar region is involved with the formation of emphysema, which is known to affect the gas exchange and ventilation to perfusion ratio (VA/Q) matching [24], which starts already in GOLD stage 1 (FEV_1-% predicted ≥ 80) [25]. Further investigation is needed to determine if the loss of lung volume causes a compensatory upregulation of NO in the peripheral lung. McCurdy et al. studied physical performance and $C_A NO$ in COPD patients. They found higher $C_A NO$ values with shorter travel distances in a walking test [7], which gives the hypothesis for compensatory upregulation credibility. Another possibility is that the uptake of the inhaled NO that is produced in the airways is not homogenous, such that some of the inhaled NO is exhaled at high flows giving a higher $C_A NO$.

In contrast to the NO from the airways, as well as the content of NO in the airway wall, the effect of smoking was not seen in $C_A NO$ or in the diffusing capacity of NO from the airway wall in this study. That $C_A NO$ is not affected by smoking has been shown previously [3]. The contrary has also been shown, but then the highest flow was too low, which allowed NO to be picked up from the airway [9,12]. In a study examining smoking cessation over a four-week period, the airway NO gradually increased, while $C_A NO$ remained unchanged [26]. This suggests that $C_A NO$ might be a useful marker since many COPD patients are still smoking or are trying to quit.

Most of our research subjects could perform the NO modelling with multiple flows. There were only two subjects in the completed group at inclusion that could not perform the lowest flow of 20 mL/s. It was more difficult at the two-year follow-up since, for 24 subjects, we had to use the linear model that excludes the low flow. Among all of the subjects, both completed and non-completed, NO modelling was missed in 22% for whatever reason (performance, analyser, or simply not done). Lazar et al. missed 7% in their stable subjects due to an inability to complete a flow of 250 mL/s and as much as 32% in the subjects that had an exacerbation at inclusion [13]. Karvonen et al. had a higher rate of successful results with the linear model compared to the HMA [27]. We can conclude that NO modelling with multiple flows cannot be accomplished in all patients.

A limitation of this study was that we were not able to follow the subjects who did not complete the study and had more severe disease. We do not know what the reasons were for the missing values, but during the follow-up period, there were more subjects that required the use of higher flows for the NO analysis. This points to a more severe disease as the possible reason. It could be seen as a limitation that different methods of estimating C_ANO were used, but they are partially based on the same measurements, and it has been found that the estimation of C_ANO with the linear and the non-linear methods do not differ [12]. To strengthen the clinical value of C_ANO, it would have been interesting to evaluate both hyperinflation and lung diffusion capacity (DLCO) from a pulmonary function perspective, and have a computerized tomography assessment of emphysema in the present study.

The strength of this study is that we have longitudinal data on estimated C_ANO over a two-year period and could analyse changes over time in relation to changes in disease burden. Another strength is that the subjects were examined in a stable disease state at all time points. Our study population involved patients from both primary and secondary care settings, making these results relevant to most of the patients. We have used validated questionnaires at all three visits and the same research nurse reviewed these questionnaires with the subjects. Finally, COPD was physician-diagnosed and verified by spirometry at the inclusion in the study.

5. Conclusions

Alveolar NO increased slightly over the follow-up period, together with a small decline in lung function. There was a lack of consistency in the alveolar NO values, with only a third of our subjects with higher C_ANO values, remaining at the same level after two years. The increase in C_ANO was found especially in those whose levels of dyspnoea increased over time.

Author Contributions: M.H. and A.M. initiated, and together with C.J., B.S., K.B., J.S. and K.L. conceptualized the TIE study. M.H., A.M., B.S., J.S. and A.P. contributed to the data analysis performed in this manuscript. M.H. had full access to the study data and wrote the initial draft. All authors have analysed and interpreted the data, contributed with critical revision of the manuscript, and approved the final version to be published. All authors have read and agreed to the published version of the manuscript.

Funding: This work was supported by the Uppsala-Örebro Regional Research Council; the Centre for Research and Development, Uppsala University/Region Gävleborg; the Centre for Clinical Research, Uppsala University; County Council Dalarna; the Swedish Heart and Lung Association; the Bror Hjerpstedt Foundation; and the Uppsala County Association Against Heart and Lung Diseases.

Institutional Review Board Statement: The protocol was approved by the Regional Review Board in Uppsala, Sweden (Dnr 2013/358) 28 April 2014.

Informed Consent Statement: A written informed consent was obtained from all subjects involved in the study. The study was conducted in accordance with the Declaration of Helsinki.

Data Availability Statement: Data cannot be made freely available as they are subject to secrecy in accordance with the Swedish Public Access to Information and Secrecy Act, but can be made available to researchers upon request (subject to a secrecy review).

Acknowledgments: The authors would like to thank all of the study participants for giving their time and providing valuable information for this study. We are grateful to Lise-Lotte Sundgren, the research nurse at the Gävle study site. The authors wish to thank Robin Quell for proofreading and editing this manuscript.

Conflicts of Interest: All authors declare no conflict of interest. J.S. is today an employee at Medical Affairs, GlaxoSmithKline (GSK), 169 29 Solna, Sweden, but when this work was done, she was a PhD student at Uppsala university and employed at Region Gävleborg. GSK has in no way influenced on the TIE study or this manuscript.

Abbreviations

B-Eos	blood eosinophils
B-Neu	blood neutrophils
BMI	body mass index
C_ANO	alveolar NO
CAT	COPD Assessments Test-scores
$C_{aw}NO$	NO content in airway wall
COPD	chronic obstructive pulmonary disease
$D_{aw}NO$	NO diffusion capacity over airway wall
F_ENO_{50}	fraction of exhaled NO at 50 mL/s
FEV_1	forced expiratory volume in 1 s
FVC	forced vital capacity
HMA	Högman Meriläinen algorithm
mMRC	modified Medical Research Council dyspnoea scale
NO	nitric oxide

References

1. Lu, Z.; Huang, W.; Wang, L.; Xu, N.; Ding, Q.; Cao, C. Exhaled nitric oxide in patients with chronic obstructive pulmonary disease: A systematic review and meta-analysis. *Int. J. Chronic Obstr. Pulm. Dis.* **2018**, *13*, 2695–2705. [CrossRef] [PubMed]
2. Rio Ramirez, M.T.; Juretschke Moragues, M.A.; Fernandez Gonzalez, R.; Alvarez Rodriguez, V.; Aznar Andres, E.; Zabaleta Camino, J.P.; Romero Pareja, R.; Esteban de la Torre, A. Value of exhaled nitric oxide (F_ENO) and eosinophilia during the exacerbations of chronic obstructive pulmonary disease requiring hospital admission. *COPD* **2018**, *15*, 369–376. [CrossRef]
3. Malinovschi, A.; Janson, C.; Holmkvist, T.; Norbäck, D.; Meriläinen, P.; Högman, M. Effect of smoking on exhaled nitric oxide and flow-independent nitric oxide exchange parameters. *Eur. Respir. J.* **2006**, *28*, 339–345. [CrossRef]
4. Mostafavi-Pour-Manshadi, S.M.; Naderi, N.; Barrecheguren, M.; Dehghan, A.; Bourbeau, J. Investigating fractional exhaled nitric oxide in chronic obstructive pulmonary disease (COPD) and asthma-COPD overlap (ACO): A scoping review. *COPD* **2018**, *15*, 377–391. [CrossRef]
5. Brindicci, C.; Ito, K.; Resta, O.; Pride, N.B.; Barnes, P.J.; Kharitonov, S.A. Exhaled nitric oxide from lung periphery is increased in COPD. *Eur. Respir. J.* **2005**, *26*, 52–59. [CrossRef]
6. Williamson, P.A.; Clearie, K.; Menzies, D.; Vaidyanathan, S.; Lipworth, B.J. Assessment of small-airways disease using alveolar nitric oxide and impulse oscillometry in asthma and COPD. *Lung* **2011**, *189*, 121–129. [CrossRef] [PubMed]
7. McCurdy, M.R.; Sharafkhaneh, A.; Abdel-Monem, H.; Rojo, J.; Tittel, F.K. Exhaled nitric oxide parameters and functional capacity in chronic obstructive pulmonary disease. *J. Breath Res.* **2011**, *5*, 016003. [CrossRef]
8. Högman, M.; Holmkvist, T.; Wegener, T.; Emtner, M.; Andersson, M.; Hedenström, H.; Meriläinen, P. Extended NO analysis applied to patients with COPD, allergic asthma and allergic rhinitis. *Respir. Med.* **2002**, *96*, 24–30. [CrossRef]
9. Lehouck, A.; Carremans, C.; De Bent, K.; Decramer, M.; Janssens, W. Alveolar and bronchial exhaled nitric oxide in chronic obstructive pulmonary disease. *Respir. Med.* **2010**, *104*, 1020–1026. [CrossRef]
10. Horvath, I.; Barnes, P.J.; Loukides, S.; Sterk, P.J.; Högman, M.; Olin, A.C.; Amann, A.; Antus, B.; Baraldi, E.; Bikov, A.; et al. A European Respiratory Society technical standard: Exhaled biomarkers in lung disease. *Eur. Respir. J.* **2017**, *49*, 1600965. [CrossRef] [PubMed]
11. Högman, M.; Lehtimäki, L.; Dinh-Xuan, A.T. Utilising exhaled nitric oxide information to enhance diagnosis and therapy of respiratory disease—Current evidence for clinical practice and proposals to improve the methodology. *Expert Rev. Respir. Med.* **2017**, *11*, 101–109. [CrossRef]
12. Högman, M.; Thornadtsson, A.; Hedenstierna, G.; Meriläinen, P. A practical approach to the theoretical models to calculate NO parameters of the respiratory system. *J. Breath Res.* **2014**, *8*, 016002. [CrossRef]
13. Lazar, Z.; Kelemen, A.; Galffy, G.; Losonczy, G.; Horvath, I.; Bikov, A. Central and peripheral airway nitric oxide in patients with stable and exacerbated chronic obstructive pulmonary disease. *J. Breath Res.* **2018**, *12*, 036017. [CrossRef]
14. Fan, X.; Zhao, N.; Yu, Z.; Yu, H.; Yin, B.; Zou, L.; Zhao, Y.; Qian, X.; Sai, X.; Qin, C.; et al. Clinical utility of central and peripheral airway nitric oxide in aging patients with stable and acute exacerbated chronic obstructive pulmonary disease. *Int. J. Gen. Med.* **2021**, *14*, 571–580. [CrossRef] [PubMed]
15. Lehtimäki, L.; Kankaanranta, H.; Saarelainen, S.; Annila, I.; Aine, T.; Nieminen, R.; Moilanen, E. Bronchial nitric oxide is related to symptom relief during fluticasone treatment in COPD. *Eur. Respir. J.* **2010**, *35*, 72–78. [CrossRef] [PubMed]
16. Högman, M.; Sulku, J.; Ställberg, B.; Janson, C.; Bröms, K.; Hedenström, H.; Lisspers, K.; Malinovschi, A. 2017 Global initiative for chronic obstructive pulmonary lung disease reclassifies half of COPD subjects to lower risk group. *Int. J. Chronic Obstr. Pulm. Dis.* **2018**, *13*, 165–173. [CrossRef]
17. Hedenström, H.; Malmberg, P.; Agarwal, K. Reference values for lung function tests in female. Regression equations with smoking variables. *Bull. Eur. Physiopathol. Respir.* **1985**, *21*, 551–557.

18. Hedenström, H.; Malmberg, P.; Fridriksson, H.V. Reference values for pulmonary function test in men: Regression equations which include tobacco smoking variables. *Upsala J. Med. Sci.* **1986**, *91*, 299–310. [CrossRef]
19. American Thoracic Society; European Respiratory Society. ATS/ERS recommendations for standardized procedures for the online and offline measurement of exhaled lower respiratory nitric oxide and nasal nitric oxide, 2005. *Am. J. Respir. Crit. Care Med.* **2005**, *171*, 912–930. [CrossRef]
20. Bestall, J.C.; Paul, E.A.; Garrod, R.; Garnham, R.; Jones, P.W.; Wedzicha, J.A. Usefulness of the Medical Research Council (MRC) dyspnoea scale as a measure of disability in patients with chronic obstructive pulmonary disease. *Thorax* **1999**, *54*, 581–586. [CrossRef]
21. Kon, S.S.; Canavan, J.L.; Jones, S.E.; Nolan, C.M.; Clark, A.L.; Dickson, M.J.; Haselden, B.M.; Polkey, M.I.; Man, W.D. Minimum clinically important difference for the COPD Assessment Test: A prospective analysis. *Lancet Respir. Med.* **2014**, *2*, 195–203. [CrossRef]
22. Kocks, J.W.; Tuinenga, M.G.; Uil, S.M.; van den Berg, J.W.; Stahl, E.; van der Molen, T. Health status measurement in COPD: The minimal clinically important difference of the clinical COPD questionnaire. *Respir. Res.* **2006**, *7*, 62. [CrossRef] [PubMed]
23. Gelb, A.F.; Flynn, T.C.; Krishnan, A.; Fraser, C.; Shinar, C.M.; Schein, M.J.; Osann, K. Central and peripheral airway sites of nitric oxide gas exchange in COPD. *Chest* **2010**, *137*, 575–584. [CrossRef]
24. Gunnarsson, L.; Tokics, L.; Lundquist, H.; Brismar, B.; Strandberg, A.; Berg, B.; Hedenstierna, G. Chronic obstructive pulmonary disease and anesthesia: Formation of atelectasis and gas exchange impairment. *Eur. Respir. J.* **1991**, *4*, 1106–1116.
25. Rodriguez-Roisin, R.; Drakulovic, M.; Rodriguez, D.A.; Roca, J.; Barbera, J.A.; Wagner, P.D. Ventilation-perfusion imbalance and chronic obstructive pulmonary disease staging severity. *J. Appl. Physiol.* **2009**, *106*, 1902–1908. [CrossRef] [PubMed]
26. Högman, M.; Holmkvist, T.; Wålinder, R.; Meriläinen, P.; Ludviksdottir, D.; Håkansson, L.; Hedenström, H. Increased nitric oxide elimination from the airways after smoking cessation. *Clin. Sci.* **2002**, *103*, 15–19. [CrossRef] [PubMed]
27. Karvonen, T.; Kankaanranta, H.; Saarelainen, S.; Moilanen, E.; Lehtimäki, L. Comparison of feasibility and estimates of central and peripheral nitric oxide parameters by different mathematical models. *J. Breath Res.* **2017**, *11*, 047102. [CrossRef]

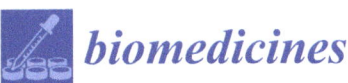

Article

Biological Sensing of Nitric Oxide in Macrophages and Atherosclerosis Using a Ruthenium-Based Sensor

Achini K. Vidanapathirana [1,2,3,†], **Jarrad M. Goyne** [1,2,3,†], **Anna E. Williamson** [1,3], **Benjamin J. Pullen** [1,2,3], **Pich Chhay** [1,3], **Lauren Sandeman** [1], **Julien Bensalem** [4], **Timothy J. Sargeant** [4], **Randall Grose** [5], **Mark J. Crabtree** [6], **Run Zhang** [7], **Stephen J. Nicholls** [2,8], **Peter J. Psaltis** [1,2,3,9] and **Christina A. Bursill** [1,2,3,*]

1. Vascular Research Centre, Lifelong Health Theme, South Australian Health and Medical Research Institute, Adelaide, SA 5000, Australia; achini.vidanapathirana@sa.gov.au (A.K.V.); jarrad.goyne@sahmri.com (J.M.G.); anna.williamson@adelaide.edu.au (A.E.W.); benjamin.pullen@sahmri.com (B.J.P.); pchh7973@uni.sydney.edu.au (P.C.); lauren.sandeman@sahmri.com (L.S.); peter.psaltis@sahmri.com (P.J.P.)
2. Australian Research Council (ARC) Centre of Excellence for Nanoscale BioPhotonics (CNBP), Adelaide, SA 5000, Australia; stephen.nicholls@monash.edu
3. School of Medicine, University of Adelaide, Adelaide, SA 5000, Australia
4. Lysosomal Health in Ageing, Hopwood Centre for Neurobiology, Lifelong Health Theme, South Australian Health and Medical Research Institute, Adelaide, SA 5000, Australia; julien.bensalem@sahmri.com (J.B.); tim.sargeant@sahmri.com (T.J.S.)
5. Cancer Program, Precision Medicine Theme, South Australian Health and Medical Research Institute, Adelaide, SA 5000, Australia; randall.grose@sahmri.com
6. Division of Cardiovascular Medicine, British Heart Foundation Centre of Research Excellence, Radcliffe Department of Medicine, University of Oxford, Oxford OX3 9DU, UK; mcrab@well.ox.ac.uk
7. Australian Institute for Bioengineering and Nanotechnology (AIBN), The University of Queensland, St. Lucia, QLD 4072, Australia; r.zhang@uq.edu.au
8. MonashHeart, Monash University, Clayton, VIC 3168, Australia
9. Department of Cardiology, Central Adelaide Local Health Network, Adelaide, SA 5000, Australia
* Correspondence: christina.bursill@sahmri.com; Tel.: +61-881-284-788
† These authors contributed equally to this work.

Abstract: Macrophage-derived nitric oxide (NO) plays a critical role in atherosclerosis and presents as a potential biomarker. We assessed the uptake, distribution, and NO detection capacity of an irreversible, ruthenium-based, fluorescent NO sensor (Ru-NO) in macrophages, plasma, and atherosclerotic plaques. In vitro, incubation of Ru-NO with human THP1 monocytes and THP1-PMA macrophages caused robust uptake, detected by Ru-NO fluorescence using mass-cytometry, confocal microscopy, and flow cytometry. THP1-PMA macrophages had higher Ru-NO uptake (+13%, $p < 0.05$) than THP1 monocytes with increased Ru-NO fluorescence following lipopolysaccharide stimulation (+14%, $p < 0.05$). In mice, intraperitoneal infusion of Ru-NO found Ru-NO uptake was greater in peritoneal CD11b$^+$F4/80$^+$ macrophages (+61%, $p < 0.01$) than CD11b$^+$F4/80$^-$ monocytes. Infusion of Ru-NO into $Apoe^{-/-}$ mice fed high-cholesterol diet (HCD) revealed Ru-NO fluorescence co-localised with atherosclerotic plaque macrophages. When Ru-NO was added ex vivo to aortic cell suspensions from $Apoe^{-/-}$ mice, macrophage-specific uptake of Ru-NO was demonstrated. Ru-NO was added ex vivo to tail-vein blood samples collected monthly from $Apoe^{-/-}$ mice on HCD or chow. The plasma Ru-NO fluorescence signal was higher in HCD than chow-fed mice after 12 weeks (37.9%, $p < 0.05$). Finally, Ru-NO was added to plasma from patients (N = 50) following clinically-indicated angiograms. There was lower Ru-NO fluorescence from plasma from patients with myocardial infarction (−30.7%, $p < 0.01$) than those with stable coronary atherosclerosis. In conclusion, Ru-NO is internalised by macrophages in vitro, ex vivo, and in vivo, can be detected in atherosclerotic plaques, and generates measurable changes in fluorescence in murine and human plasma. Ru-NO displays promising utility as a sensor of atherosclerosis.

Keywords: nitric oxide; sensors; macrophages; atherosclerosis

Citation: Vidanapathirana, A.K.; Goyne, J.M.; Williamson, A.E.; Pullen, B.J.; Chhay, P.; Sandeman, L.; Bensalem, J.; Sargeant, T.J.; Grose, R.; Crabtree, M.J.; et al. Biological Sensing of Nitric Oxide in Macrophages and Atherosclerosis Using a Ruthenium-Based Sensor. *Biomedicines* **2022**, *10*, 1807. https://doi.org/10.3390/biomedicines10081807

Academic Editor: Mats Eriksson

Received: 24 May 2022
Accepted: 25 July 2022
Published: 27 July 2022

Publisher's Note: MDPI stays neutral with regard to jurisdictional claims in published maps and institutional affiliations.

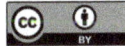

Copyright: © 2022 by the authors. Licensee MDPI, Basel, Switzerland. This article is an open access article distributed under the terms and conditions of the Creative Commons Attribution (CC BY) license (https://creativecommons.org/licenses/by/4.0/).

1. Introduction

Nitric oxide (NO) is a gaseous messenger molecule known for its significant regulatory role in almost every cell and it plays a crucial role in maintaining optimum function of the cardiovascular system [1]. NO has a well-established role as a vasodilator produced at nanomolar concentrations in vascular endothelial cells produced by phosphorylation regulated endothelial nitric oxide synthase (eNOS) [2,3]. In addition, activated macrophages within the vascular tissues produce relatively higher levels of NO via activation of inducible nitric oxide synthase (iNOS) [4,5]. Macrophages can be resident or derived from different sources, such as from monocytes or smooth muscle cells, and play a critical role in the development and progression of atherosclerosis [6]. These immune cells can be utilised as a target for detection of the presence of plaque. Derangement of NOS regulation and changes in soluble NO levels in specific tissues are associated with different cardiovascular pathologies, such as hypertension, myocardial infarction, peripheral vascular disease, stroke, and cardiogenic/septic shock [2,7]. In particular, alterations in NO metabolism and presence of reactive nitrogen species are associated with inflammation, a determinant of plaque vulnerability in atherosclerosis [8,9]. Therefore, NO has the potential to be used as marker of early detection of atherosclerosis and to predict the prognosis. Despite such clinical significance, only sub-optimal or surrogate measurements are available as research tools to detect NO in cardiovascular diseases and continue to be used despite reporting variable findings [10,11]. Although methods for detecting NO production by macrophages have been reported [11], they have not been applied to the context of cardiovascular disease.

Light-based methods, such as fluorescence and luminescence detection, represent a more feasible and applicable solution to understand the mechanisms of NO metabolism in biomedical studies, compared to existing radioisotope-based methods. To date, most NO sensor applications have been used in cell-free media conditions, cell lysates or in in vitro cell cultures to demonstrate NO sensor capabilities [11,12]. There are very limited in vivo studies that have tested NO detection probes with non-invasive methods, such as photoacoustic imaging [13]. None of these studies has focused on in vivo detection of NO in atherosclerotic plaque or in blood using fluorescent sensors. Accurate sensing of NO in macrophages and atherosclerosis has the potential to facilitate improved understanding of the role of NO in atherosclerosis and may be applied as a future point-of-care test for the early detection and monitoring of atherosclerosis.

The ruthenium-based NO sensor with the chemical composition of $[Ru(bpy)_2(dabpy)]^{2+}$ (Ru-NO) is converted to its active form $[Ru(bpy)_2(T-bpy)]^{2+}$ in the presence of NO, leading to an increase in luminescence [14]. It has previously been validated as an extracellular sensor of secreted NO from endothelial cells [15]. In this study, we aimed to assess the uptake and distribution of the Ru-NO sensor in macrophages in vitro and in in vivo murine models of atherosclerosis as well as to test the utility of using Ru-NO sensor fluorescence to track atherosclerosis in mouse and human plasma. We report that Ru-NO has potential future applications as a research tool to study NO metabolism and macrophage function in atherosclerosis and other cardiovascular diseases.

2. Materials and Methods

2.1. Ruthenium Based NO Sensor (Ru-NO)

The synthesis and preliminary application of the ruthenium-based NO sensor complex bis(2,2'-bipyridine)(4-(3,4-diaminophenoxy)-2,2'-bipyridine)ruthenium(II)hexafluorophosphate ($[(Ru(bpy)_2(dabpy)][PF6]_2$) has been previously described [14]. Serial dilutions from a 100 mM working solution of Ru-NO made in 0.1% dimethyl sulfoxide (DMSO) in phosphate-buffered saline (PBS) were used for in vitro, ex vivo, and in vivo studies with working solutions at a 10–50 µM concentration.

2.2. In Vitro Studies

2.2.1. Human Monocytes and Macrophages

THP1-monocytes were obtained from American Type Culture Collection (ATCC) and grown in RPMI medium with 10% foetal bovine serum (FBS), 1% L-glutamine, and 1% Penicillin-Streptomycin (Sigma-Aldrich, Sydney, Australia). Cells were seeded in a six-well plate at a concentration of 2×10^5 and treated with 200 nM phorbol-12-myristate-13-acetate (PMA) for three days to stimulate differentiation of monocytes to macrophages, as previously described [16]. Macrophages were used two days after changing to PMA-free media. THP1 monocytes and THP1-PMA macrophages were treated with 10 or 50 µM Ru-NO for 24 h for assessments of Ru-NO uptake using flow cytometry, confocal microscopy, and mass cytometry (Supplementary Methods S1–S3). In parallel, a sample of macrophages were permeabilised using 0.3% saponin in PBS, gently vortexed, and centrifuged at $800 \times g$ for 10 min. The permeabilised cells were reassessed for the presence/absence of fluorescence signal. THP1 monocytes and THP1-PMA macrophages were also treated in some experiments with 40 µM Ru-NO and 10 µg/mL lipopolysaccharide (LPS) for 18 h [17]. Changes in the Ru-NO fluorescence intensity (λ_{ex} = 488 nm, λ_{em} = 780/60 nm) in treated cells were assessed using flowcytometry.

2.2.2. Bone Marrow Derived Mouse Macrophages (BMDMs)

BMDMs were isolated from the tibial/femoral bone marrow of C57BL/6J mice, cultured and differentiated [18]. Briefly, the extracted BMDMs were seeded in DMEM F12, 5% FBS, 25 ng/mL macrophage colony-stimulating factor (MCSF), L-glutamine, and penicillin–streptomycin. MCSF (50 ng/mL) was added on Day 5 and granulocyte-MCSF (GMCSF) (50 ng/mL) was added on Day 6 for differentiation. During the differentiation process, the cells were treated with 50 µM Ru-NO for 24 h on Day 8 with or without LPS (100 ng/mL) and interferon gamma (IFNγ, 10 ng/mL) for 16 h. Ru-NO fluorescence within the BMDMs was then analysed using flowcytometry and mass cytometry or used for analysis of iNOS protein expression by Western blotting (Supplementary Methods S4).

2.3. In Vivo Studies in Mice

All animal care and handling procedures were approved by the Animal Ethics Committee of the South Australian Health and Medical Research Institute (SAHMRI, protocol SAM310) and performed in accordance with the Australian Code for the Care and Use of Animals for Scientific Purposes (2013). C57BL/6J and $Apoe^{-/-}$ null (homozygous$^{-/-}$) male mice were bred in-house and housed at the SAHMRI Bio-resources animal facility. Food and water were provided *ad libitum*. A pilot study was first conducted to determine the optimum concentration of Ru-NO for in vivo studies and to assess sensor biodistribution and toxicity (Supplementary Methods S5). At the end of Ru-NO administration, mice were humanely killed using a single administration of 5% isoflurane via inhalation, followed by terminal cardiac puncture and exsanguination.

2.3.1. Peritoneal Macrophages

We tested the uptake and sensor capabilities of Ru-NO in peritoneal macrophages. C57BL/6J male mice of 4–12 weeks were injected with 2.4 µM/kg of Ru-NO intraperitoneally and humanely killed 24 h post-infusion using a single administration of 5% isoflurane via inhalation. Peritoneal cells were collected via peritoneal wash/lavage as previously described [19]. Briefly, ice cold PBS was injected into the peritoneal cavity, massaged gently, and peritoneal fluid collected. These steps were repeated twice to obtain the maximum number of cells. Some cells (3×10^4) were concentrated onto a microscopic slide via a Cytospin™ 4 Cytocentrifuge (Thermo Fisher Scientific, Scoresby, VIC, Australia) and later imaged by confocal microscopy. The remaining peritoneal lavage cells were analysed using flow cytometry to detect Ru-NO fluorescence following incubation with antibodies against myeloid/macrophage markers F4/80 (Australian Biosearch, Karrinyup, WA, Australia) and CD11b (BD Biosciences, Adelaide, Australia) to characterise cell populations.

2.3.2. Murine Model of Atherosclerosis

Apolipoprotein E$^{-/-}$ ($Apoe^{-/-}$) mice at 6 weeks of age were fed a high-cholesterol diet (HCD, 21% fat, 0.15% cholesterol) for 12 weeks to develop mid-stage plaques. A cohort of $Apoe^{-/-}$ mice that remained on chow for the same time period were included in parallel. Ru-NO (2.4 µM/kg) was injected intravenously 24 h and 5 min before being humanely killed using a single administration of 5% isoflurane via inhalation. Blood was collected through cardiac puncture in EDTA tubes and the aorta, liver, heart, and spleen were harvested and analysed for Ru-NO sensor uptake by flow cytometry. Cross sections of plaque-containing aortic sinuses from optimal cutting temperature compound (OCT, Tissue-Tek)-embedded hearts were fixed post culling and incubated with an antibody against CD68 (1:1000, rat anti-CD68, clone FA-11, #MCA1957GA, Bio-Rad) followed by a fluorescently conjugated secondary antibody (1:2000, Donkey anti-Rat IgG with Alexa Fluor 488, #A-21208) (Invitrogen, Thornton, NSW, Australia) before imaging under confocal microscopy.

2.4. Ex Vivo Assessment of Ru-NO Sensor Uptake
2.4.1. Aorta, Spleen, and Liver Cells

$Apoe^{-/-}$ mice were fed HCD or normal chow for 16 weeks. Aortas, livers, and spleens were digested (Supplementary Methods S5), then incubated with PBS or 40 µM Ru-NO (in duplicate) at 37 °C for 60 min. Cells were then washed and analysed using flowcytometry to detect Ru-NO fluorescence following incubation with antibodies against CD11b and F4/80 (myeloid cells/macrophages) and CD31 (endothelial cells).

2.4.2. Blood

From $Apoe^{-/-}$ mice fed a HCD or normal diet, 100–150 µL blood was collected via tail bleed, at timepoints of 4, 8, 12, and 16 weeks. Aliquots of 50 µL were immediately added to two tubes containing equal volumes of (1) 40 µM Ru-NO or (2) 40 µM Ru-NO + NO scavenger 2-(4-carboxyphenyl)-4,4,5,5-tetramethylimidazoline-1-oxyl-3-oxide (cPTIO; 200 µM, final concentration [20]), both in PBS. The blood samples were left on ice for 30 min, centrifuged at 7000 rpm for 3 min to isolate plasma then kept on ice before being snap frozen at a consistent time point 100 min after collection. Ru-NO fluorescence was read in thawed plasma samples using a SynergyMx Microplate Reader (BioTek) at λ_{ex} = 450 nm and λ_{em} = 615 nm and the fluorescence values at 615 nm were taken for the analysis. The difference (delta, Δ) between Ru-NO only and Ru-NO + cPTIO fluorescence was calculated to determine the NO-specific signal.

2.5. Clinical Blood Samples

Peripheral arterial blood samples were obtained from 50 human subjects who underwent clinically indicated coronary angiography at the Royal Adelaide Hospital, Adelaide, Australia, as approved by the Human Research Ethics Committee of the Central Adelaide Local Health Network, Adelaide, Australia (CALHN HREC # 13579). Informed, written consent was obtained from subjects in accordance with the Declaration of Helsinki and all procedures were performed in accordance with the National Statement on Ethical Conduct in Human Research (2007) in Australia. A 5 mL blood sample was obtained from a radial artery sheath from each patient prior to diagnostic cardiac catheterisation and a 1 mL aliquot of the blood sample was immediately added to a tube containing an equal volume of PBS with the Ru-NO sensor, bringing it to a final concentration of 40 µM of Ru-NO. Another 1 mL aliquot of the same blood sample was also immediately added to a tube containing an equal volume of PBS with the Ru-NO sensor and cPTIO (200 µM, final concentration). Blood added with PBS only and cPTIO only in equal volumes were used as background controls for fluorescence. Following the addition of the sensor/scavenger, the blood samples were left on ice for 30 min, centrifuged at 2600 rpm for 10 min to isolate the plasma, then left on ice before snap freezing one hour after collection. Ru-NO fluorescence was read at λ_{ex} = 450 nm and λ_{em} = 615 nm and the fluorescence values at 615 nm were taken for the analysis.

2.6. Statistical Analysis

GraphPad Prism software (GraphPad Software, Inc. La Jolla, San Diego, CA, USA) was used for data analysis. The normality of the distribution was tested using Shapiro–Wilk normality test. The fluorescence values between Ru-NO and PBS treated cells were compared using a paired or unpaired t-test as relevant. A one-way ANOVA was used to compare three or more groups with the p-values for significant differences derived using a Tukey's post-hoc test for multiple comparisons. The two-tailed p-value for significance was <0.05. All data are reported as mean $\pm$ standard error of the mean (SEM).

3. Results

3.1. Ru-NO Is Detectable In Vitro in THP1 Monocytes and Macrophages

In vitro, THP1 monocytes and PMA-differentiated macrophages were able to take up the Ru-NO sensor following incubation. This was identified using CyTOF mass spectrometry for detection of elemental Ruthenium; specifically, the ^{102}Ru isotope (Figure 1A,B). THP1-PMA macrophages demonstrated approximately two-fold higher Ru-NO sensor uptake compared with THP1 monocytes at both 10 µM (MFI: THP1 monocytes 4.03; THP1-PMA macrophages 9.2, +128%) and 50 µM (MFI: THP1 monocytes 28.12; THP1-PMA macrophages 58.46, +108%). Intracellular Ru-NO fluorescence was also demonstrated in THP1-PMA macrophages using confocal microscopy (Figure 1C). Ru-NO fluorescence was also detected in both THP1 monocytes and THP1-PMA macrophages using flow cytometry (Figure 1D,E). The mean fluorescence intensity (MFI) was greater than six-fold higher in THP1-PMA macrophages compared with THP1 monocytes (THP1 monocytes: 81.1 ± 24.7 vs. THP1-PMA macrophages: 652.6 ± 39.9) and the fluorescence in macrophages was further enhanced by the addition of lipopolysaccharide (+13.8%, $p < 0.05$, Figure 1F). The Ru-NO fluorescence disappeared following permeabilisation, further confirming that the Ru-NO sensor is internalised and the fluorescence signal is specific to the sensor (Figure 1G).

3.2. Detection of Ru-NO in Murine Macrophages

The Ru-NO sensor fluorescence was also detected in CD11b$^+$ F4/80$^+$ BMDMs from healthy adult C57BL/6 mice (Figure 2A,B). A longer incubation period with the Ru-NO sensor from 1 h to 4 h was found to significantly increase the fluorescence signal. Using Western Blotting, we next confirmed an increase in iNOS protein expression in BMDMs following stimulation with LPS and IFNγ (Figure 2C and Supplementary Figure S1). Polarised M1- and M2-like macrophages were next tested for their ability to take up the Ru-NO sensor and respond to inflammatory stimuli. In contrast with our findings in human macrophages and despite the induction in iNOS, it was found that stimulation with LPS + IFNγ for 1 h and 4 h reduced the Ru-NO fluorescence signal in the CD86$^+$ (M1-like) macrophages (Figure 2D) and CD206$^+$ (M2-like) macrophages (Figure 2E). We then determined if the LPS + IFNγ stimulation was affecting cell number or the uptake of the Ru-NO sensor. We found that LPS + IFNγ stimulation increased the proportion of M1-like cells and, conversely, decreased the number of M2-like cells (Figure 2E,F). These effects of LPS + IFNγ were independent of the presence of the Ru-NO sensor, occurring also in the PBS-treated controls. Using mass cytometry, less ^{102}Ru was found in BMDMs stimulated with LPS + IFNγ (Figure 2G), indicating an impairment of Ru-NO sensor uptake with inflammatory stimulation.

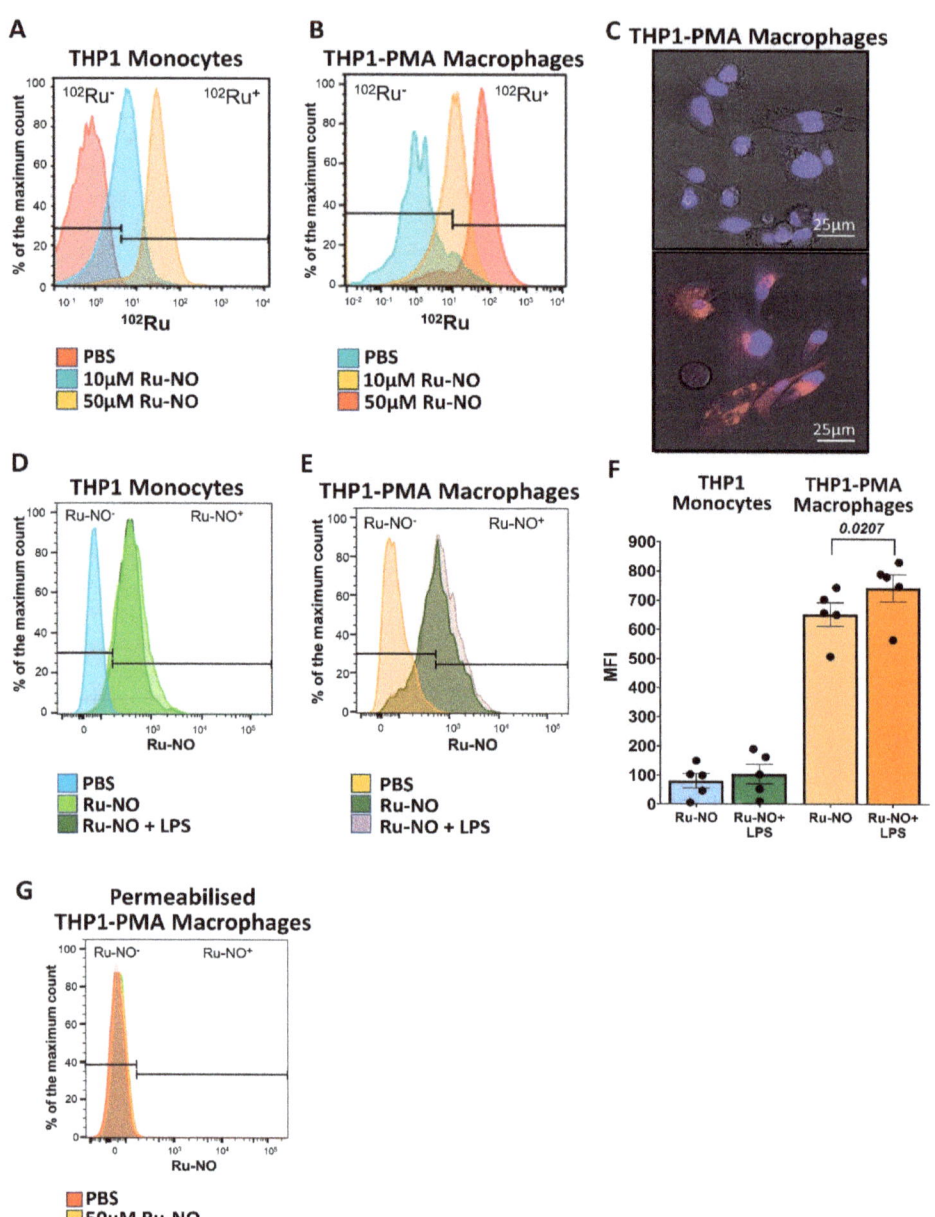

Figure 1. **Ru-NO sensor uptake and detection in human THP1 monocytes and THP1-PMA macrophages.** THP1 monocytes and macrophages were exposed to the Ru-NO sensor to assess sensor uptake and fluorescence detection. The histograms of ^{102}Ru in (**A**) THP1 monocytes and (**B**) macrophages exposed to 10 and 50 μM of Ru-NO as assessed by Mass Cytometry (CyTOF). (**C**) Confocal microscopic images of THP1-PMA macrophages treated with PBS (top) and 50 μM Ru-NO (bottom) (red: Ru-NO, and blue: DAPI). Representative flow cytometry histograms of Ru-NO fluorescence in (**D**) THP1 monocytes and (**E**) THP1-PMA macrophages with/without LPS stimulation (**F**) with analyses. (**G**) Lack of Ru-NO fluorescence detection in permeabilised THP1-PMA macrophages by flow cytometry. Mean ± SEM of the mean fluorescence intensity (MFI) of independent experiments, and p values derived from a paired t-test (n = 5 replicates).

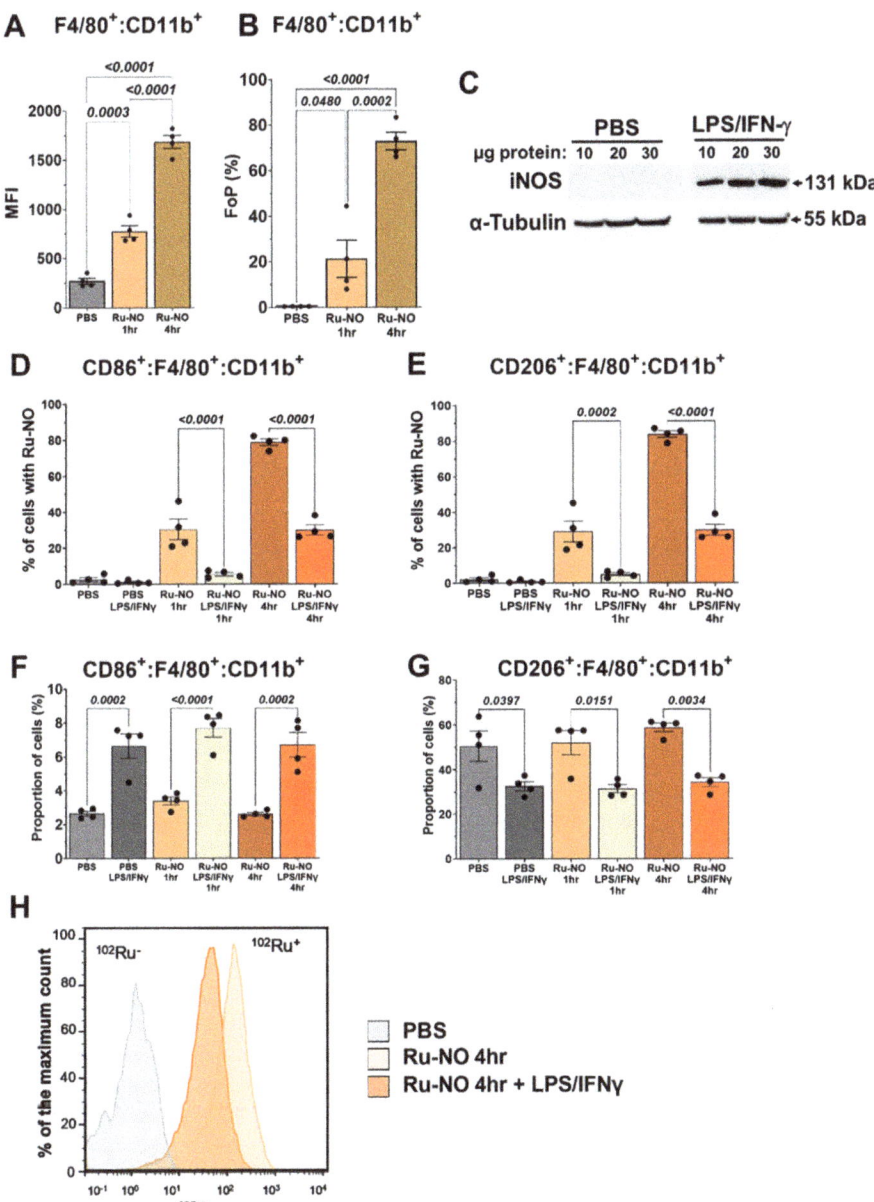

Figure 2. Ru-NO sensor uptake and detection in murine M1- and M2-like macrophages. Mouse bone marrow derived macrophages (BMDMs) were assessed for Ru-NO uptake using flowcytometry. (**A**) Mean Fluorescence Intensity (MFI) and (**B**) Frequency of Parental (FoP) of PBS and Ru-NO exposed CD11b⁺F4/80⁺ BMDMs in the absence of inflammation/polarisation. (**C**) Western Blot analysis of iNOS expression in BMDMs with/without LPS + IFN-γ stimulation. The percentage of cells with Ru-NO uptake in (**D**) M1-like and (**E**) M2-like macrophages with/without LPS + IFN-γ. The proportion of (**F**) M1-like (CD86⁺) and (**G**) M2-like (CD206⁺) macrophages with/without LPS + IFN-γ stimulation. (**H**) Mass cytometry histogram for Ruthenium uptake in BMDM with/without LPS + IFN-γ stimulation. Mean ± SEM, p values derived from a one-way ANOVA with Tukey post-hoc test (n = 3, performed in quadruplicate) repeated experiments.

3.3. In Vivo Toxicity, and Detection and Distribution of Ru-NO

A pilot study was conducted in C57BL/6J mice to determine optimum intravenous concentration and exposure time for the Ru-NO sensor. Toxicity testing revealed that infusion of Ru-NO was well tolerated without any adverse events in vivo at 0.6–2.4 µM/kg. Twenty-four hours following administration of 2.4 µM/kg Ru-NO, tissue Ru-NO fluorescence was detected in liver by flow cytometry, greater than for livers of mice infused with PBS (7.1 ± 4.1% of all liver cells, n = 3–5). Ru-NO fluorescence was also present in kidney (+10.7 ± 3.25%) and spleen (+3.2 ± 2.0%), and, to a very modest extent, in aorta (+0.16 ± 0.15%), compared to PBS-infused control mice (Supplementary Figure S2). Sensor uptake was minimal/negligible in these organs at a dose of 0.6 µM/kg (data not shown). Fluorescence was also negligible in bone marrow, lungs, heart, and plasma after 24 h of either 0.6 and 2.4 µM/kg of Ru-NO infusions (data not shown). Time-course studies using the selected dose of 2.4 µM/kg of Ru-NO sensor injected 5 min, 2, 4, 6, and 24 h before euthanasia revealed that Ru-NO fluorescence was maximum at the 24 h time point in the liver (6.6 ± 4.1%) and kidney (9.5 ± 3.2%), whereas the maximum Ru-NO fluorescence was detected at the 6 h timepoint in the spleen (28.3 ± 15.6) and the aorta (6.4 ± 4.7%) (Supplementary Figure S3).

3.4. Detection of Ru-NO in Peritoneal Macrophages

Confocal microscopy demonstrated an intracellular fluorescence signal in peritoneal macrophages 24 h following intraperitoneal injection of Ru-NO (Figure 3A). When analysed using flow cytometry, we observed a substantial increase in viable fluorescent cells in the Ru-NO exposed peritoneal lavage cells, when compared to PBS injected controls (Figure 3B). There were no differences in overall cell viability or distribution with either PBS or Ru-NO administration to the peritoneum (data not shown). Two distinct populations of cells, (1) myeloid cells (F4/80$^-$D11b$^+$) and (2) macrophages (F4/80$^+$CD11b$^+$), were identified in all samples (Figure 3C). When compared to the PBS-treated group (Figure 3D), both CD11b$^+$F4/80$^-$ myeloid cells and CD11b$^+$F4/80$^+$ macrophage populations showed robust Ru-NO fluorescence (Figure 3E). The macrophage population demonstrated the highest Ru-NO sensor uptake with consistently higher MFI, when compared to PBS controls (Figure 3F). Within the Ru-NO treated mice, the fluorescence from the Ru-NO sensor was significantly higher in CD11b$^+$F4/80$^+$ macrophages (MFI: 515.9 ± 121.4; Frequency of Parent, FoP: 61.2 ± 10.6%), demonstrating macrophage-specific uptake of Ru-NO when compared to non-myeloid cells (MFI: 20.5 ± 6.2; FoP: 0.3 ± 0.1%) and myeloid cells (MFI: 202 ± 114.6; FoP: 30.0 ± 9.4%, Figure 3G,H).

3.5. Ru-NO in In Vivo Atherosclerotic Plaque Macrophages

We next investigated whether Ru-NO sensor fluorescence was detectable in atherosclerotic plaques in *Apoe*$^{-/-}$ mice fed HCD for 12 weeks. Following infusion of the Ru-NO sensor we were able to detect the presence of Ru-NO fluorescence in atherosclerotic plaques in aortic sinus cryosections by confocal microscopy. Immunofluorescent staining for CD68 revealed that the Ru-NO fluorescence signal localised with CD68$^+$ plaque macrophages (Figure 4A–F). Consistent with this, flow cytometry analyses of aortic cell suspensions from these mice found that the aortic CD11b$^+$F4/80$^+$ macrophage population had a significantly higher in vivo Ru-NO sensor uptake/fluorescence (MFI: 125 ± 33.9; FoP: 65.1 ± 19.1%) compared to CD11b$^+$F4/80$^-$ myeloid cells (MFI: 6.6 ± 5.8; FoP: 6.5 ± 5.1%) and CD11b$^-$F4/80$^-$ non-myeloid cells (MFI: 4.3 ± 0.8; FoP: 0.62 ± 0.23% Figure 4G,H).

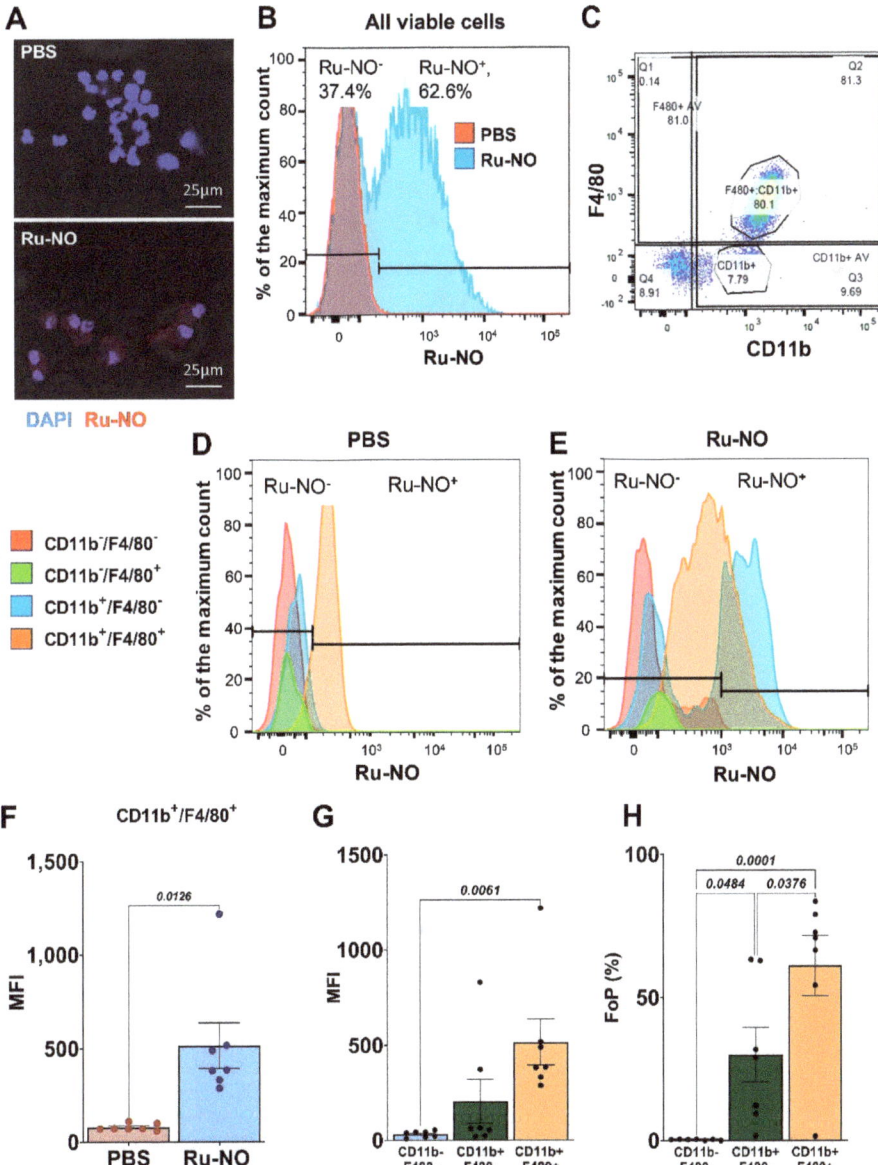

Figure 3. Ru-NO uptake and detection in peritoneal macrophages (**A**) Representative confocal microscopy images of Ru-NO intracellular fluorescence signal in peritoneal cells 24 h following intraperitoneal injection of PBS (top) and 40 μM Ru-NO (bottom). (**B**) Representative flow cytometry histograms of peritoneal lavage cells following intraperitoneal infusion of PBS and Ru-NO. (**C**) Representative plot of the distribution of cells with F4/80 and CD11b markers. Representative flow cytometry histograms identifying four populations based on F4/80 and CD11b markers and sensor uptake in (**D**) PBS and (**E**). Ru-NO exposed peritoneal lavage cells. (**F**) Mean fluorescence intensity (MFI) of PBS and Ru-NO exposed CD11b$^+$F4/80$^+$ peritoneal lavage cells. (**G**) MFI and (**H**) frequency of parental (FoP) analyses of Ru-NO fluorescence in non-myeloid cells (CD11b$^-$F4/80$^-$), myeloid cells (CD11b$^+$F4/80$^-$) and macrophages (CD11b$^+$F4/80$^+$). Mean ± SEM, p values derived from a t test or one-way ANOVA with Tukey post-hoc test (n = 7 repeated experiments).

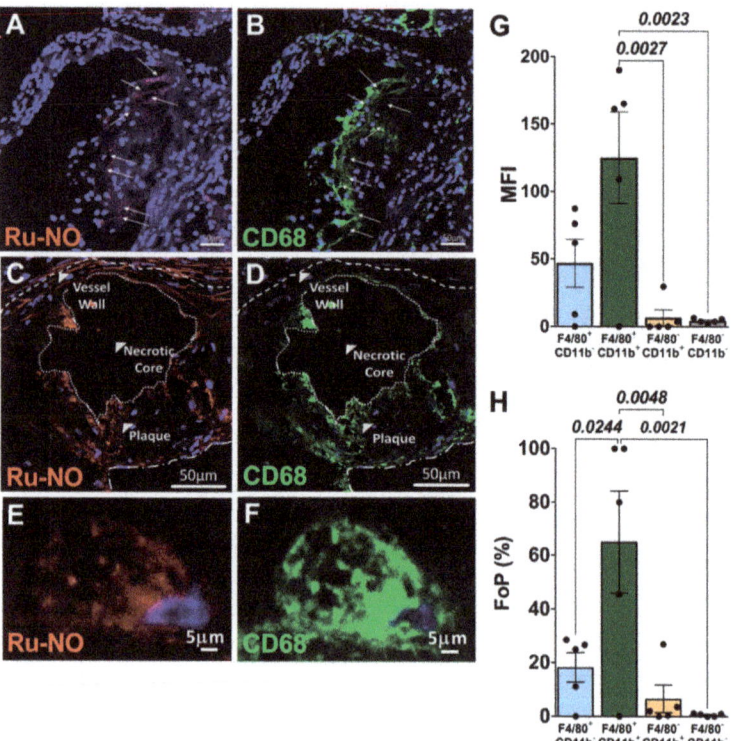

Figure 4. In vivo detection of Ru-NO in mouse atherosclerotic plaque. Detection of Ru-NO fluorescence in aortic sinus plaque following intravenous administration of Ru-NO (40 µM) to $Apoe^{-/-}$ mice fed a high-cholesterol diet (HCD) for 12 weeks and imaged using confocal microscopy. (**A,C,E**): Distribution of the Ru-NO (red) in cellular areas of the plaques with nuclear stain DAPI (blue) with increasing magnification. (**B,D,F**): Comparison with plaque macrophage location (CD68+, green). (**G**) Mean fluorescence intensity (MFI) and (**H**). frequency of parental (FoP) of aortic cell suspensions for the detection on Ru-NO fluorescence in non-myeloid cells (CD11b+F4/80−), myeloid cells (CD11b+F4/80−) and macrophages (CD11b+F4/80+) in HCD-fed mice post-Ru-NO infusion. Mean ± SEM, *p* values derived from a repeated measures one-way ANOVA with Tukey post-hoc test (n = 5 animals).

3.6. Ru-NO in Ex Vivo Cell Suspensions of Atherosclerotic Mice

Ex vivo testing of Ru-NO uptake in cell suspensions from the aorta, liver, and spleen of $Apoe^{-/-}$ mice fed on HCD or normal chow for 20 weeks was then conducted using flow cytometry. In the aortic cell suspensions, a distinct CD11b+F4/80+ macrophage population was identified (Figure 5A) and 36.8% of these cells displayed Ru-NO uptake (Figure 5B). The Ru-NO uptake/fluorescence was then analysed among the myeloid (CD11b+F4/80−), macrophage (CD11b+F4/80+) and endothelial cell (CD11b− F4/80− CD31+) populations. In the mice fed normal chow, the aortic macrophage population displayed the highest fluorescence compared to myeloid cells and endothelial cells (Figure 5C,D). The same Ru-NO uptake/fluorescence patterns were observed in aortic cell suspensions from the HCD fed group (Figure 5E,F). We found a significant increase in the FoP (Figure 5G) and the MFI (Figure 5H) in macrophages from those mice injected with the Ru-NO sensor, compared to the PBS controls in both the HCD and normal chow-fed groups. Interestingly, there were no differences in aortic macrophage Ru-NO fluorescence between normal chow-fed and HCD mice. When we then compared the proportion of aortic macrophages in the chow-fed and HCD mice, it was revealed that the proportion of macrophages in all viable cells was significantly decreased (60.8%) in the HCD group, compared to the normal chow group (Figure 5I). This pattern remained consistent following ex vivo exposure to Ru-NO (Figure 5J).

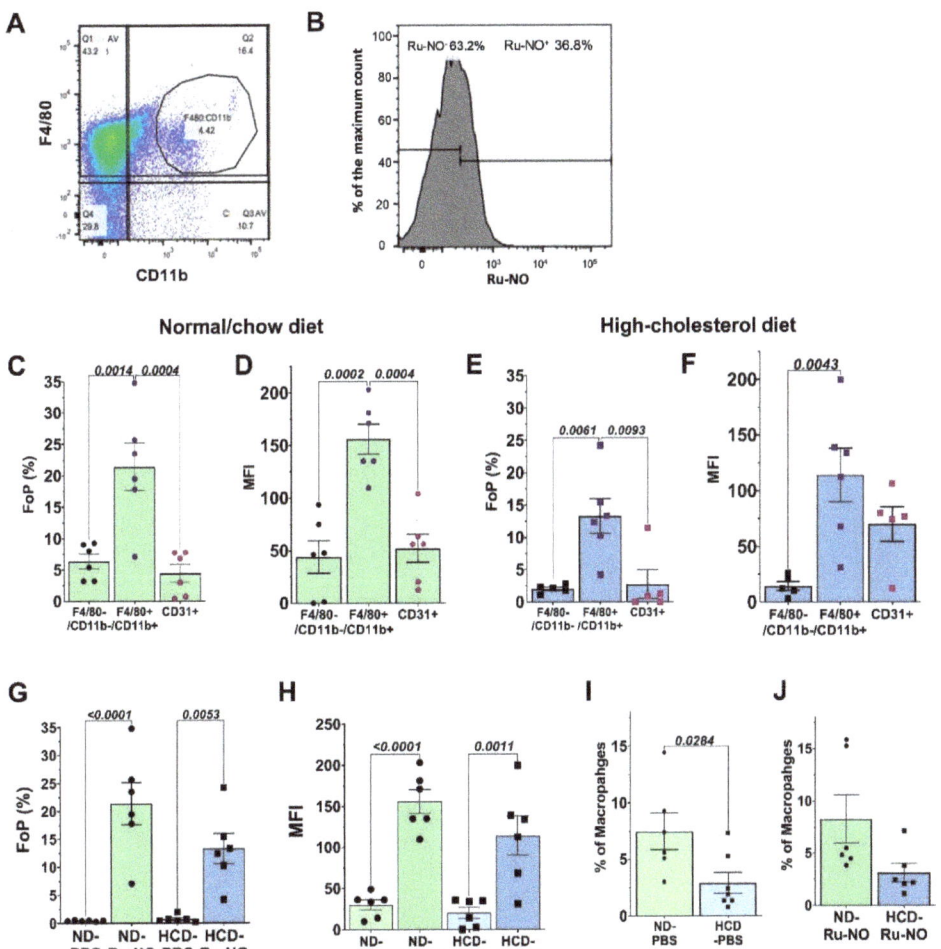

Figure 5. Ex vivo uptake of Ru-NO by macrophages in aortic cell suspensions from atherosclerotic mice. (A) Representative plot for the distributions of aortic cell suspensions incubated with antibodies against CD11b and F4/80 markers. (B) Representative histogram demonstrating the shift in Ru-NO fluorescence in aortic cell suspensions. (C) Frequency of parental (FoP) and (D) mean fluorescence intensity (MFI) for Ru-NO fluorescence in myeloid cells (CD11b$^+$F4/80$^-$), macrophages (CD11b$^+$F4/80$^+$) and endothelial cells (CD31$^+$) in aortic cell suspensions from chow-fed mice. (E). FoP and (F) MFI for Ru-NO fluorescence in aortic cell suspensions in high-cholesterol diet (HCD)-fed group. (G) FoP and (H) MFI in CD11b$^+$F4/80$^+$ macrophages comparing aortic cell suspensions from chow and HCD-fed groups with ex vivo addition of PBS or Ru-NO. Proportion of macrophages in all viable cells that had been incubated with (I) PBS and (J) Ru-NO. Mean ± SEM, p values derived from one-way ANOVA with Tukey post-hoc test for multiple comparisons across different groups (n = 5–6 mice/group).

Comparative assessments for the liver and spleen cells were also conducted (Supplementary Figures S4 and S5). In comparison to the aorta, a relatively higher percentage of macrophages took up the Ru-NO sensor in the spleen (+52.9%) and a relatively lower percentage uptake was reported with the liver cell suspensions (−29.3%). In contrast to the aorta, both spleen and liver cell suspensions contained a higher proportion of macrophages in all viable cells from the HCD group. The uptake patterns in the spleen and liver were, however, similar to the aorta in that the macrophages had the highest uptake/fluorescence of the sensor than myeloid and endothelial cell populations. There remained a lack of change between the Ru-NO sensor uptake between HCD and normal diet fed groups.

3.7. Ru-NO in Mouse Blood in Atherosclerosis

We next tested the utility of the Ru-NO sensor to track atherosclerosis progression using blood samples. Serial, four-weekly tail-vein blood samples from atherosclerotic mice were added ex vivo with Ru-NO with/without the NO scavenger cPTIO. Plasma fluorescence was then quantified using spectrophotometry. At every time point, the sample with only Ru-NO reported a significantly higher fluorescence reading compared Ru-NO + cPTIO sample in both HCD and normal diet-fed mice (Figure 6A,B). This indicates the presence of background fluorescence in blood that can be identified by the inclusion of the Ru-NO + cPTIO sample. There was a trend for an increase in Δfluorescence readings (specific NO signal) from the Ru-NO samples with increasing age and time on the HCD (Figure 6C) and chow diets (Figure 6D). When comparing the chow and HCD-fed mice, the Δfluorescence reading was significantly higher in the HCD group (+37.9%, $p < 0.05$) at the 12-week timepoint, when compared to chow fed mice (Figure 6E).

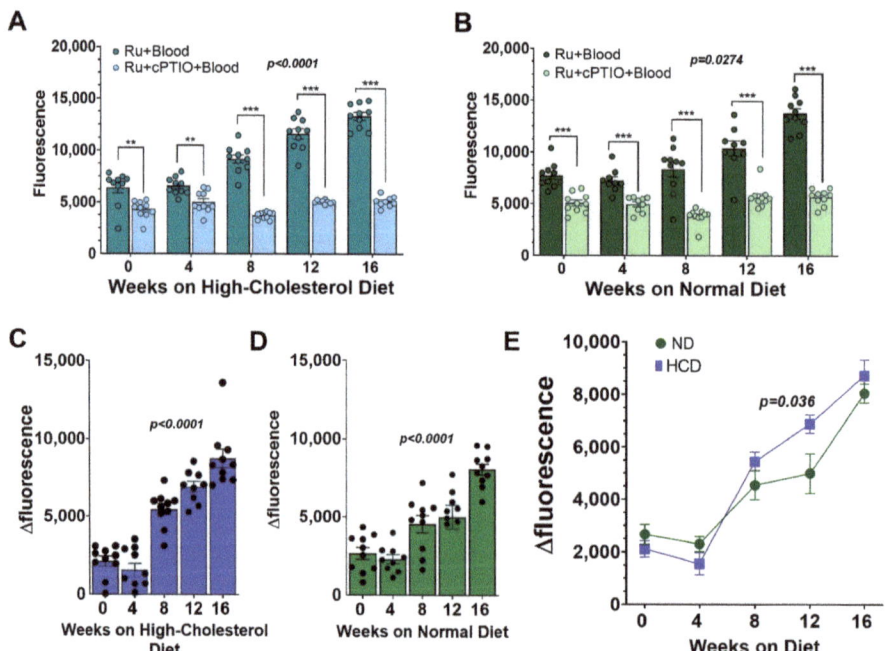

Figure 6. Plasma Ru-NO fluorescence is higher in mice after 12 weeks of high-cholesterol diet than with chow feeding. Spectrophotometric readings of Ru-NO fluorescence in plasma from blood samples collected every four weeks added with Ru-NO or Ru-NO + cPTIO (NO scavenger) in mice fed (**A**) high-cholesterol diet (HCD) and (**B**) chow for 16 weeks. Δfluorescence (Ru-NO–Ru-NO + cPTIO) specific NO signal in plasma from mice fed (**C**) HCD and (**D**) chow with (**E**): combined analyses directly comparing the signal between HCD- and chow-fed mice. Mean ± SEM, ** $p < 0.01$ and *** $p < 0.001$ using two-way ANOVA with Tukey post-hoc test for multiple comparisons across different groups. The p values in (**A–D**) for the linear trend were also calculated (n = 9–10 mice/group).

3.8. Ru-NO Changes in Clinical Blood Samples

Peripheral arterial blood samples from patients presenting for an angiogram were spiked with Ru-NO with/without NO scavenger cPTIO. Plasma fluorescence was quantified using spectrophotometry. The relevant demographic and clinical details are reported in Supplementary Table S1. We identified three categories of patients based on the angiogram findings and clinical manifestations: (1) no or minor coronary artery disease (CAD), <20% narrowing in the vessels, n = 19; (2) stable CAD: >20% narrowing in the vessels without myocardial infarction, n = 20 and; (3) myocardial infarction: >70% narrowing in the vessels with ST elevation myocardial infarction (STEMI) or non-STEMI, n = 11. In all categories, the plasma samples added with Ru-NO only reported a significantly higher reading compared to samples added with Ru-NO + cPTIO, irrespective of the plaque burden or clinical manifestation (Figure 7A). The plasma Δfluorescence reading of the specific NO signal for each patient revealed an upward non-significant trend in the stable CAD group, compared to the no CAD group. Interestingly, the plasma Δfluorescence was significantly lower in the myocardial infarction group, compared to the stable CAD group (-30.7%, $p < 0.01$, Figure 7B).

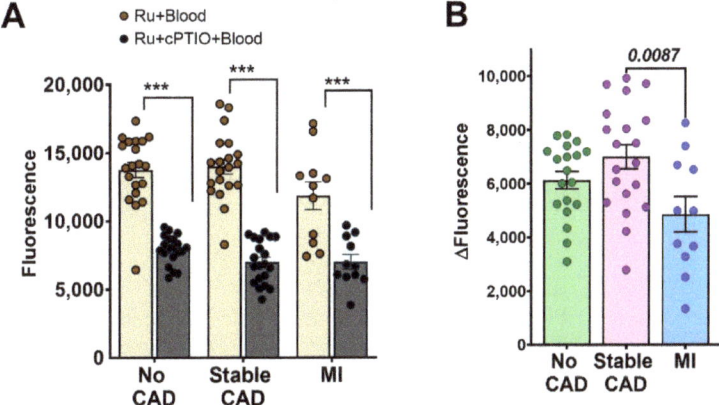

Figure 7. Ru-NO in blood samples from patients with coronary artery disease. Plasma Ru-NO fluorescence was quantified using spectrophotometry in peripheral arterial blood samples from patients presenting for an angiogram that were divided into groups of either (1) no or minor coronary artery disease (CAD, <20% narrowing of the vessels, n = 19), (2) stable CAD (<20% narrowing of the vessels without myocardial infarction, n = 20), or (3) with myocardial infarction (MI, >70% narrowing of the vessels with myocardial infarction, n = 11). (**A**) Plasma fluorescence from blood samples added with Ru-NO or Ru-NO + cPTIO (NO scavenger). (**B**) The Δfluorescence (Ru-NO–Ru-NO + cPTIO) NO specific signal from patient blood samples. Mean + SEM, *** $p < 0.01$ using one-way ANOVA with Tukey post-hoc test for multiple comparisons across different groups.

4. Discussion

In this study, we demonstrated the NO detection capabilities of a Ruthenium-based NO sensor, Ru-NO [14,15], in macrophages, plasma, and atherosclerosis. We show that the Ru-NO sensor is internalised within macrophages and provides NO detection in vitro, ex vivo, and in vivo, including in macrophages in atherosclerotic plaques and aortas. In addition, the Ru-NO sensor was able to detect NO in murine plasma across different stages of atherosclerosis. This was supported by detection of NO in human blood samples from patients with stable and unstable CAD. Using our systematic stepwise approach, we demonstrate bench-to-bedside translation of the Ru-NO sensor, with potential application as a research tool for the measurement of NO in macrophages and as a point-of-care test for atherosclerosis.

The sensitivity and specificity of the Ru-NO sensor was first validated in cell-free media conditions [14] and then in vitro in endothelial cells [15]. It was reported to display comparative responses with commercially available, conventional sensors, such as DAF-FM-diacetate (4-Amino-5-methylamino−2′,7′-difluorofluorescein diacetate) and the Griess assay [15]. The Ru-NO sensor demonstrated relatively higher stability compared to these sensors/assays with no evidence of cytotoxicity at 10–50 µM concentrations in human umbilical vein endothelial cells [15]. We, therefore, used the same concentration range of the Ru-NO sensor in the current study in vitro, ex vivo, and in vivo. In vascular endothelial cells, the Ru-NO sensor was not internalised and, therefore, functioned as an extracellular sensor for the detection of endogenous changes in NO [15]. In contrast, the current study found that the Ru-NO sensor was able to be internalised by macrophages, probably due to their greater phagocytotic capabilities [21].

In our in vitro studies, Ru-NO was internalised by both human THP1 monocytes and THP1-PMA macrophages, as demonstrated by changes in the proportion of cells with Ru-NO fluorescence and confirmed by the absence of these changes with cell permeabilisation. These observations were further supported by confocal microscopy and mass cytometry. Both THP1 monocytes and THP1-PMA macrophages demonstrated concentration-dependent increases in Ru-NO uptake, while THP1-PMA macrophages reported two-fold higher levels of intracellular ^{102}Ru compared with THP1 monocytes using mass cytometry. Mass cytometry (CyTOF) detects and quantifies the presence of elemental Ruthenium in the cells, but does not differentiate NO-bound and unbound forms of the sensor. However, our Ru-NO fluorescence data also show higher Ru-NO sensor uptake and/or higher NO levels in THP1-PMA macrophages than THP1 monocytes that was further enhanced in inflammatory conditions. There are several mechanisms that may underly these quantifiable differences in Ru-NO fluorescence. Macrophages are more phagocytic than monocytes [21] and, therefore, may internalise more Ru-NO, which is supported by the CyTOF findings. The Ru-NO sensor only emits a fluorescence signal at specified wavelengths when bound to and activated by NO [14]. This is supported by the PBS controls that had minimal autofluorescence. The Ru-NO fluorescence is, therefore, likely to predominantly represent NO-bound sensor levels inside cells. Previously, in endothelial cells we found similar changes in extracellular NO in response to endogenous stimuli that were compatible with changes in phosphorylated eNOS [15]. Together, these studies support the application of Ru-NO as a sensor to detect both intra and extracellular NO in different cell types associated with vascular function and disease.

Macrophages polarise into M1 and M2-like phenotypes following physiological or pathological stimuli and the M1/M2 distribution within plaques is predictive of the prognosis of atherosclerosis [22]. Increased activity of iNOS-producing NO is evident in M1-like (pro-inflammatory) and some sub-sets of M2-like cells [23]. We found that under non-inflammatory conditions, murine unpolarised (M0) F4/80$^+$/CD11b$^+$ BMDMs displayed time-dependent increases in Ru-NO fluorescence from 1 h to 4 h. This observation reflects either increased sensor uptake or NO accumulation over time. Following inflammatory stimulation, an expected increase in the proportion of CD86$^+$ (M1-type, pro-inflammatory) BMDMs and a decrease in CD206$^+$ (M2-type) BMDMs occurred. These changes in macrophage phenotype were independent of the presence or duration of exposure to Ru-NO, suggesting that the Ru-NO sensor does not affect macrophage differentiation or cell viability. Unexpectedly, LPS + IFNγ stimulation reduced Ru-NO uptake/fluorescence in CD86$^+$ M1-like BMDMs, despite an increase in the proportion of this cell population. Interestingly, this response was opposite to that of human THP1 macrophages. Previous studies testing different NO sensors have predominately used the murine macrophage RAW264 cell line, which report sensor uptake in undifferentiated macrophages via microscopy. These studies have not demonstrated parallel changes in iNOS activity or reported changes in sensor uptake in the presence of inflammatory stimuli [11,24]. These reports and our observations suggest a cell-species dependent effect in which inflammation has varying effects on Ru-NO uptake into macrophages. There were no differences in Ru-NO fluorescence between the M1 and M2 macrophages. It may have been expected that Ru-NO fluorescence would be higher in the M1-like macrophages, however, variable expression of iNOS in M1, M2 and other sub-types of macrophages has been reported [23] and may explain this lack of change. In summary, our in vitro findings identify Ru-NO as a sensor that can detect NO in macrophages irrespective of cell polarity or inflammation.

In this study we conducted important pilot testing in non-atherosclerotic C57BL6/J mice to determine the biodistribution, optimal dose, time course, and toxicity of the Ru-NO sensor. No adverse toxicological effects were observed. The absence of a Ru-NO fluorescence signal in blood, with low and variable amounts of Ru-NO sensor signal in the liver and kidney 24 h post-systemic infusion, indicates variation in the metabolism and clearance rates of the Ru-NO sensor. This was supported by the time-course studies, in which the highest Ru-NO fluorescence signal occurred in excretory/metabolic organs, such as the kidney and liver at the 24 h time point. In contrast, at the 6 h time point, the highest Ru-NO signal was in the spleen and aorta. This signal declined after 24 h, suggesting there is minimum tissue retention in an uninflamed state in non-atherosclerotic mice. Relatively rapid excretion with minimal tissue retention has significant advantages. Studies with other fluorescence sensors that are retained long-term within tissues following intravenous administration have reported adverse sub-cellular changes [25].

We demonstrated that the Ru-NO sensor can be taken up in vivo into peritoneal macrophages. Peritoneal macrophages from mice injected with the Ru-NO sensor demonstrated a clear shift in fluorescence intensity, compared to PBS controls, suggesting negligible autofluorescence at these wavelengths in vivo. The internalisation of the Ru-NO sensor is a positive attribute as it enables the study of NO using flow cytometry in cell suspensions. Background autofluorescence can, thereby, be kept to a minimum and not be affected by the constituents of culture media for example. Our peritoneal studies found both macrophages and myeloid cells took up the Ru-NO sensor. Consistent with our initial in vitro studies, macrophages had significantly higher uptake/fluorescence of the Ru-NO sensor, compared to myeloid cells and $F4/80^-/CD11b^-$ non-myeloid cells. Once again this could be due to higher levels of iNOS and NO production in macrophages or their greater phagocytic properties. We demonstrate, however, the important utility of the Ru-NO sensor to track macrophage-driven diseases in vivo.

We next tested the Ru-NO sensor in atherosclerotic $Apoe^{-/-}$ mice for its ability to detect changes in NO levels in plaque, other organs (liver and spleen) and in blood with increasing development of atherosclerosis. We tested plaque-prone regions of the aorta for Ru-NO sensor uptake. Confocal microscopy on aortic sinus sections revealed a robust signal for Ru-NO sensor fluorescence in plaque that co-localised predominantly with $CD68^+$ macrophages. We were able to confirm this observation using flow cytometry on atherosclerotic aortic cell suspensions in which there was also robust aortic macrophage uptake/fluorescence of the Ru-NO sensor following infusion. This signal was far higher than in the non-atherosclerotic C57BL6 mice of the pilot studies, supporting that it has potential utility for detecting disease. While similar findings were found when the Ru-NO sensor was spiked into aortic cell suspensions, Ru-NO fluorescence from aortic macrophages was not different between mice fed the HCD and those on chow. These findings may suggest that the advancement of atherosclerosis in the HCD mice promoted macrophage apoptosis/necrosis, thereby decreasing the number of macrophages able to take up the Ru-NO sensor. This is supported by our analyses that show the total number of viable aortic macrophages on HCD was lower than chow-fed aortas. Endothelial uptake was minimal/negligible compared to monocytes and macrophages. These observations are compatible with our previous findings that were confirmed with ICP-MS analysis [15]. When comparing other NO sensors, endogenous changes in macrophage NO have been previously reported in vitro with a Coumarin-based sensor [24]. In vivo studies in mice with LPS-induced inflammation have used a photoacoustic sensor to image NO in subcutaneous tissue [13]. Intravenous administration of NO sensors has also led to detection in the liver [26]. To our knowledge, the current study is the first demonstration of NO sensing in vivo in plaque macrophages using a NO-specific fluorescence sensor. As demonstrated in previous studies with iNOS imaging [27], NO can, therefore, potentially be utilised as a marker of disease activity. With its specificity, macrophage NO-specific binding, and multimodality imaging potential, Ru-NO presents as a good candidate to detect vulnerable plaque.

As an alternate application, we tested the ability of the Ru-NO sensor to track longitudinal changes in NO levels in serial blood samples from mice fed HCD for 16 weeks and assess if it associated with atherosclerotic disease progression. The mouse plasma samples showed increases in the Δfluorescence NO-specific signal with age and time on HCD/chow. It may have been expected that plasma NO levels from HCD mice would have consistently carried a higher signal than the chow-fed mouse plasma but this was not the case. A significantly higher NO signal did not occur until 12 weeks of HCD and this difference disappeared after 16 weeks of HCD. This suggests there is a certain window in which the Ru-NO sensor can detect changes in atherosclerosis. The chow-fed mice will also develop plaque but after 12 weeks of HCD the plaque is likely to be sufficiently large enough for a detectably different NO signal to be generated from plaque macrophages [28,29]. The lack of change after 16 weeks indicates that the plaques may then have been heading to a stage in which there is significant macrophage apoptosis that lowers iNOS-derived NO production. This hypothesis is consistent with our findings in human plasma from patients with different clinical presentations of CAD. Interestingly, we found the Δfluorescence NO-specific signal in the plasma from myocardial infarction patients was significantly lower than from the plasma of patients with stable CAD. This may reflect that unstable plaque has a substantial level of macrophage apoptosis/necrosis that renders them unable to generate iNOS-derived NO.

Plasma NO can be derived from multiple sources with contributions from both eNOS [3], iNOS [30], nNOS [31], non-enzymatic sources (e.g., dietary nitrites) [32], and ischaemic conditions [30]. Plasma NO concentrations in our study are, therefore, representative of NO production in the whole cardiovascular system from multiple sources in response to the progression of atherosclerosis. It is possible our NO plasma findings in mice and human samples are a reflection of a reduction in eNOS-derived NO. It may also be a manifestation of dysfunctional nitric oxide activity that causes a predisposition to myocardial infarction [33,34]. There is currently no consensus on what NO levels associate with atherosclerosism [35]. Previous studies have reported mixed findings with a decrease in eNOS-mediated expression of NO and reduced nitrite and nitrate levels in HCD mice [36], whereas others have found increased iNOS activity with inflammation [35].

Limitations: There are several limitations that may confound the interpretation of the findings of the current study. Detailed distribution studies using radiolabelled Ruthenium were not performed; instead, we used fluorescence as an indicator of the sensor, which would emit a signal only in the presence of NO. Due to the human ethical implications and potential exposure concerns, we could not include Ru-NO in the blood collection syringe, which may have been optimal for a point-of-care test to minimise the time between the blood draw and sensor contact. This limitation is critical when quantifying a volatile molecule such as NO, which could be addressed in future larger clinical studies using this sensor.

5. Conclusions

In conclusion, we report a stepwise in vitro, ex vivo, and in vivo approach for the detection of NO using a molecular sensor. Compared to other multimodality imaging techniques for NO, we identify several positive characteristics of Ru-NO, such as toxicological tolerance at reasonable concentrations, minimal retention in tissues, a bright fluorescent signal for detection with different modalities, and sensitivity to atherosclerosis-related endogenous changes in NO. Due to its molecular size, Ru-NO uptake can be used as a marker of macrophage activity within the vessel wall at the onset and during the progression of atherosclerosis. Most importantly, the application of Ru-NO in blood as a point-of care test has the potential to be further developed, modified, and designed as a clinical tool for early detection of unstable plaque and monitoring of NO-related cardiovascular disease.

Supplementary Materials: The following supporting information can be downloaded at: https://www.mdpi.com/article/10.3390/biomedicines10081807/s1, Figure S1: Unedited gels from Western blot assessments presented in Figure 2C; Figure S2: Biodistribution of Ru-NO in vivo following intravenous; Figure S3: Time course of Ru-NO fluorescence in vivo after intravenous infusion. Figure S4: Ex vivo uptake of Ru-NO by macrophages in liver cell suspensions from atherosclerotic mice. Figure S5: Ex vivo uptake of Ru-NO by macrophages in spleen cell suspensions from atherosclerotic mice. Table S1: Demographic and Clinical information of patient blood samples for the analyses with the Ru-NO sensor.

Author Contributions: Conceptualization, A.K.V., P.J.P. and C.A.B.; methodology, A.K.V., J.M.G., T.J.S., A.E.W., M.J.C., B.J.P., P.C., L.S., R.Z. and R.G.; formal analysis, A.K.V. and J.M.G.; data curation, J.M.G., A.E.W., B.J.P. and R.G.; writing—original draft preparation, A.K.V. and C.A.B.; writing—review and editing, A.K.V., J.B., S.J.N., P.J.P. and C.A.B.; supervision, S.J.N., P.J.P. and C.A.B.; project administration, A.K.V. and C.A.B.; funding acquisition, S.J.N. All authors have read and agreed to the published version of the manuscript.

Funding: This work was supported by the Centre of Excellence for Nanoscale BioPhotonics, through the Australian Research Council (ARC, CE140100003). C.A.B. is supported by the Heart Foundation Lin Huddleston Fellowship. P.J.P. is supported by a Career Development Fellowship from the National Health and Medical Research Council of Australia (CDF 1161506) and Future Leader Fellowship from the National Heart Foundation (NHF, FLF100412) of Australia. B.J.P's funding is supported by an Australian Postgraduate Award.

Institutional Review Board Statement: The study was conducted in accordance with the Declaration of Helsinki, and approved by the Institutional Ethics Committee of the Central Adelaide Local Health Network (protocol code CALHN HREC #13579, approved October 2020). The animal study protocol was approved by the Institutional Ethics Committee of South Australian Health and Medical Research Institute (protocol code SAM310, approved December 2017).

Informed Consent Statement: Informed consent was obtained from all subjects involved in the study. Written informed consent has been obtained from the patient(s) to publish this paper.

Data Availability Statement: Not applicable.

Conflicts of Interest: The authors declare no conflict of interest.

References

1. Infante, T.; Costa, D.; Napoli, C. Novel Insights Regarding Nitric Oxide and Cardiovascular Diseases. *Angiology* **2021**, *72*, 411–425. [CrossRef] [PubMed]
2. Farah, C.; Michel, L.Y.M.; Balligand, J.-L. Nitric oxide signalling in cardiovascular health and disease. *Nat. Rev. Cardiol.* **2018**, *15*, 292–316. [CrossRef] [PubMed]
3. Förstermann, U.; Münzel, T. Endothelial nitric oxide synthase in vascular disease: From marvel to menace. *Circulation* **2006**, *113*, 1708–1714. [CrossRef] [PubMed]
4. Luoma, J.S.; Strålin, P.; Marklund, S.L.; Hiltunen, T.P.; Särkioja, T.; Ylä-Herttuala, S. Expression of extracellular SOD and iNOS in macrophages and smooth muscle cells in human and rabbit atherosclerotic lesions: Colocalization with epitopes characteristic of oxidized LDL and peroxynitrite-modified proteins. *Arterioscler. Thromb. Vasc. Biol.* **1998**, *18*, 157–167. [CrossRef]
5. Vico, T.C.; Marchini, T.; Ginart, S.; Lorenzetti, M.A.; Areán, J.S.A.; Calabró, V.; Garcés, M.; Ferrero, M.C.; Mazo, T.; D'Annunzio, V.; et al. Mitochondrial bioenergetics links inflammation and cardiac contractility in endotoxemia. *Basic Res. Cardiol.* **2019**, *114*, 38. [CrossRef]
6. Flynn, M.C.; Pernes, G.; Lee, M.K.S.; Nagareddy, P.R.; Murphy, A.J. Monocytes, Macrophages, and Metabolic Disease in Atherosclerosis. *Front. Pharmacol.* **2019**, *10*, 666. [CrossRef] [PubMed]
7. Ceron, C.S.; do Vale, G.T.; Simplicio, J.A.; Ricci, S.T.; De Martinis, B.S.; de Freitas, A.; Tirapelli, C.R. Chronic ethanol consumption increases vascular oxidative stress and the mortality induced by sub-lethal sepsis: Potential role of iNOS. *Eur. J. Pharmacol.* **2018**, *825*, 39–47. [CrossRef]
8. Hansson, G.K.; Libby, P.; Tabas, I. Inflammation and plaque vulnerability. *J. Intern. Med.* **2015**, *278*, 483–493. [CrossRef]
9. Bäck, M.; Yurdagul, A., Jr.; Tabas, I.; Öörni, K.; Kovanen, P.T. Inflammation and its resolution in atherosclerosis: Mediators and therapeutic opportunities. *Nat. Rev. Cardiol.* **2019**, *16*, 389–406. [CrossRef]

10. Chen, K.; Pittman, R.N.; Popel, A.S. Nitric oxide in the vasculature: Where does it come from and where does it go? A quantitative perspective. *Antioxid. Redox Signal.* **2008**, *10*, 1185–1198. [CrossRef]
11. Vidanapathirana, A.K.; Psaltis, P.J.; Bursill, C.A.; Abell, A.D.; Nicholls, S.J. Cardiovascular bioimaging of nitric oxide: Achievements, challenges, and the future. *Med. Res. Rev.* **2021**, *41*, 435–463. [CrossRef]
12. Bryan, N.S.; Grisham, M.B. Methods to detect nitric oxide and its metabolites in biological samples. *Free Radic. Biol. Med.* **2007**, *43*, 645–657. [CrossRef]
13. Reinhardt, C.J.; Zhou, E.Y.; Jorgensen, M.D.; Partipilo, G.; Chan, J. A Ratiometric Acoustogenic Probe for in Vivo Imaging of Endogenous Nitric Oxide. *J. Am. Chem. Soc.* **2018**, *140*, 1011–1018. [CrossRef] [PubMed]
14. Zhang, R.; Ye, Z.; Wang, G.; Zhang, W.; Yuan, J. Development of a ruthenium(II) complex based luminescent probe for imaging nitric oxide production in living cells. *Chem. A Eur. J.* **2010**, *16*, 6884–6891. [CrossRef]
15. Vidanapathirana, A.K.; Pullen, B.J.; Zhang, R.; Duong, M.; Goyne, J.M.; Zhang, X.; Bonder, C.S.; Abell, A.D.; Bursill, C.A.; Nicholls, S.J.; et al. A Novel Ruthenium-based Molecular Sensor to Detect Endothelial Nitric Oxide. *Sci. Rep.* **2019**, *9*, 1720. [CrossRef] [PubMed]
16. Daigneault, M.; Preston, J.A.; Marriott, H.M.; Whyte, M.K.; Dockrell, D.H. The identification of markers of macrophage differentiation in PMA-stimulated THP-1 cells and monocyte-derived macrophages. *PLoS ONE* **2010**, *5*, e8668. [CrossRef]
17. Shin, J.-S.; Choi, H.-E.; Seo, S.; Choi, J.-H.; Baek, N.-I.; Lee, K.-T. Berberine Decreased Inducible Nitric Oxide Synthase mRNA Stability through Negative Regulation of Human Antigen R in Lipopolysaccharide-Induced Macrophages. *J. Pharmacol. Exp. Ther.* **2016**, *358*, 3–13. [CrossRef] [PubMed]
18. Bailey, J.D.; Shaw, A.; McNeill, E.; Nicol, T.; Diotallevi, M.; Chuaiphichai, S.; Patel, J.; Hale, A.; Channon, K.M.; Crabtree, M.J. Isolation and culture of murine bone marrow-derived macrophages for nitric oxide and redox biology. *Nitric Oxide* **2020**, *100–101*, 17–29. [CrossRef] [PubMed]
19. Ray, A.; Dittel, B.N. Isolation of Mouse Peritoneal Cavity Cells. *JoVE* **2010**, *35*, 1488. [CrossRef]
20. Cáceres, L.; Paz, M.L.; Garcés, M.; Calabró, V.; Magnani, N.D.; Martinefski, M.; Adami, P.V.M.; Caltana, L.; Tasat, D.; Morelli, L.; et al. NADPH oxidase and mitochondria are relevant sources of superoxide anion in the oxinflammatory response of macrophages exposed to airborne particulate matter. *Ecotoxicol. Environ. Saf.* **2020**, *205*, 111186. [CrossRef] [PubMed]
21. Uribe-Querol, E.; Rosales, C. Phagocytosis: Our Current Understanding of a Universal Biological Process. *Front. Immunol.* **2020**, *11*, 1066. [CrossRef]
22. de Gaetano, M.; Crean, D.; Barry, M.; Belton, O. M1- and M2-Type Macrophage Responses Are Predictive of Adverse Outcomes in Human Atherosclerosis. *Front. Immunol.* **2016**, *7*, 275. [CrossRef]
23. Chistiakov, D.A.; Bobryshev, Y.V.; Orekhov, A.N. Changes in transcriptome of macrophages in atherosclerosis. *J. Cell. Mol. Med.* **2015**, *19*, 1163–1173. [CrossRef] [PubMed]
24. Sadek, M.M.; Barzegar Amiri Olia, M.; Nowell, C.J.; Barlow, N.; Schiesser, C.H.; Nicholson, S.E.; Norton, R.S. Characterisation of a novel coumarin-based fluorescent probe for monitoring nitric oxide production in macrophages. *Bioorg. Med. Chem.* **2017**, *25*, 5743–5748. [CrossRef]
25. Ramírez-García, G.; Gutiérrez-Granados, S.; Gallegos-Corona, M.A.; Palma-Tirado, L.; d'Orlyé, F.; Varenne, A.; Mignet, N.; Richard, C.; Martínez-Alfaro, M. Long-term toxicological effects of persistent luminescence nanoparticles after intravenous injection in mice. *Int. J. Pharm.* **2017**, *532*, 686–695. [CrossRef] [PubMed]
26. Iverson, N.M.; Barone, P.W.; Shandell, M.; Trudel, L.J.; Sen, S.; Sen, F.; Ivanov, V.; Atolia, E.; Farias, E.; McNicholas, T.P.; et al. In vivo biosensing via tissue-localizable near-infrared-fluorescent single-walled carbon nanotubes. *Nat. Nanotechnol.* **2013**, *8*, 873–880. [CrossRef]
27. Terashima, M.; Ehara, S.; Yang, E.; Kosuge, H.; Tsao, P.S.; Quertermous, T.; Contag, C.H.; McConnell, M.V. In vivo bioluminescence imaging of inducible nitric oxide synthase gene expression in vascular inflammation. *Mol. Imaging Biol. MIB Off. Publ. Acad. Mol. Imaging* **2011**, *13*, 1061–1066. [CrossRef]
28. Giannetto, A.; Esposito, E.; Lanza, M.; Oliva, S.; Riolo, K.; Di Pietro, S.; Abbate, J.M.; Briguglio, G.; Cassata, G.; Cicero, L.; et al. Protein Hydrolysates from Anchovy (*Engraulis encrasicolus*) waste: In Vitro and in Vivo Biological Activities. *Mar. Drugs* **2020**, *18*, 86. [CrossRef]
29. Abbate, J.M.; Macrì, F.; Arfuso, F.; Iaria, C.; Capparucci, F.; Anfuso, C.; Ieni, A.; Cicero, L.; Briguglio, G.; Lanteri, G. Antiatherogenic effect of 10% supplementation of Anchovy (*Engraulis encrasicolus*) Waste Protein Hydrolysates in ApoE-Deficient Mice. *Nutrients* **2021**, *13*, 2137. [CrossRef] [PubMed]
30. Kibbe, M.; Billiar, T.; Tzeng, E. Inducible nitric oxide synthase and vascular injury. *Cardiovasc. Res.* **1999**, *43*, 650–657. [CrossRef]
31. Ally, A.; Powell, I.; Ally, M.M.; Chaitoff, K.; Nauli, S.M. Role of neuronal nitric oxide synthase on cardiovascular functions in physiological and pathophysiological states. *Nitric Oxide* **2020**, *102*, 52–73. [CrossRef]
32. Weitzberg, E.; Lundberg, J.O. Nonenzymatic nitric oxide production in humans. *Nitric Oxide* **1998**, *2*, 1–7. [CrossRef] [PubMed]
33. Bolli, R. Cardioprotective Function of Inducible Nitric Oxide Synthase and Role of Nitric Oxide in Myocardial Ischemia and Preconditioning: An Overview of a Decade of Research. *J. Mol. Cell. Cardiol.* **2001**, *33*, 1897–1918. [CrossRef] [PubMed]
34. Erdmann, J.; Stark, K.; Esslinger, U.B.; Rumpf, P.M.; Koesling, D.; de Wit, C.; Kaiser, F.J.; Braunholz, D.; Medack, A.; Fischer, M.; et al. Dysfunctional nitric oxide signalling increases risk of myocardial infarction. *Nature* **2013**, *504*, 432–436. [CrossRef]

35. Gliozzi, M.; Scicchitano, M.; Bosco, F.; Musolino, V.; Carresi, C.; Scarano, F.; Maiuolo, J.; Nucera, S.; Maretta, A.; Paone, S.; et al. Modulation of Nitric Oxide Synthases by Oxidized LDLs: Role in Vascular Inflammation and Atherosclerosis Development. *Int. J. Mol. Sci.* **2019**, *20*, 3294. [CrossRef] [PubMed]
36. Eccleston, H.B.; Andringa, K.K.; Betancourt, A.M.; King, A.L.; Mantena, S.K.; Swain, T.M.; Tinsley, H.N.; Nolte, R.N.; Nagy, T.R.; Abrams, G.A.; et al. Chronic exposure to a high-fat diet induces hepatic steatosis, impairs nitric oxide bioavailability, and modifies the mitochondrial proteome in mice. *Antioxid. Redox Signal.* **2011**, *15*, 447–459. [CrossRef]

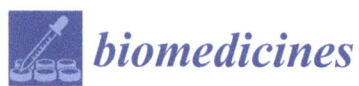

Review

Kidney Renin Release under Hypoxia and Its Potential Link with Nitric Oxide: A Narrative Review

Weiwei Kong [1,2], Yixin Liao [3], Liang Zhao [4], Nathan Hall [5], Hua Zhou [6], Ruisheng Liu [5], Pontus B. Persson [7] and Enyin Lai [1,2,7,*]

[1] Kidney Disease Center of First Affiliated Hospital, Zhejiang University School of Medicine, Hangzhou 310003, China; weiweikong@zju.edu.cn
[2] Department of Physiology, School of Basic Medical Sciences, Zhejiang University School of Medicine, Hangzhou 310003, China
[3] Department of Obstetrics and Gynaecology, Nanfang Hospital, Southern Medical University, Guangzhou 510515, China; yinxin1225@126.com
[4] Department of Nephrology, Children's Hospital, Zhejiang University School of Medicine, National Clinical Research Center for Child Health, Hangzhou 310052, China; liang.zhao@zju.edu.cn
[5] Department of Molecular Pharmacology & Physiology, Morsani College of Medicine, University of South Florida, Tampa, FL 33612, USA; nathanhall@usf.edu (N.H.); ruisheng@usf.edu (R.L.)
[6] Department of Nephrology, Shengjing Hospital of China Medical University, Shenyang 110004, China; huazhou_cmu@163.com
[7] Institute of Translational Physiology, Charité–Universitätsmedizin Berlin, 10117 Berlin, Germany; pontus.persson@charite.de
* Correspondence: laienyin@zju.edu.cn

Abstract: The renin–angiotensin system (RAS) and hypoxia have a complex interaction: RAS is activated under hypoxia and activated RAS aggravates hypoxia in reverse. Renin is an aspartyl protease that catalyzes the first step of RAS and tightly regulates RAS activation. Here, we outline kidney renin expression and release under hypoxia and discuss the putative mechanisms involved. It is important that renin generally increases in response to acute hypoxemic hypoxia and intermittent hypoxemic hypoxia, but not under chronic hypoxemic hypoxia. The increase in renin activity can also be observed in anemic hypoxia and carbon monoxide-induced histotoxic hypoxia. The increased renin is contributed to by juxtaglomerular cells and the recruitment of renin lineage cells. Potential mechanisms regulating hypoxic renin expression involve hypoxia-inducible factor signaling, natriuretic peptides, nitric oxide, and Notch signaling-induced renin transcription.

Keywords: renin; hypoxia; HIFs; juxtaglomerular cells; nitric oxide

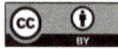

1. Introduction

The renin–angiotensin system (RAS) is a hormonal system responsible for blood pressure homeostasis and electrolyte balance. This systemic RAS consists of several key components: renin, angiotensinogen (AGT), angiotensin I (Ang I), angiotensin-converting enzymes (ACEs), angiotensin II (Ang II), angiotensin II type 1 receptors (AT1Rs), and angiotensin II type 2 receptors (AT2Rs) [1,2]. Renin metabolizes AGT, liberating Ang I. ACEs, which are released from endothelial cells, convert Ang I to Ang II. Then, Ang II acts on two types of receptors, including AT1Rs and AT2Rs. The actions of Ang II on AT1Rs lead to increased sodium retention, vasoconstriction, stimulation of thirst and desire for salt, increased sympathetic nervous system activity, and aldosterone release. Ang II actions on AT2Rs are counter to those on AT1Rs, where AT2R stimulation leads to anti-inflammatory, antifibrotic, and vasodilatory effects. In addition to the classic axis, another axis through ACE2/Ang-(1–7)/MAS has been found. ACE homolog ACE2 can form Ang-(1–7) directly or indirectly from either the decapeptide Ang I or from Ang II. By acting through the receptor MAS, Ang-(1–7) promotes vasodilation, antiproliferation, and antihypertrophy [3–5]. Apart from the systemic RAS, local RASs have been found in various organ systems. Local RASs exhibit multiple physiological effects in addition to and distinct from those of the circulating RAS. In addition to hemodynamic actions, multiple and novel functions of local RASs have been found, including the regulation of cell growth, differentiation, proliferation and apoptosis, reactive oxygen species (ROS) generation, tissue inflammation and fibrosis, and hormonal secretion [4,5].

Hypoxia is a state that arises when the cellular demand for molecular oxygen exceeds supply. It often occurs in tissue and organs with microcirculation injury and hypoperfusion [6]. Under some hypoxia conditions, the RAS is activated and the level of Ang II increases [7–9]. In return, Ang II binding on AT1Rs increases the constriction of both afferent and efferent arterioles, which can aggravate hypoxia [10]. Oxidative stress is a condition that results in the excessive production of oxygen radicals beyond the antioxidant capacity. Both Ang II and hypoxia can induce oxidative stress, which decreases oxygen supply and increases oxygen demand. Finally, the progression of renal injury by oxidative stress further aggravates hypoxia and the activation of RAS. The complexity of the relationship between RAS, hypoxia, and oxidative stress is a vicious cycle [11]. The amount of renin in the bloodstream is a key step in determining Ang II levels and RAS activity [12]. Thus, the pathophysiological change in renin secretion under hypoxia plays a crucial role in the complex correlation between the RAS and hypoxia. To provide the latest evidence for future research and practice, this study critically reviewed the role of kidney renin under hypoxia. Two electronic databases, PubMed and Web of Science, were searched and the main keywords were 'hypoxia' AND 'renin'.

2. Renin Expression in Kidneys

From the embryonic stage, renin expression is located in renin precursor cells (RPCs) [13,14]. During kidney development, RPCs gradually disappear, mostly differentiating into renal vascular smooth muscle cells (VSMCs), mesangial cells, and interstitial pericytes. At the same time, the expression of renin in tubular cells also disappears. After kidney development is complete, only a small number of renin-expressing cells are maintained and restricted to the juxtaglomerular apparatus (JG) in adult mammals. They synthesize and release renin in response to a decrease in renal perfusion pressure, a decrease in the concentration of sodium chloride in the macula densa, or activation of β adrenergic receptors [15,16]. The number of JG cells is quite small in adult mammals, accounting for only about 0.01% of total kidney cells. Under normal circumstances, the release of renin by those few cells generally suffices for maintaining blood pressure and fluid–electrolyte balance [17,18]. Although renin-expressing cells are classically regarded as JG cells in adults, some studies have established that an increase in renin-expressing cells can be derived from the renin lineage cells. This process is termed recruitment. The renin lineage cells in kidneys are not fully differentiated but retain a degree of developmental plasticity or molecular memory, allowing them to re-express renin. Under homeostatic threats, the renin lineage cells like VSMCs, mesangial cells, and interstitial peritubular pericytes are transformed to synthesize renin [19–21].

3. The Change in Renin under Hypoxia

Oxygen is a significant microenvironmental factor that acts as a terminal electron acceptor in oxidative phosphorylation reactions to produce adenosine triphosphate (ATP). Hypoxia is an insufficient supply of oxygen to tissues, which results in abnormal cell metabolism and function [22,23]. According to the etiology of hypoxia, hypoxia can be classified as hypoxemic hypoxia, anemic hypoxia, stagnant hypoxia, or histotoxic hypoxia. According to the time of hypoxia, hypoxia can also be divided into chronic hypoxia and acute hypoxia. Chronic hypoxia includes sustained hypoxia and intermittent hypoxia [24]. Here, we summarise the changes in systemic renin under different hypoxia conditions (Table 1).

For hypoxemic hypoxia, studies have confirmed that plasma renin activity (PRA) increases after acute hypoxia treatment under different oxygen concentrations. PRA increases from 2.3 ± 0.4 ng/mL/h to 4.9 ± 0.8 ng/mL/h after 8% oxygen breathing for 20 min and increases from 2.8 ± 0.4 ng/mL/h to 8.4 ± 1.8 ng/mL/h after 5% oxygen breathing for 20 min [25]. A 12% oxygen breathing treatment for 20 min in rats increases PRA from 3.08 ± 0.68 ng/mL/h to 8.36 ± 1.8 ng/mL/h [26]. Sustained hypoxia (10% oxygen) leads to a decrease in renal renin gene expression to 76% of that of a control after two weeks of treatment and 49% of a control after four weeks of treatment [27,28]. Intermittent hypoxia is composed of hypoxia–normoxia cycles. Hypoxia–normoxia cycles are controlled by individually ventilated cages, which can rapidly change the fraction of inspired oxygen (FiO_2) in seconds [29]. In Fletcher's research, the hypoxia–normoxia cycle was 2 min per cycle and the lowest FiO_2 level reached 2% or 3%. After 35 days of intermittent hypoxia treatment, PRA increased about fourfold compared with the control group [30]. Saxena's team set a longer intermittent hypoxia cycle of 6 min and the lowest FiO_2 level was 10%. The PRA also increased after 1 day and 7 days of intermittent hypoxia treatment [31]. In summary, acute hypoxemic hypoxia or intermittent hypoxemic hypoxia both induce an increase in renin activity but sustained hypoxemic hypoxia negatively regulates renin activity.

Obstructive sleep apnea (OSA) is a common type of intermittent hypoxemic hypoxia in clinics that is characterized by recurrent episodes of oxygen desaturation and reoxygenation [32]. A meta-analysis conducted on 13 studies found that elevated aldosterone levels were observed in OSA patients with hypertension compared to normotensive OSA patients. Hypertensive disorders are strongly linked with an overactive RAS because the activation of RAS can regulate the body's hemodynamic equilibrium, circulating volume, and electrolyte balance. The activation of RAS has been implicated in playing a pathophysiological role in the relationship between OSA and hypertension, particularly resistant hypertension [33].

Another special type of hypoxemic hypoxia occurs at high altitudes. With increasing altitude, the partial pressure of oxygen in the ambient air decreases. Humans ascending to high altitudes inhale fewer oxygen molecules per breath [34]. The effect on plasma renin activity depends on the time spent at high altitudes. Two studies have moved the objects of observation from sea level to high altitudes and have tested the change in renin at different time points. A short time at high altitudes causes a decrease in RAS, which seems to be protective against plasma Ang II and could lead to vasoconstriction and sodium retention. After a prolonged stay at high altitudes, plasma renin activity increases but remains reduced compared to at sea level. The different change in renin at high altitudes compared to classical hypoxemic hypoxia may be related to complex modifications in systemic vascular dysfunction. In addition to the exposure to hypoxia, high altitudes cause a significant increase in aortic stiffness, blood pressure, heart rate, and cardiac output. RAS is not to be the determining factor for vascular changes because the inhibition of RAS did not show any difference in parameters reflecting the viscoelastic properties of large arteries at high altitudes [35,36]. Both hypoxia and systemic vascular dysfunction can influence a change in RAS, which may be the reason for a different change in renin at high altitudes compared to classical hypoxia. Another study compared high-altitude natives and sea-level natives. It found that the level of PRA was higher in high-altitude natives compared with sea-level natives [37]. In this study design, the higher PRA may be influenced by hypoxia but is also affected by cardiopulmonary maladaptation, race, diet, and lifestyle.

Erythrocytes are essential for the delivery of oxygen to organs. Anemia causes a whole-body oxygen shortage, which belongs to anemic hypoxia [38]. Kenichiro Miyauchi's team utilized inherited super anemic mutant (ISAM) mice to modulate anemia-related hypoxia. Under anemic hypoxia, the levels of renin expression increased in the kidneys [39]. Exposure to carbon monoxide is one kind of histotoxic hypoxia. Kramer et al. found that exposure to carbon monoxide increased PRA approximately three to four times and boosted renin mRNA levels approximately two times compared to the control group [40]. Stagnant hypoxia is usually accompanied by changes in hemodynamics, which may play a more dominant role in regulation than hypoxia. Thus, it is hard to evaluate the renin changes that are contributed to by the insufficient supply of oxygen under the condition of stagnant hypoxia.

Table 1. The change in renin under hypoxia.

			Change in Renin Activity/Expression	Reference
Acute hypoxemic hypoxia				
20 min	Beagle dogs	5 and 8% O_2	Increased	[25]
20 min	SD rats	12% O_2	Increased	[26]
Chronic sustained hypoxemic hypoxia				
2/4 w	Wistar rats	10% O_2	Decreased	[27,28]
Chronic intermit hypoxemic hypoxia				
35 d	Wistar rats	2–3% O_2 2 min/cycle	Increased	[30]
1 d	SD rats	10% O_2 6 min/cycle	Increased	[31]
7 d	SD rats	10% O_2 6 min/cycle	Increased	[31]
Special type of hypoxemic hypoxia				
Obstructive sleep apnea			Increased	[33]
High altitude natives (vs sea level natives)			Higher	[37]
6 days stay at high altitude (vs basal at sea level)			Decreased	[35]
Acute exposure to high altitudes (vs basal at sea level)			Decreased	[36]
2 weeks stay at high altitudes (vs basal at sea level)			Decreased	[36]
Anemic hypoxia				
Inherited super anemic mutant mice			Increased	[39]
Histotoxic hypoxia				
6 h	SD rats	0.1% Carbon monoxide	Increased	[40]

4. Sources of Renin under Hypoxia

This part summarizes two sources of renin expression under hypoxia, including the activation of JG cells and the recruitment of renin lineage cells (Figure 1).

The activation of JG cells under hypoxia: JG cells store renin in dense core secretory granules and can become hypergranulated when renin secretion increases [41]. To study the change in hypoxia on JG cells, Goldfarb first used a hypoxia chamber but found no changes in the morphology of JG cell granularity under the hypoxia condition of one-half atmospheric pressure for 12 h [42]. Furthermore, Oliver et al. found that hypoxia-treated rats exhibited poor intake of food and sodium compared to control rats. Since serum sodium levels can influence renin secretion, they improved the research design by adding sodium supplements. In Olivers study, a supplemental injection of sodium chloride was used daily to avoid the effect of sodium deprivation. The hypoxia condition was constructed by maintaining an oxygen content of 7% to 8%. Finally, they verified that hypoxia induces the hypergranulation of JG cells [43]. The in vivo preliminarily experiment revealed that hypoxia leads to the granularity of JG cells, but the in vitro experiment did not present similar results. In the primary culture of renal JG cells, hypoxia treatment (1% or 3% oxygen for 6 or 20 h) did not affect renin activity [40]. The difference between in vivo and in vitro studies indicates that the link between renin secretion and hypoxia may be indirect, reflecting the demand for some kind of systemic signaling link. The sympathetic nervous system may be one of the potential linking mechanisms. Renin secretion is the downstream effector of the sympathetic nervous system, and afferent nerve signals are required during the stimulation process. An in vitro culture of JG cells is a state of renal denervation, which is not regulated by the sympathetic nervous system [44]. Circulating catecholamine may be another potential medium related to hypoxia and renin secretion. Previous evidence showed that circulating catecholamines such as noradrenaline and adrenalin are stimulated under some hypoxia conditions and catecholamine-induced receptor activation significantly stimulates both renin secretion and gene expression. Local renal factors, such as the renal baroreceptor mechanism or the macula densa mechanism, may be a step in the systemic signaling link, but are not yet clearly understood [45–49].

Re-expression of renin under hypoxia: RPCs and their descendants are the center of nephrogenesis. With kidney development, RPCs gradually disappear and most of these RPCs differentiate into renal VSMCs, mesangial cells, interstitial pericytes, and renal tubular cells. Such renin lineage cells in adults retain their ability to transdifferentiate into the original state to re-express renin [50]. Renin lineage cells transformed into their pre-differentiated state to re-express the renin gene is a process known as recruitment [51].

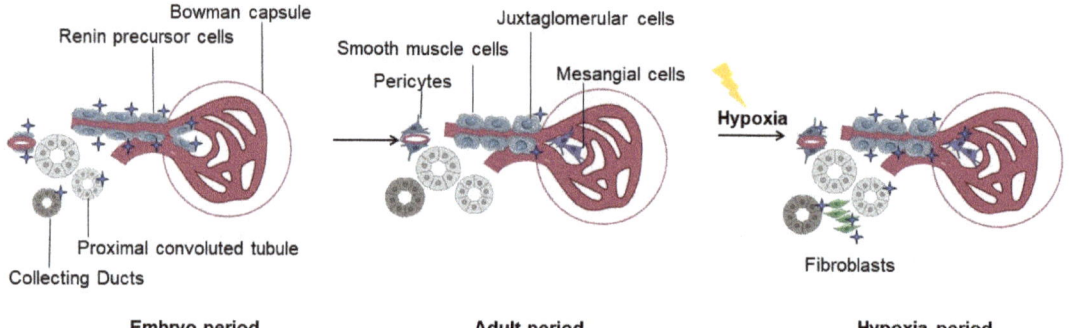

Figure 1. The expression of renin in kidneys under hypoxia. From the embryonic stage, renin expression is located along vascular and around collecting ducts and proximal tubules. As the kidneys develop, renin precursor cells gradually disappear and most of them differentiate into intrinsic renal cells (like pericytes, mesangial cells, and smooth muscle cells). Renin-expressing tubular cells in the embryonic stage also disappear in the adult period. After kidney development is complete, only a small number of renin-expressing cells are maintained and are restricted to the juxtaglomerular (JG) apparatus in adult mammals. The expression of renin increases under hypoxia, which is observed in both JG cells and other intrinsic renal cells. The descendants of renin precursor cells can transform into their pre-differentiated states to re-express the renin gene. Also, renin-expressing tubular cells in the embryonic stage can re-express renin in response to hypoxia.

The recruitment process in renin lineage cells was found in anemic hypoxia. Miyauchi et al. found that renin activity increases in an anemia model of ISAM mice. As expected, the expression of renin 1 structural (*Ren1*) mRNA was consistently detected in JG cells in both the ISAM mice and the control mice. But, the *Ren1* expression in renal interstitial cells could be detected in ISAM mice, but not in control mice. In situ hybridization analysis found that interstitial cells with *Ren1* positive were fibroblasts with the characteristic of being positive pericyte markers [39]. It was preliminarily shown that renin-expressing fibroblasts were transdifferentiated from recruitment pericytes. Unilateral ureteral obstruction (UUO) is a classic model of chronic obstructive kidney disease, with the characteristic of tubulointerstitial fibrosis. Tubulointerstitial fibrosis affects oxygen diffusion and supply, leading to tissue hypoxia [52]. The recruitment process was also found in the UUO model. RenCreER (Ren1cCreERxRs-tdTomato) transgenic mice were applied to the fate map of *Ren1*+ cells in the UUO model, in which *Ren1*+ progenitors were permanently labeled during a period of tamoxifen induction. There was only a marginal increase in *Ren1*+ cells in the JG areas. However, the number of *Ren1*+ cells in interstitial areas increased significantly from day 7 after UUO. The labeled *Ren1*+ cells initially co-expressed the pericyte markers and appeared around peritubular capillaries. On day 14 post-UUO, the majority of labeled cells were away from blood vessels and transdifferentiated into myofibroblasts. $Ren1^+$ cells around interstitial areas in a UUO model possibly participated in vessel remodeling in the early period and ultimately underwent transitions into myofibroblast-like cells, which might favor fibrosis rather than repair. Interestingly, the recruitment of $Ren1^+$ cells in UUO cannot retain renin protein, which was indicated by the fact that renin protein staining was negative in interstitial areas [53]. Similarly, another study found that recruitment pericytes in interstitial areas cannot store renin [54]. Renin storage is a crucial part of renin secretion. Thus, it is currently recognized that recruitment cells can express the renin gene, but is unknown whether the recruitment cells can lead to renin secretion. Future studies are needed to give us the answer.

5. Potential Mechanisms Regulating Renin under Hypoxia

Here, we summarized the potential mechanisms for regulating renin expression or secretion under hypoxia. Notch signaling and nitric oxide (NO) are potential up-regulation mechanisms, while hypoxia-inducible factors (HIFs) and natriuretic peptides are efforts to downregulate renin (Figure 2).

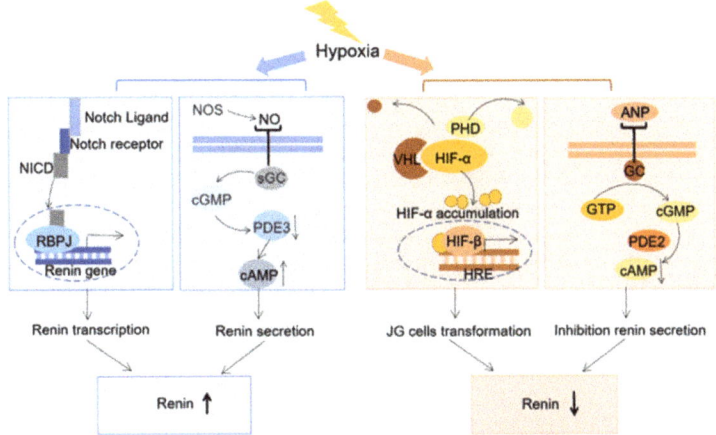

Figure 2. Possible mechanism regulating renin expression under hypoxia. Notch signaling is activated under hypoxia and then the Notch intracellular domain (NICD) translocates into nuclear and binds with the co-effector recombination signal sequence binding protein J kappa (REBPJ) to form the transcription complex. The transcription complex has a specific binding sequence and binds with the promoter of the renin gene, which finally induces renin transcription. Nitric oxide (NO) is essential to regulate renin secretion. Hypoxia can promote NO production by increasing nitric oxide synthase (NOS), especially neuronal-type NOS (nNOS), transcription. Increased NO can stimulate soluble guanylate cyclase (sGC) and increase cyclic guanosine monophosphate (cGMP). Then, cGMP-mediated inhibition of phosphodiesterase (PDE) 3 prevents cAMP degradation and stimulates renin secretion. The activation of hypoxia-inducible factor (HIF) signaling is a hypoxia protection mechanism. Under normoxic conditions, HIF-α subunits are hydroxylated by the prolyl 4-hydroxylase domain (PHD) and then degraded by the von Hippel–Lindau tumor suppressor protein (VHL). Under hypoxia, the hydroxylation of HIF-α by VHL is inhibited and HIF-α/HIF-β heterodimers bind to the HIF-responsive element (HRE), thereby promoting the transcription of downstream genes. The activation of HIF signaling in JG cells leads to a reprogramming of cells against hypoxia by increasing erythropoietin (EPO) secretion and reducing renin secretion. Atrial natriuretic peptide (ANP) is hypoxia-responsive and has an inhibitory role for renin secretion. its mechanism starts from binding with the guanylyl cyclase (Gc) receptor, then stimulates the cGMP/PDE2 pathway, and subsequently degrades the cyclic adenosine monophosphate (cAMP).

Hypoxia-inducible factors (HIFs) regulating renin expression: HIFs are key transcription factors in the response to hypoxia [55]. HIFs consist of one HIF-α subunit and one HIF-β subunit. There are three isoforms of the HIF-α subunit (HIF-1α, HIF-2α, and HIF-3α), among which HIF-1α and HIF-2α are critical in the response to hypoxia [56,57]. Under normoxic conditions, HIF-α subunits are hydroxylated by the prolyl 4-hydroxylase domain (PHD) and then degraded by the von Hippel–Lindau tumor suppressor protein (VHL) [58,59]. Under hypoxia, the hydroxylation of HIF-α is inhibited and HIF-α combines with HIF-β to form HIF-α/HIF-β heterodimers. Subsequently, the HIF-α/HIF-β heterodimers bind to the HIF-responsive element (HRE), thereby promoting the transcription of downstream genes [60,61]. Recently, researchers found that HIF-α accumulation under normoxia leads to a change in hormone expression in JG cells. The deletion of both PHD2 and PHD3 upregulates HIF-α accumulation, which is accompanied by reduced renin expression and promoted erythropoietin (EPO) expression in both JG cells and interstitial cells [54]. Similarly, HIF overexpression induced by PHD inhibitors also increases EPO levels in peripheral blood [62,63]. Furthermore, Kurt et al. developed a mouse model involving the specific deletion of VHL in renin-expressing cells. The mouse model shows downregulated renin activity in the baseline condition. Also, the mice-specific deletion of VHL also has an attenuated expansion in renin-expressing cells, even under the stimulation of the RAS (a low-salt diet combined with an ACE inhibitor). The deletion of VHL in renin-expressing cells activates EPO expression [64].

The switch of hormone expression in JG cells under the HIF signaling activation is associated with changes in morphological and gene expression profiles. Electron microscopy reveals that control JG cells have cuboid-like morphological features with an accumulation of prominent electron-dense renin storage vesicles. However, JG cells with the specific deletion of VHL have flat and elongated morphological features with no classical electron-dense granules. Additionally, gene expression profiles show a loss of typical markers of renin cells and an increase in fibroblast markers in pVHL-deficient JG cells [65,66]. Till now, both pharmaceutical-treated mice and transgenic mice with HIF-α accumulation under normoxia have shown increased expression of EPO and decreased expression of renin under normoxia. Such changes in renin-expressing cells help alleviate hypoxia because increased EPO expression may enhance oxygen delivery and decreased renin expression can lead to vasorelaxation. This change is in accordance with the protective role of HIFs in hypoxia.

Potential role of Notch signaling in renin expression: The Notch signaling pathway is critical for normal cell proliferation and differentiation. It is composed of receptors, ligands, and the final common effector. The binding of the Notch ligand to its cellular receptor causes the latter to cleave and release the Notch intracellular domain (NICD), which is subsequently translocated into the nucleus. In the nucleus, the NICD binds to the transcription factor recombination signal sequence binding protein J kappa (RBPJ), and then RBPJ as a transcription factor induces downstream gene transcription [67,68].

We supposed a potential link between Notch and renin expression under hypoxia by reviewing previous studies. Firstly, the link between Notch signaling and hypoxia has been reported. Notch signaling is activated under hypoxia, which is supported by the increased expression of NICD and the downstream gene of Notch signaling under hypoxia [69]. In addition, the promotion role of Notch signaling in renin expression has also been reported. The deletion of *RBPJ* in renin lineage cells reveals a significant decrease in the number of renin-positive cells [70]. Also, the expression of two crucial genes that indicate the endocrine phenotype of JG cells, Ren1 and aldo-keto reductase family 1, and member B7 (Akr1b7), substantially diminishes after *RBPJ* deletion [71]. Further, renin gene transcription can be promoted by Notch signaling. As revealed by chromatin immunoprecipitation, the final common effector of Notch signaling RBPJ can bind with the promoter of the renin gene [72]. Furthermore, the mutation of four core nucleotides at the RBPJ binding site of the renin promoter is sufficient to suppress renin expression [71]. Through the above review, an indirect link between Notch signaling and renin expression under hypoxia has been revealed. We indicate that Notch signaling is activated under hypoxia; then, NICD/RBPJ forms the transcription complex and binds with the promoter of the renin gene, which finally induces renin transcription. Jagged1 is one of the five cell surface ligands of the Notch signaling pathway. The classic Jagged1-Notch interaction provokes a cascade of proteolytic cleavages, which transport the NICD into the nucleus [73]. However, the specifically conditional deletion of Jagged1 within renin-expressing cells does not result in downregulated renin expression in JG cells [74]. This indicates that renin transcription regulated by Notch signaling is not dependent on the ligand of Jagged1. Which ligands participate in this process needs to be further studied.

The potential role of NO in promoting renin secretion: NO is a short-lived, endogenously produced signaling molecule that plays multiple roles in mammalian physiology. NO is formed from its precursor l-arginine by a family of nitric oxide synthase (NOS), which has three identified isoforms: neuronal type NOS (nNOS), endothelial type NOS (eNOS), and inducible type NOS (iNOS). Different isoforms are expressed depending on the organs, tissues, and cells [75,76].

The role of NO in renin secretion under hypoxia is not clear, but a potential link between NO and renin expression under hypoxia is revealed by reviewing previous studies. In theory, NO can participate in both inhibitory and stimulatory pathways of renin secretion. NO can stimulate soluble guanylate cyclase (sGC) and increase cyclic guanosine monophosphate (cGMP). Then, cGMP-mediated protein kinase (PKG II) and phosphodiesterase (PDE) 2 are involved in the inhibition of renin secretion, whereas the cGMP-mediated inhibition of PDE3 prevents cyclic adenosine monophosphate (cAMP) degradation and stimulates renin secretion. Thus, NO can have dual effects on renin release. The controversial regulation ability of NO on renin secretion could be partly explained by different sources of NO. Increased NO from eNOS activation is always accompanied by elevated renal perfusion and shear stress, which is probably involved in the inhibition of renin release by the activation of PKG II. Another source of NO for JG cells is nNOS, which is involved in the activation of renin secretion by inhibiting PDE3 activity [77]. However, current research data have established that the overall effect of NO on renin secretion is stimulatory [14]. The increase in renin secretion observed in response to a low salt concentration was markedly attenuated in the presence of the nonspecific NOS inhibitor (NG-nitro-l-arginine). Similar results were obtained in vivo, where increased renin secretion in response to loop diuretics was attenuated by concomitant NOS inhibition. The availability of NO is also required for the recruitment of renin-expressing cells, in particular, for the recruitment of preglomerular VSMCs [78]. The promotion of NO on renin may be related to the source of NO under hypoxia. eNOS, nNOS, and eNOS all contribute to NO under hypoxia, but nNOS is the main source of NO under hypoxia [79]. NO derived from nNOS can stimulate cGMP, which further mediates the activation of renin secretion by inhibiting PDE3 activity [77].

Hydrogen sulfide (H2S) is an endogenously produced gas with known antioxidant and neuroprotective properties. H2S has a complex interaction with NO, which can upregulate eNOS expression, increase NO bioavailability by reducing oxidative stress, and enhance downstream NO signaling by inhibiting PDE5A activity [80]. Like NO, enhanced H2S production has been proposed as a universal response to hypoxic stress. The increase in H2S has an inhibitory role in the pathological signaling of RAS. H2S has been reported to downregulate cAMP by inhibiting adenylate cyclase activity, thereby regulating renin release [81–83].

Natriuretic peptides: Natriuretic peptides are hormones secreted from the heart to promote Na$^+$ excretion in the kidneys. Currently, there are three known peptides in the natriuretic peptides family: atrial natriuretic peptide (ANP), B-type natriuretic peptide (BNP), and C-type natriuretic peptide (CNP) [84]. ANP is hypoxia-responsive and its circulating levels are increased by decreased clearance due to downregulation of the natriuretic peptide receptor-C in hypoxia [85]. The increased ANP has an inhibition role for renin secretion in JG cells. The inhibition role of ANP on renin may be related to an increase in cGMP [86]. Further, it was shown that the inhibitory effects of ANP on renin are mediated by the cGMP/PDE2 pathway, which promotes cAMP degradation [87].

6. Renin in Renal Local RASs under Hypoxia

In the classical definition, RAS is a peptidergic system with endocrine characteristics. Current results have changed our view of RASs and introduced the concept of "local" or "tissue" RASs. For inter-renal RASs, the observation of renin was reported in collecting ducts, proximal tubules and the bowman capsule. The inter-renal RAS also has a complex interaction with systemic RASs. Ang II produced in systemic RASs acts in a feed-forward manner to stimulate local renin synthesis. Furthermore, some components of local RASs, such as renin or angiotensinogen, may be taken up from the systemic RAS in circulation. Such local RASs and their interaction with the systemic RAS make the story of RAS complex [5].

Hypoxia occurs commonly in chronic kidney diseases because tubulointerstitial fibrosis impairs oxygen diffusion and supply [88]. The activation of the intrarenal RAS in the CKD model has been evaluated by immunoreactivities for Ang II in the tubulointerstitial area. The activation score of interstitial Ang II correlated with plasma creatinine concentration, glomerulosclerosis, fibrosis, and cell infiltration in interstitial inflammation [89]. UUO, characterized by tubulointerstitial fibrosis, showed increases in renal renin content, ACE activity, and Ang II concentration on the first day after surgery. Angiotensin II receptor antagonists ameliorate renal tubulointerstitial fibrosis caused by UUO, which suggests a pathogenic role of the intrarenal RAS in renal fibrosis [90,91]. NO also has a regulatory role in the local RAS, but the regulation is complicated. Curnow's team found that different levels of NO bioavailability have different regulation roles in renin synthesis in the collecting duct: low NO bioavailability enhances the synthesis and secretion of renin in collecting duct; high level of NO promotes the accumulation of renin intracellularly, but does not increase renin secretion in collecting duct [92].

7. Future Prospects

In recent years, our understanding of the physiological and pathological activity of renin under hypoxia has gradually deepened. The results obtained from several related studies have shed light on questions regarding the change in renin under hypoxia. Both systemic and local renin show an increase in most hypoxia conditions. The increase in renin expression under hypoxia comes from the activation of JG cells and the recruitment of renin lineage cells. The possible regulation mechanisms of renin activity under hypoxia include HIF signaling, Notch signaling, NO, and natriuretic peptides.

However, some questions remain unanswered. For example, renin expression, but not renin secretion, was reported in recruitment cells. A recent study also found that the re-expression of renin in recruitment cells cannot store renin. Thus, whether the re-expression of renin in recruitment cells is accompanied by renin secretion is still unknown. In addition, Notch signaling and NO-induced renin secretion under hypoxia are two potential mechanisms that may explain the increased activity of renin under hypoxia. We reviewed relevant articles and highlighted possible links, but no study directly confirms the role of Notch signaling and NO in renin secretion under hypoxia. Another problem is that evidence of decreased renin activity regulated by HIF signaling comes mainly from the HIF overexpression model under normoxia but not hypoxia. The question of whether HIF overexpression in normoxia can explain the change in renin activity in hypoxia remains to be further verified. Prorenin was previously considered to be the inactive precursor of renin, but recent findings show that prorenin has a more complex regulation on RAS via prorenin receptors. Related research about prorenin under hypoxia is still rare and studies in this field should be carried out in the future. This review focused on the change in kidney renin but did not cover the downstream of renin, like aldosterone or Ang-(1–7), because the downstream signaling of renin is complicated. For one thing, RAS is not limited to the classical axis. For another, the classical downstream aldosterone also has a renin-independent activation pathway. Current studies cannot tell us the full map of RAS under hypoxia. Thus, we expect future studies to provide us with the answers to these questions.

Author Contributions: W.K.: conceptualization. W.K., Y.L., L.Z. and H.Z.: resources. W.K.: writing. N.H. and R.L.: language editing. P.B.P. and E.L.: reviewing and editing. All authors contributed to the article. All authors have read and agreed to the published version of the manuscript.

Funding: This work was supported by grants to Weiwei Kong from the Natural Foundation of Zhejiang LQ21H050004 and National Natural Foundation of China 82000635, to En Yin Lai and Pontus B. Persson from Deutsche Forschungsgemeinschaft (German Research Foundation) Project 394046635-SFB 1365, and to Liang Zhao from the Joint Funds of the Zhejiang Provincial Natural Science Foundation of China under grant no. LHDMZ23H050002.

Data Availability Statement: No new data were created or analyzed in this study. Data sharing is not applicable to this article.

Conflicts of Interest: The authors declare no conflict of interest. The funders had no role in the design of the study; in the collection, analyses, or interpretation of data; in the writing of the manuscript; or in the decision to publish the results.

References

1. Mirabito Colafella, K.M.; Bovée, D.M.; Danser, A.H.J. The renin-angiotensin-aldosterone system and its therapeutic targets. *Exp. Eye Res.* **2019**, *186*, 107680. [CrossRef] [PubMed]
2. Vargas Vargas, R.A.; Varela Millán, J.M.; Fajardo Bonilla, E. Renin–angiotensin system: Basic and clinical aspects-A general perspective. *Endocrinol. Diabetes Nutr.* **2022**, *69*, 52–62. [CrossRef] [PubMed]
3. Ardaillou, R. Angiotensin II receptors. *J. Am. Soc. Nephrol.* **1999**, *10* (Suppl. S11), S30–S39.
4. Santos, R.A.S.; Sampaio, W.O.; Alzamora, A.C.; Motta-Santos, D.; Alenina, N.; Bader, M.; Campagnole-Santos, M.J. The ACE2/Angiotensin-(1-7)/MAS Axis of the Renin–angiotensin system: Focus on Angiotensin-(1-7). *Physiol. Rev.* **2018**, *98*, 505–553. [CrossRef]
5. Paul, M.; Poyan Mehr, A.; Kreutz, R. Physiology of local renin–angiotensin systems. *Physiol. Rev.* **2006**, *86*, 747–803. [CrossRef] [PubMed]
6. Shu, S.; Wang, Y.; Zheng, M.; Liu, Z.; Cai, J.; Tang, C.; Dong, Z. Hypoxia and Hypoxia-Inducible Factors in Kidney Injury and Repair. *Cells* **2019**, *8*, 207. [CrossRef]
7. Zhou, T.-B.; Ou, C.; Rong, L.; Drummen, G.P. Effect of all-trans retinoic acid treatment on prohibitin and renin-angiotensin-aldosterone system expression in hypoxia-induced renal tubular epithelial cell injury. *J. Renin-Angiotensin-Aldosterone Syst.* **2014**, *15*, 243–249. [CrossRef]
8. Nicholl, D.; Hanly, P.; Zalucky, A.; Handley, G.; Sola, D.; Ahmed, S.J.S. Nocturnal hypoxemia severity influences the effect of CPAP therapy on renal renin-angiotensin-aldosterone system activity in humans with obstructive sleep apnea. *Sleep* **2021**, *44*, zsaa228. [CrossRef]
9. Raff, H.; Sandri, R.B.; Segerson, T.P. Renin, ACTH, and adrenocortical function during hypoxia and hemorrhage in conscious rats. *Am. J. Physiol.* **1986**, *250*, R240–R244. [CrossRef]
10. Feng, M.G.; Navar, L.G. Angiotensin II-mediated constriction of afferent and efferent arterioles involves T-type Ca^{2+} channel activation. *Am. J. Nephrol.* **2004**, *24*, 641–648. [CrossRef]
11. Nangaku, M.; Fujita, T. Activation of the renin–angiotensin system and chronic hypoxia of the kidney. *Hypertens. Res.* **2008**, *31*, 175–184. [CrossRef] [PubMed]
12. Chaszczewska-Markowska, M.; Sagan, M.; Bogunia-Kubik, K. The renin-angiotensin-aldosterone system (RAAS)—Physiology and molecular mechanisms of functioning. *Postep. Hig. I Med. Dosw.* **2016**, *70*, 917–927. [CrossRef] [PubMed]
13. Kurtz, A. Renin release: Sites, mechanisms, and control. *Annu. Rev. Physiol.* **2011**, *73*, 377–399. [CrossRef]
14. Castrop, H.; Höcherl, K.; Kurtz, A.; Schweda, F.; Todorov, V.; Wagner, C. Physiology of kidney renin. *Physiol. Rev.* **2010**, *90*, 607–673. [CrossRef] [PubMed]
15. Damkjær, M.; Isaksson, G.L.; Stubbe, J.; Jensen, B.L.; Assersen, K.; Bie, P. Renal renin secretion as regulator of body fluid homeostasis. *Pflug. Arch. Eur. J. Physiol.* **2013**, *465*, 153–165. [CrossRef] [PubMed]
16. Kurtz, A. Control of renin synthesis and secretion. *Am. J. Hypertens.* **2012**, *25*, 839–847. [CrossRef] [PubMed]
17. Gomez, R.A.; Sequeira-Lopez, M.L.S. Renin cells in homeostasis, regeneration and immune defence mechanisms. *Nat. Rev. Nephrol.* **2018**, *14*, 231–245. [CrossRef]
18. Guessoum, O.; de Goes Martini, A.; Sequeira-Lopez, M.L.S.; Gomez, R.A. Deciphering the Identity of Renin Cells in Health and Disease. *Trends Mol. Med.* **2021**, *27*, 280–292. [CrossRef]
19. Assmus, A.M.; Mullins, J.J.; Brown, C.M.; Mullins, L.J. Cellular plasticity: A mechanism for homeostasis in the kidney. *Acta Physiol.* **2020**, *229*, e13447. [CrossRef]

20. Kurtz, A. How can juxtaglomerular renin-producing cells support the integrity of glomerular endothelial cells? *Pflug. Arch. Eur. J. Physiol.* **2019**, *471*, 1161–1162. [CrossRef]
21. Pippin, J.W.; Sparks, M.A.; Glenn, S.T.; Buitrago, S.; Coffman, T.M.; Duffield, J.S.; Gross, K.W.; Shankland, S.J. Cells of renin lineage are progenitors of podocytes and parietal epithelial cells in experimental glomerular disease. *Am. J. Pathol.* **2013**, *183*, 542–557. [CrossRef] [PubMed]
22. Samanta, D.; Prabhakar, N.R.; Semenza, G.L. Systems biology of oxygen homeostasis. *Wiley Interdiscip. Rev. Syst. Biol. Med.* **2017**, *9*, e1382. [CrossRef] [PubMed]
23. Persson, P.B.; Bondke Persson, A. Oxygen-to little, too much or just right. *Acta Physiol.* **2018**, *223*, e13076. [CrossRef] [PubMed]
24. Mallat, J.; Rahman, N.; Hamed, F.; Hernandez, G.; Fischer, M.O. Pathophysiology, mechanisms, and managements of tissue hypoxia. *Anaesth. Crit. Care Pain Med.* **2022**, *41*, 101087. [CrossRef]
25. Liang, C.S.; Gavras, H. Renin–angiotensin system inhibition in conscious dogs during acute hypoxemia. Effects on systemic hemodynamics, regional blood flows, and tissue metabolism. *J. Clin. Investig.* **1978**, *62*, 961–970. [CrossRef]
26. Neylon, M.; Marshall, J.; Johns, E.J. The role of the renin–angiotensin system in the renal response to moderate hypoxia in the rat. *J. Physiol.* **1996**, *491 Pt 2*, 479–488. [CrossRef]
27. Schweda, F.; Schweda, A.; Pfeifer, M.; Blumberg, F.C.; Kammerl, M.C.; Holmer, S.R.; Riegger, G.A.; Krämer, B.K. Role of endothelins for the regulation of renal renin gene expression. *J. Cardiovasc. Pharmacol.* **2000**, *36*, S187–S190. [CrossRef]
28. Schweda, F.; Blumberg, F.C.; Schweda, A.; Kammerl, M.; Holmer, S.R.; Riegger, G.A.; Pfeifer, M.; Krämer, B.K. Effects of chronic hypoxia on renal renin gene expression in rats. *Nephrol. Dial. Transplant.* **2000**, *15*, 11–15. [CrossRef]
29. Da Silva, M.P.; Magalhães, K.S.; de Souza, D.P.; Moraes, D.J.A. Chronic intermittent hypoxia increases excitability and synaptic excitation of protrudor and retractor hypoglossal motoneurones. *J. Physiol.* **2021**, *599*, 1917–1932. [CrossRef]
30. Fletcher, E.C.; Bao, G.; Li, R. Renin activity and blood pressure in response to chronic episodic hypoxia. *Hypertension* **1999**, *34*, 309–314. [CrossRef]
31. Saxena, A.; Little, J.T.; Nedungadi, T.P.; Cunningham, J.T. Angiotensin II type 1a receptors in subfornical organ contribute towards chronic intermittent hypoxia-associated sustained increase in mean arterial pressure. *Am. J. Physiol. Heart Circ. Physiol.* **2015**, *308*, H435–H446. [CrossRef] [PubMed]
32. Loh, H.H.; Lim, Q.H.; Chai, C.S.; Goh, S.L.; Lim, L.L.; Yee, A.; Sukor, N. Influence and implications of the renin-angiotensin-aldosterone system in obstructive sleep apnea: An updated systematic review and meta-analysis. *J. Sleep Res.* **2023**, *32*, e13726. [CrossRef] [PubMed]
33. Jin, Z.N.; Wei, Y.X. Meta-analysis of effects of obstructive sleep apnea on the renin-angiotensin-aldosterone system. *J. Geriatr. Cardiol.* **2016**, *13*, 333–343. [CrossRef]
34. Sharma, V.; Varshney, R.; Sethy, N.K. Human adaptation to high altitude: A review of convergence between genomic and proteomic signatures. *Hum. Genom.* **2022**, *16*, 21. [CrossRef] [PubMed]
35. Keynes, R.J.; Smith, G.W.; Slater, J.D.; Brown, M.M.; Brown, S.E.; Payne, N.N.; Jowett, T.P.; Monge, C.C. Renin and aldosterone at high altitude in man. *J. Endocrinol.* **1982**, *92*, 131–140. [CrossRef] [PubMed]
36. Revera, M.; Salvi, P.; Faini, A.; Giuliano, A.; Gregorini, F.; Bilo, G.; Lombardi, C.; Mancia, G.; Agostoni, P.; Parati, G. Renin-Angiotensin-Aldosterone System Is Not Involved in the Arterial Stiffening Induced by Acute and Prolonged Exposure to High Altitude. *Hypertension* **2017**, *70*, 75–84. [CrossRef]
37. Antezana, A.M.; Richalet, J.P.; Noriega, I.; Galarza, M.; Antezana, G. Hormonal changes in normal and polycythemic high-altitude natives. *J. Appl. Physiol.* **1995**, *79*, 795–800. [CrossRef]
38. Mistry, N.; Mazer, C.D.; Sled, J.G.; Lazarus, A.H.; Cahill, L.S.; Solish, M.; Zhou, Y.Q.; Romanova, N.; Hare, A.G.M.; Doctor, A.; et al. Red blood cell antibody-induced anemia causes differential degrees of tissue hypoxia in kidney and brain. *Am. J. Physiol. Regul. Integr. Comp. Physiol.* **2018**, *314*, R611–R622. [CrossRef]
39. Miyauchi, K.; Nakai, T.; Saito, S.; Yamamoto, T.; Sato, K.; Kato, K.; Nezu, M.; Miyazaki, M.; Ito, S.; Yamamoto, M.; et al. Renal interstitial fibroblasts coproduce erythropoietin and renin under anaemic conditions. *EBioMedicine* **2021**, *64*, 103209. [CrossRef]
40. Kramer, B.K.; Ritthaler, T.; Schweda, F.; Kees, F.; Schricker, K.; Holmer, S.R.; Kurtz, A. Effects of hypoxia on renin secretion and renal renin gene expression. *Kidney Int. Suppl.* **1998**, *67*, S155–S158. [CrossRef] [PubMed]
41. Berka, J.L.; Alcorn, D.; Coghlan, J.P.; Fernley, R.T.; Morgan, T.O.; Ryan, G.B.; Skinner, S.L.; Weaver, D.A. Granular juxtaglomerular cells and prorenin synthesis in mice treated with enalapril. *J. Hypertens.* **1990**, *8*, 229–238. [CrossRef] [PubMed]
42. Goldfarb, B.; Tobian, L. The interrelationship of hypoxia, erythropoietin, and the renal juxtaglomerular cell. *Proc. Soc. Exp. Biol. Med.* **1962**, *111*, 510–511. [CrossRef]
43. Oliver, W.J.; Brody, G.L. Effect of prolonged hypoxia upon granularity of rneal juxtaglomerular cells. *Circ. Res.* **1965**, *16*, 83–88. [CrossRef] [PubMed]
44. Czyzyk-Krzeska, M.F.; Trzebski, A. Respiratory-related discharge pattern of sympathetic nerve activity in the spontaneously hypertensive rat. *J. Physiol.* **1990**, *426*, 355–368. [CrossRef]
45. Riquier-Brison, A.D.M.; Sipos, A.; Prókai, Á.; Vargas, S.L.; Toma, L.; Meer, E.J.; Villanueva, K.G.; Chen, J.C.M.; Gyarmati, G.; Yih, C.; et al. The macula densa prorenin receptor is essential in renin release and blood pressure control. *Am. J. Physiol. Ren. Physiol.* **2018**, *315*, F521–F534. [CrossRef] [PubMed]

46. Haase, M.; Dringenberg, T.; Allelein, S.; Willenberg, H.S.; Schott, M. Excessive Catecholamine Secretion and the Activation of the Renin-Angiotensin-Aldosterone-System in Patients with Pheochromocytoma: A Single Center Experience and Overview of the Literature. *Horm. Metab. Res.* **2017**, *49*, 748–754. [CrossRef] [PubMed]
47. Rico, A.J.; Prieto-Lloret, J.; Gonzalez, C.; Rigual, R. Hypoxia and acidosis increase the secretion of catecholamines in the neonatal rat adrenal medulla: An in vitro study. *Am. J. Physiol. Cell Physiol.* **2005**, *289*, C1417–C1425. [CrossRef] [PubMed]
48. Steele, S.L.; Ekker, M.; Perry, S.F. Interactive effects of development and hypoxia on catecholamine synthesis and cardiac function in zebrafish (*Danio rerio*). *J. Comp. Physiol. B* **2011**, *181*, 527–538. [CrossRef] [PubMed]
49. Nakagawa, P.; Sigmund, C.D. Under Pressure: A Baroreceptor Mechanism in the Renal Renin Cell Controlling Renin. *Circ. Res.* **2021**, *129*, 277–279. [CrossRef]
50. Hickmann, L.; Steglich, A.; Gerlach, M.; Al-Mekhlafi, M.; Sradnick, J.; Lachmann, P.; Sequeira-Lopez, M.L.S.; Gomez, R.A.; Hohenstein, B.; Hugo, C.; et al. Persistent and inducible neogenesis repopulates progenitor renin lineage cells in the kidney. *Kidney Int.* **2017**, *92*, 1419–1432. [CrossRef]
51. Gomez, R.A.; Belyea, B.; Medrano, S.; Pentz, E.S.; Sequeira-Lopez, M.L. Fate and plasticity of renin precursors in development and disease. *Pediatr. Nephrol.* **2014**, *29*, 721–726. [CrossRef] [PubMed]
52. Martinez-Klimova, E.; Aparicio-Trejo, O.E.; Tapia, E.; Pedraza-Chaverri, J. Unilateral Ureteral Obstruction as a Model to Investigate Fibrosis-Attenuating Treatments. *Biomolecules* **2019**, *9*, 141. [CrossRef] [PubMed]
53. Stefanska, A.; Eng, D.; Kaverina, N.; Pippin, J.W.; Gross, K.W.; Duffield, J.S.; Shankland, S.J. Cells of renin lineage express hypoxia inducible factor 2alpha following experimental ureteral obstruction. *BMC Nephrol.* **2016**, *17*, 5. [CrossRef] [PubMed]
54. Broeker, K.A.E.; Fuchs, M.A.A.; Schrankl, J.; Lehrmann, C.; Schley, G.; Todorov, V.T.; Hugo, C.; Wagner, C.; Kurtz, A. Prolyl-4-hydroxylases 2 and 3 control erythropoietin production in renin-expressing cells of mouse kidneys. *J. Physiol.* **2022**, *600*, 671–694. [CrossRef] [PubMed]
55. Fitzpatrick, S.F. Immunometabolism and Sepsis: A Role for HIF? *Front. Mol. Biosci.* **2019**, *6*, 85. [CrossRef]
56. Suzuki, N.; Gradin, K.; Poellinger, L.; Yamamoto, M. Regulation of hypoxia-inducible gene expression after HIF activation. *Exp. Cell Res.* **2017**, *356*, 182–186. [CrossRef]
57. Choudhry, H.; Harris, A.L. Advances in Hypoxia-Inducible Factor Biology. *Cell Metab.* **2018**, *27*, 281–298. [CrossRef]
58. Fallah, J.; Rini, B.I. HIF Inhibitors: Status of Current Clinical Development. *Curr. Oncol. Rep.* **2019**, *21*, 6. [CrossRef]
59. Nicholson, H.E.; Tariq, Z.; Housden, B.E.; Jennings, R.B.; Stransky, L.A.; Perrimon, N.; Signoretti, S.; Kaelin, W.G., Jr. HIF-independent synthetic lethality between CDK4/6 inhibition and VHL loss across species. *Sci. Signal.* **2019**, *12*, eaay0482. [CrossRef]
60. Malkov, M.I.; Lee, C.T.; Taylor, C.T. Regulation of the Hypoxia-Inducible Factor (HIF) by Pro-Inflammatory Cytokines. *Cells* **2021**, *10*, 2304. [CrossRef]
61. Urrutia, A.A.; Guan, N.; Mesa-Ciller, C.; Afzal, A.; Davidoff, O.; Haase, V.H. Inactivation of HIF-prolyl 4-hydroxylases 1, 2 and 3 in NG2-expressing cells induces HIF2-mediated neurovascular expansion independent of erythropoietin. *Acta Physiol.* **2021**, *231*, e13547. [CrossRef] [PubMed]
62. Maxwell, P.H.; Eckardt, K.U. HIF prolyl hydroxylase inhibitors for the treatment of renal anaemia and beyond. *Nat. Rev. Nephrol.* **2016**, *12*, 157–168. [CrossRef] [PubMed]
63. Sakashita, M.; Tanaka, T.; Nangaku, M. Hypoxia-Inducible Factor-Prolyl Hydroxylase Domain Inhibitors to Treat Anemia in Chronic Kidney Disease. *Contrib. Nephrol.* **2019**, *198*, 112–123. [CrossRef] [PubMed]
64. Kurt, B.; Paliege, A.; Willam, C.; Schwarzensteiner, I.; Schucht, K.; Neymeyer, H.; Sequeira-Lopez, M.L.; Bachmann, S.; Gomez, R.A.; Eckardt, K.U.; et al. Deletion of von Hippel-Lindau protein converts renin-producing cells into erythropoietin-producing cells. *J. Am. Soc. Nephrol. JASN* **2013**, *24*, 433–444. [CrossRef] [PubMed]
65. Gerl, K.; Miquerol, L.; Todorov, V.T.; Hugo, C.P.; Adams, R.H.; Kurtz, A.; Kurt, B. Inducible glomerular erythropoietin production in the adult kidney. *Kidney Int.* **2015**, *88*, 1345–1355. [CrossRef] [PubMed]
66. Gerl, K.; Steppan, D.; Fuchs, M.; Wagner, C.; Willam, C.; Kurtz, A.; Kurt, B. Activation of Hypoxia Signaling in Stromal Progenitors Impairs Kidney Development. *Am. J. Pathol.* **2017**, *187*, 1496–1511. [CrossRef]
67. Monticone, G.; Miele, L. Notch Pathway: A Journey from Notching Phenotypes to Cancer Immunotherapy. *Adv. Exp. Med. Biol.* **2021**, *1287*, 201–222. [CrossRef]
68. Sprinzak, D.; Blacklow, S.C. Biophysics of Notch Signaling. *Annu. Rev. Biophys.* **2021**, *50*, 157–189. [CrossRef]
69. Zhang, Y.; He, K.; Wang, F.; Li, X.; Liu, D. Notch-1 signaling regulates astrocytic proliferation and activation after hypoxia exposure. *Neurosci. Lett.* **2015**, *603*, 12–18. [CrossRef]
70. Castellanos Rivera, R.M.; Monteagudo, M.C.; Pentz, E.S.; Glenn, S.T.; Gross, K.W.; Carretero, O.; Sequeira-Lopez, M.L.; Gomez, R.A. Transcriptional regulator RBPJ regulates the number and plasticity of renin cells. *Physiol. Genom.* **2011**, *43*, 1021–1028. [CrossRef]
71. Castellanos-Rivera, R.M.; Pentz, E.S.; Lin, E.; Gross, K.W.; Medrano, S.; Yu, J.; Sequeira-Lopez, M.L.; Gomez, R.A. Recombination signal binding protein for Ig-κJ region regulates juxtaglomerular cell phenotype by activating the myo-endocrine program and suppressing ectopic gene expression. *J. Am. Soc. Nephrol. JASN* **2015**, *26*, 67–80. [CrossRef] [PubMed]
72. Brunskill, E.W.; Sequeira-Lopez, M.L.; Pentz, E.S.; Lin, E.; Yu, J.; Aronow, B.J.; Potter, S.S.; Gomez, R.A. Genes that confer the identity of the renin cell. *J. Am. Soc. Nephrol. JASN* **2011**, *22*, 2213–2225. [CrossRef] [PubMed]

73. Grochowski, C.M.; Loomes, K.M.; Spinner, N.B. Jagged1 (JAG1): Structure, expression, and disease associations. *Gene* **2016**, *576*, 381–384. [CrossRef] [PubMed]
74. Belyea, B.C.; Xu, F.; Sequeira-Lopez, M.L.; Ariel Gomez, R. Loss of Jagged1 in renin progenitors leads to focal kidney fibrosis. *Physiol. Rep.* **2015**, *3*, e12544. [CrossRef]
75. Pappas, G.; Wilkinson, M.L.; Gow, A.J. Nitric oxide regulation of cellular metabolism: Adaptive tuning of cellular energy. *Nitric Oxide* **2023**, *131*, 8–17. [CrossRef]
76. Förstermann, U.; Sessa, W.C. Nitric oxide synthases: Regulation and function. *Eur. Heart J.* **2012**, *33*, 829–837. [CrossRef]
77. Gambaryan, S.; Mohagaonkar, S.; Nikolaev, V.O. Regulation of the renin-angiotensin-aldosterone system by cyclic nucleotides and phosphodiesterases. *Front. Endocrinol.* **2023**, *14*, 1239492. [CrossRef]
78. Neubauer, B.; Machura, K.; Kettl, R.; Lopez, M.L.; Friebe, A.; Kurtz, A. Endothelium-derived nitric oxide supports renin cell recruitment through the nitric oxide-sensitive guanylate cyclase pathway. *Hypertension* **2013**, *61*, 400–407. [CrossRef]
79. Jeffrey Man, H.S.; Tsui, A.K.; Marsden, P.A. Nitric oxide and hypoxia signaling. *Vitam. Horm.* **2014**, *96*, 161–192. [CrossRef]
80. Oza, P.P.; Kashfi, K. The Triple Crown: NO, CO, and H(2)S in cancer cell biology. *Pharmacol. Ther.* **2023**, *249*, 108502. [CrossRef]
81. Feng, J.; Lu, X.; Li, H.; Wang, S. The roles of hydrogen sulfide in renal physiology and disease states. *Ren. Fail.* **2022**, *44*, 1289–1308. [CrossRef] [PubMed]
82. Lu, M.; Liu, Y.H.; Goh, H.S.; Wang, J.J.; Yong, Q.C.; Wang, R.; Bian, J.S. Hydrogen sulfide inhibits plasma renin activity. *J. Am. Soc. Nephrol. JASN* **2010**, *21*, 993–1002. [CrossRef] [PubMed]
83. Liu, Y.H.; Lu, M.; Xie, Z.Z.; Hua, F.; Xie, L.; Gao, J.H.; Koh, Y.H.; Bian, J.S. Hydrogen sulfide prevents heart failure development via inhibition of renin release from mast cells in isoproterenol-treated rats. *Antioxid. Redox Signal.* **2014**, *20*, 759–769. [CrossRef] [PubMed]
84. Gallo, G.; Rubattu, S.; Autore, C.; Volpe, M. Natriuretic Peptides: It Is Time for Guided Therapeutic Strategies Based on Their Molecular Mechanisms. *Int. J. Mol. Sci.* **2023**, *24*, 5131. [CrossRef] [PubMed]
85. Chen, Y.F. Atrial natriuretic peptide in hypoxia. *Peptides* **2005**, *26*, 1068–1077. [CrossRef] [PubMed]
86. Kurtz, A. Transmembrane signalling of atrial natriuretic peptide in rat renal juxtaglomerular cells. *Klin. Wochenschr.* **1986**, *64* (Suppl. S6), 37–41.
87. MacFarland, R.T.; Zelus, B.D.; Beavo, J.A. High concentrations of a cGMP-stimulated phosphodiesterase mediate ANP-induced decreases in cAMP and steroidogenesis in adrenal glomerulosa cells. *J. Biol. Chem.* **1991**, *266*, 136–142. [CrossRef]
88. Nangaku, M. Chronic hypoxia and tubulointerstitial injury: A final common pathway to end-stage renal failure. *J. Am. Soc. Nephrol.* **2006**, *17*, 17–25. [CrossRef]
89. Mitani, S.; Yabuki, A.; Taniguchi, K.; Yamato, O. Association between the intrarenal renin–angiotensin system and renal injury in chronic kidney disease of dogs and cats. *J. Vet. Med. Sci.* **2013**, *75*, 127–133. [CrossRef]
90. Pimentel, J.L., Jr.; Montero, A.; Wang, S.; Yosipiv, I.; El-Dahr, S.; Martínez-Maldonado, M. Sequential changes in renal expression of renin–angiotensin system genes in acute unilateral ureteral obstruction. *Kidney Int.* **1995**, *48*, 1247–1253. [CrossRef]
91. Ishidoya, S.; Morrissey, J.; McCracken, R.; Reyes, A.; Klahr, S. Angiotensin II receptor antagonist ameliorates renal tubulointerstitial fibrosis caused by unilateral ureteral obstruction. *Kidney Int.* **1995**, *47*, 1285–1294. [CrossRef] [PubMed]
92. Curnow, A.C.; Gonsalez, S.R.; Gogulamudi, V.R.; Visniauskas, B.; Simon, E.E.; Gonzalez, A.A.; Majid, D.S.A.; Lara, L.S.; Prieto, M.C. Low Nitric Oxide Bioavailability Increases Renin Production in the Collecting Duct. *Front. Physiol.* **2020**, *11*, 559341. [CrossRef] [PubMed]

Disclaimer/Publisher's Note: The statements, opinions and data contained in all publications are solely those of the individual author(s) and contributor(s) and not of MDPI and/or the editor(s). MDPI and/or the editor(s) disclaim responsibility for any injury to people or property resulting from any ideas, methods, instructions or products referred to in the content.

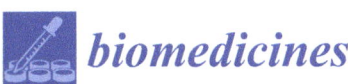

Review

The Multiple Faces of Nitric Oxide in Chronic Granulomatous Disease: A Comprehensive Update

Juan Agustín Garay [1,†], Juan Eduardo Silva [1,2,†], María Silvia Di Genaro [1,2] and Roberto Carlos Davicino [1,2,*]

1. División de Inmunología, Facultad de Química, Bioquímica y Farmacia, Universidad Nacional de San Luis, San Luis 5700, Argentina
2. Instituto Multidisciplinario de Investigaciones Biológicas (IMIBIO), Consejo Nacional de Investigaciones Científicas y Técnicas (CONICET), San Luis 5700, Argentina
* Correspondence: rcdavici@unsl.edu.ar
† These authors contributed equally to this work.

Abstract: Nitric oxide (NO), a signaling molecule, regulates multiple biological functions, including a variety of physiological and pathological processes. In this regard, NO participates in cutaneous inflammations, modulation of mitochondrial functions, vascular diseases, COVID-19, neurologic diseases, and obesity. It also mediates changes in the skeletal muscle function. Chronic granulomatous disease (CGD) is a primary immunodeficiency disorder characterized by the malfunction of phagocytes caused by mutations in some of the genes encoding subunits of the superoxide-generating phagocyte NADPH (NOX). The literature consulted shows that there is a relationship between the production of NO and the NADPH oxidase system, which regulates the persistence of NO in the medium. Nevertheless, the underlying mechanisms of the effects of NO on CGD remain unknown. In this paper, we briefly review the regulatory role of NO in CGD and its potential underlying mechanisms.

Keywords: nitric oxide; disease; chronic granulomatous disease

1. Introduction

Nitric oxide (NO) is an endogenous gaseous signaling molecule produced by Nitric Oxide Synthase (NOS) through the oxidation of L-arginine [1], which is highly active and mediates many physiological processes. Due to its chemical characteristic, NO diffuses freely across cell membranes, interacts with intracellular targets to activate signal transduction pathways, and plays different roles in biological systems [2], including vasodilation and signal transmission in neurons [3]. NO can also activate cellular and humoral immunity and has antibacterial properties. Additionally, it activates the proliferation of keratinocytes, the antioxidant system, and the proliferation and synthetic activity of fibroblasts [3].

Three isozymes of nitric oxide synthase (NOS) have been widely studied: endothelial nitric oxide synthase (eNOS), neuronal nitric oxide synthase (nNOS), and inducible nitric oxide synthase (iNOS) [4]. eNOS is mostly found in endothelial cells and is in charge of keeping the tone of the blood vessels. Numerous cell types, including neurons, heart muscle, and endothelial cells, contain its three primary isoforms. iNOS is typically located in macrophages [5] and can produce toxic amounts of NO, representing an important component in the antimicrobial, antiparasitic, and antineoplasic activity of these cells [4].

NO is a promiscuous signaling molecule with active participation in health and disease. In this regard, its critical role in the modulation of inflammatory circuits in cutaneous tissue [6], the regulation of mitochondrial O_2 consumption [7], the mediation of vascular relaxation through the second messenger cyclic guanosine monophosphate [1], and the adjustment of skeletal muscle contractile function have been demonstrated [8]. During SARS-CoV-2 infection, NO has played a protective role through four mechanisms: regulating blood flow, initiating anti-inflammatory responses, promoting anti-coagulation effects, and exerting antiviral properties [9]. Further, iNOS-derived NO can induce insulin

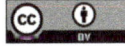

resistance and glucose intolerance [10]. It is a well-known neuromodulator agent that participates in fear-like behavior [2], major depression pathogenesis [11], and memory consolidation processes exerting a context-dependent dual role [12,13]. On the other hand, NO is generated by almost all myocardial cell types and controls cardiac function through both vascular-dependent and -independent mechanisms [14]. It has been seen that the amount of NO in coronary heart disease is decreased [15] and that this could be due to a lower bioavailability of L-arginine [16]. In fact, there are therapies that restore optimal levels of NO to prevent heart failure [17].

Chronic granulomatous disease (CGD) is a hereditary illness in which phagocytic leukocytes fail to produce reactive oxygen species (ROS), such as superoxide anion (O_2^-) and antimicrobial oxidants. Catalase positive bacteria cause recurring infections in CGD patients [18]. It has been suggested that the CGD and NO are linked. In this regard, Tsuji et al. (2012) showed that polymorphonuclear neutrophils (PMNs) from CGD patients increase nitric oxide after phagocytes stimulation [18]. In this review, we focus on the current evidence that shows the intervention of NO in the physiopathology of CGD.

2. Chronic Granulomatous Disease (CGD) and NADPH Oxidase (NOX)

Chronic granulomatous disease is a primary immunodeficiency (PID) which affects 1 in 120,000–250,000 live births [19]. Patients with CGD present recurrent clinical manifestations [20] (Table 1). CGD is characterized by a defect in the bactericidal and fungicidal activity of phagocytes due to mutations in the enzyme complex nicotinamide adenine dinucleotide phosphate (NADPH) oxidase (NOX). This is an oxidase machinery that takes electrons from NADPH in the cytoplasm, generated by the hexose monophosphates hunt, and transfers them onto oxygen in the vacuole to produce O_2^- [21] (Figure 1). The catalytic component of the phagocyte NADPH oxidase has six human homologs: NOX1, NOX3, NOX4, NOX5, DUOX1, and DUOX2. The homologs are collectively referred to as the NOX family of NADPH oxidases, together with the NOX2/gp91phox component found in the phagocyte NADPH oxidase assembly. NOX is a multidomain complex that requires different protein combinations for assembly in order to function [22].

Table 1. Clinical manifestations of CGD.

Cutaneous Manifestations	Gastrointestinal Manifestations	Autoimmune Manifestations	Infections	Ophthalmic Manifestations
Photosensitive malar rash Discoid lupus erythematosus Recurrent aphthous Seborrheic dermatitis Infections Abscesses recurring on skin	Colitis/Diarrhea Inflammatory bowel disease Stomatitis Autoimmune hepatitis Granulomatous enteritis Recurrent liver infections Liver abscess	Lupus, Lupus-like síndrome Arthritis Oral ulcers Raynaud's phenomenon IgA nephropathy	Staphylococcus aureus Aspergillus fumigatus, Nocardia Burkholderia cepacia Serratia marcescens	Chorioretinitis

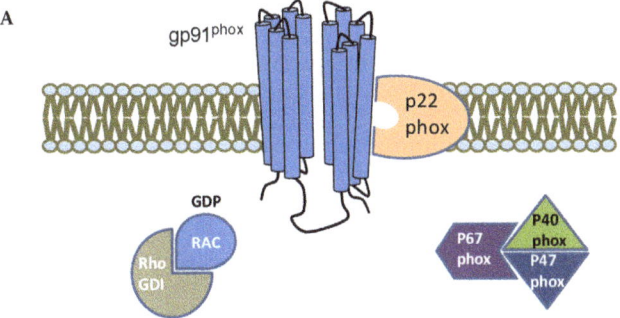

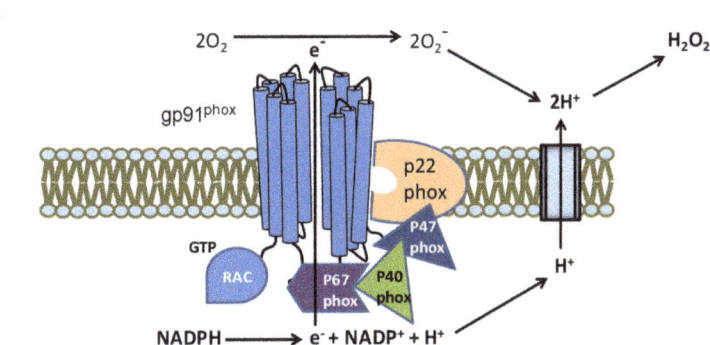

Figure 1. The NADPH oxidase (NOX) activation complex in the cytoplasmic membrane of a phagocyte is depicted in a schematic form. (**A**) The oxidase complex is inactive in the absence of stimuli, with gp91phox and p22phox attached to cell membranes and p67phox, p47phox, and p40phox in the cytosol. (**B**) The cytosolic p47phox subunit is phosphorylated in response to inflammatory stimuli, which activates NADPH oxidase and causes the assembly of all cytosolic components (p67phox, p40phox) to p22phox/gp91phox. Rac is also bound in conjunction with this. The active enzymatic complex moves electrons from the cytosol to phagosome lumen, where oxygen (O_2) is changed into superoxide anion and then hydrogen peroxide (H_2O_2).

3. Innate Immunity

The immune system has been traditionally classified into two categories: the adaptive immune system and the innate immune system [23]. Innate immunity consists of a series of physical, chemical, and anatomical barriers [24] that act as the first line of defense against all types of infectious agents, including extra [25] and intracellular [26] bacteria, viruses [27], fungi [28], protozoa [29], and helminths [30].

While adaptive immunity consists of two basic cell types, B lymphocytes and T lymphocytes, innate immunity has a more diverse cellular composition. In this regard, the innate immune system presents both hematopoietic and non-hematopoietic cells within the tissue barriers [31,32]. Innate hematopoietic cells are becoming important in health and disease [33]. There are several studies on innate immune cells of the myeloid lineage, being the most representative cells the neutrophils, eosinophils, basophils, mast, monocytes, macrophages, and dendritic cells [34].

The cellular components of innate immunity have a series of extra and intracellular molecules that allow an initial recognition of the pathogen [35]. In addition, they have a series of microstatic and microbicidal effector mechanisms to contain the infection during the first hours and days, thus triggering specific immune responses [33]. Therefore, innate immunity presents a series of humoral and cellular effector mechanisms. Humoral mechanisms include activation of the complement, coagulation cascade, lactoferrin secretion, and defensins [36]. Regarding cell-based effector mechanisms, phagocytosis together with cell-mediated cytotoxicity are predominant. Phagocytes are cells capable of perform phagocytosis, which sense a series of events triggered by the presence of molecular patterns associated with pathogens and/or molecular patterns associated with damage. The sequence of events includes migration, adhesion, diapedesis, and phagocytosis [36]. It is now acknowledged that phagocytosis is a cellular process that is not only involved in the immune response against pathogens but also in the preservation of homeostasis since it participates in the clearance of cell debris [37]. It is a highly regulated process favored by ligand-receptor recognition processes with subsequent engulfment of particles within the so-called phagosome [38]. The phagosome undergoes a series of maturation processes and drastic biochemical changes known as respiratory burst.

It is now recognized that innate immunity is not only a mere effector of adaptive immunity but also contributes to the optimization and course of the immune response by providing the appropriate cytokine microenvironment for the differentiation of T lymphocytes into a specific phenotype [39]. Cytokine networks established by innate immunity play a central role in the pathogenesis of various diseases with immunopathological bases [40]. The effectors and regulatory functions of innate immunity in immunodeficiency have also been studied. The condition known as CGD serves as a typical example (Primary Immunodeficiency) [41] which presents susceptibility to recurrent infections and the development of autoimmunity [42].

4. Immunomodulatory Properties of NO

NO has a variety of functions in immunity, including its role as immunoregulator, apoptosis modulator, and as toxic agent against infectious organisms. [43]. In this context, iNOS is the most relevant source of immunomodulatory NO, and its expression is upregulated through multiple proinflammatory signals [44,45] via NF-kB as a master inflammation regulator [46,47]. Despite their minor role, eNOS and nNOS may be important sources of NO at inflammation sites [48], and their expression is mediated by Ca^{2+} in response to multiple ligands [49].

Today, the microbicidal capacity of NO is well known [50,51] and many pathogens have developed immune response evasion mechanisms based on the inhibition of NO generation [52]. Thus, therapies based on NO-releasing agents are currently being developed to treat aggressive infections in humans [53].

In addition to its classic cytotoxic effects, NO plays a crucial role in the immune response regulation, establishing a link between innate immunity and adaptive immunity [54]. Experiments using iNOS-deficient mice showed that NO regulates adaptive immunity by restricting T cell proliferation, attenuating IFN-γ production, and differentiation to a Th1 phenotype [55], thus postulating NO as a self-regulation mediator [56]. Furthermore, NO is a potent immunoregulator in other T cell lineages, such as Th17 cells [57] and CD8(+) T cells [58]. Recently, the ability of NO to shape innate immune cell metabolic programs has been documented [59,60].

5. Relationship between NO and NADPH Oxidase

Both NOS and ROS species, generated by the concerted action of iNOS and NADPH oxidase, are known to play complementary roles in disease, such as progression of tumor growth [61,62], maintenance of intestinal bacterial homeostasis [63], microglial toxicity [64], or control of infections by opportunistic pathogens [65]. Furthermore, it has been shown that not only NO acts as a signaling molecule but that ROS- derived from NADPH oxidase-also has a regulatory function with associated signaling pathways [66,67]. It has been suggested that NADPH oxidase presents a higher hierarchy in the signaling of inflammatory circuits and that it controls the production of NO by modulating the expression of iNOS [67–70]. However, it has also been reported that iNOS activity is capable of regulating the function of the NADPH oxidase complex [71,72]. It seems that both enzymes influence each other, becoming more relevant depending on the context.

Given the demonstrated protective and regulatory role of NADPH oxidase [73–75], it is expected that patients with CGD present a complex series of immunopathological mechanisms besides immune deficiency. Patients with CGD showed an imbalance in their redox state with an increase in antioxidant activity, depletion of antioxidant metabolite levels, and higher lipoperoxidation scores together with a higher proportion of protein and nucleic acid oxidation products [76].

It has been largely reported that CGD patients can produce NO, so the activity of NOS isoforms is not completely dependent on the presence and activity of NADPH oxidase [77]. Thus, it has been shown that the NADPH oxidase system regulates the persistence of NO in the medium upon consumption, being the main enzymatic complex of phagocytes capable of regulating NO levels [78]. These findings suggest that CGD patients could present higher basal levels of NO or at least present problems in the regulation of its activity. Consistent with this, a spontaneous increase in NO production has been reported in in vitro cell models of CGD patients used as a negative control [79].

6. Impact of NO in the Pathophysiology of CGD

6.1. Susceptibility to Bacterial and Fungal Infections

CGD manifests with recurrent bacterial and fungal infections that can appear from infancy to adulthood. Males have been reported to be the most affected. The typical organs suffering from infections are the lungs, lymph nodes, skin, bones, and liver. In countries where the bacillus Calmette–Guerin (BCG) vaccine is routinely applied, the initial manifestation of CGD may be local or regional becegeitis [20]. Patients with CGD present a greater susceptibility to pyogenic and granulomatous infections, with a myriad of pathogens as possible causal agents [80]. In addition, the greater susceptibility to infections can not only be explained by the deficiency in the formation of ROS but particularly the neutrophils of patients with CGD present defects in the generation of NETs [21].

6.2. Granuloma Formation

CGD is a disease with the frequent formation of microscopic structures called granulomas. They are characterized by a predominance of macrophages transformed into epithelioid cells. Immune granulomas occur as a consequence of the development of an adaptive immune response, in which cellular immunity participates with the activation of TCD4$^+$ Th1 lymphocytes (delayed hypersensitivity or type IV), which is induced in response to the presence of life-threatening intracellular pathogens [81]. Previous studies have found that granulomas derived from glycoantigens (e.g., *Staphylococcus aureus* capsule antigens) present in murine models of CGD are generated in a NO-dependent manner from dendritic cells. Interestingly, mice with CGD respond excessively to the presence of glycoantigens, generating granulomas via activation and proliferation of CD4+ T lymphocytes. This is because the overactivity of NO in dendritic cells facilitates the processing of glycoantigens by inducing deamination-depolymerization processes and their subsequent presentation under an MHC-II context (HLA-DM) [82]. On the other hand, it has been determined that dendritic cells from CGD patients fail to alkalinize their phagosomes and present problems in the cross-presentation of antigens due to excessive protein degradation [83]. Treatment of murine CGD models with 1400W, an iNOS inhibitor, not only attenuates NO production but also reduces the size and number of glycoantigen-induced granulomas in such models [82].

6.3. Chronic Inflammation

Several studies using three different murine models of CGD have elucidated that NOX-2 deficient mononuclear phagocytes are responsible for the hyperinflammation present in the disease. In addition, IL-1β has been shown to be the main pro-inflammatory cytokine released by these cells, and thus IL-1β antagonists could be used as anti-inflammatories in CGD patients [84]. The presence of high levels of IL-1β in patients with CGD implies the existence of factors that trigger the formation of the inflammasome required for the maturation and secretion of numerous proinflammatory cytokines, including IL-1β. ROS generation during the respiratory burst is one of the conventional signals required for inflammasome assembly, such as the NALP-3-like inflammasome. However, patients and murine models deficient in NADPH oxidase show activation of caspase-1 and secretion of IL-1β against inflammatory stimuli, indicating that a functional phagocyte oxidase is not essential in the inflammatory response of monocytes derived from CGD patients [85]. This implies that there could be other species generated during the respiratory burst that compensate or replace ROS in the assembly of the inflammasome. However, NO does not seem to be it, since previous studies have shown its inhibitory nature on the formation and function of the NALP-3 type inflammasome [86]. It is known that the activation of the autophagosomal pathway limits the activity of the inflammasome by ubiquitination and subsequent degradation [87]. Failure of the autophagy pathway to stop inflammasome activity has been suggested to be an essential component of diseases with chronic inflammation [88]. CGD is a disease with a significant prevalence of chronic inflammation with aberrant activity of the inflammasome and, paradoxically, with unbalanced NO production. As part of its numerous regulatory functions, NO can inhibit autophagosome formation and activity [89]. In this regard, the inhibitory effect of autophagy mediated by NO could predominate over its inhibitory effect on inflammasome activity, resulting in the generation of IL-1β, but studies are required.

6.4. Neurological Symptoms

Although neurological symptoms are not very frequent in CGD patients [90], neurological lesions such as demyelinating lesions, infiltrations of pigmented macrophages [91], vasculitis, hemorrhages, and infarcts in different neuronal structures [92] have been reported. Although it is recognized that inhibition of NADPH oxidase activity is involved in neuroprotective effects [72], it has also been acknowledged that it has a physiological role as a source of neuronal superoxide anion in response to the activation of the NMDA receptor (NMDAR), a glutamate receptor involved in processes of synaptic plasticity, learning, developmental plasticity, and neuronal death [93]. In a retrospective study of 26 CGD patients, 23% were found to have an IQ of 70 or less, indicating cognitive deficits [94]. In line with this, it has been shown that a NADPH oxidase deficiency is related to mild impairments in hippocampus-dependent memory, spatial memory deficit, and impaired context-dependent fear memory in murine CGD models [95].

It is well known that the activation of NMDARs induces the production of NO in the brain [96]. Thus, NO acts as a mediator of glutamate activator of the NMDARs in several nervous circuits, regulating processes such as hearing [97] and angiogenesis [98]. Interestingly, an absence of NADPH oxidase expression in different nerve centers as well as different degrees of impaired cognitive performance has been observed in nNOS-deficient mice [99], showing a relationship between both enzymes in cognitive processes. As has been proved, NO presents a well-established role as a vital mediator in the consolidation of memory and learning [100]. However, it has been reported that the inhibition of NO production has protective effects against memory and learning loss in specific pathological processes [13,101]. Even so, the benefits of the inhibition of NO production in memory processes and synaptic plasticity are due to the specific labeling of microglial or astrocyticic NOS [102]. Instead, the documented benefits of NO in cognition, learning, memory, and neurodevelopment appear to be mediated by neuronal nNOS in response to glutamate in long-term potentiation processes [103]. In addition, the correlation between nNOS activity and NMDAR activation is maintained in pathological processes such as Calcium-mediated excitotoxicity [72,104]. In the same process, it has been observed that NADPH oxidase inhibition prevents neuronal death and attenuates excitotoxic effects, suggesting a synergy in the activity of nNOS and NADPH oxidase [105,106]. However, more studies are required to explore the hierarchical relationship between both enzymes on the signaling pathways derived from the activation of NMDARs and its consequence in the synaptic plasticity of CGD patients.

6.5. Mechanisms of Hypersensitivity in Respiratory and Gastrointestinal Symptoms

Together with the susceptibility to the formation of granulomas present in CGD patients, through type IV hypersensitivity mechanisms, other clinical outcomes have been reported in these patients as a consequence of abnormalities in their immune system functions. A relationship has been found between hypersensitivity pneumonitis (HP) as an initial manifestation of CGD, especially in children [107–109]. The classification of HP as an interstitial lung disease describes it as an intricate immunological response of the lung parenchyma to repeated inhalation of a sensitized allergen. HP causes a combination of type-III and type-IV hypersensitivity reactions in the lung parenchyma. After initial sensitization, the offending antigen or chemical first induces a type III (immune complex-mediated) hypersensitive reaction. As long as the antigen is present, the reaction becomes a delayed (type IV) hypersensitivity reaction [110]. Interestingly, Shirai et al. (2010) described a 57-year-old male patient with HP, who presented alveolar NO concentration increased [111]. In addition, excessive NO production by alveolar macrophages plays a predominant role in lung damage due to oxidative stress in this disease [112]. Similarly, iNOS-derived NO plays an active role in the inflammatory processes of Crohn's disease [113] and inflammatory bowel disease [114] both clinical presentations found in CGD [115,116].

6.6. Autoimmune Diseases

It is known that immunodeficiencies are related to autoimmune diseases in situations where deregulated immune responses against certain pathogens [117] occur. It has been reported that both autoimmune diseases and complications derived from an intense inflammatory state are more frequent in patients with CGD than in the rest of the population. In this regard, some findings suggest that the NADPH oxidase enzyme could be playing a critical role in the regulation of the adaptive immune response [117,118]. Thus, autoimmune diseases associated with CGD include discoid lupus, systemic lupus erythematosus, rheumatoid arthritis, idiopathic thrombocytopenic purpura [117], dermatomyositis, sacroiliitis, and autoimmune hepatitis [119], and the relationship between ROS and regulatory T responses is well known. Likewise, there is evidence suggesting a link between the ROS production and the induction of regulatory T (Treg) cells [120]. In this regard, Kraaij et al. (2010) showed that Treg cells can be induced by macrophages through a ROS-dependent mechanism [121]. Considering that Treg cells play a crucial role in the regulation of autoimmune responses [122] and that deficiency in ROS production is the hallmark of CGD, it is suggested that autoimmune diseases linked to CGD could be related, at least in part, to a decreased regulatory immune response associated with Treg cells. On the other hand, it is known that for the induction of Treg cells, interaction with an Antigen Presenting Cell (APC) is required [122]. Therefore, an impaired response of APC (macrophages and DCs) could be involved not only in the abnormal development of regulatory responses but also in the hyperinflammation state observed in both, CGD patients and animal models. However, the mechanisms by which the absence of ROS induces this failure in APC functions are still unclear. Additionally, results highlight the important role DCs play in inducing the CGD hyperinflammatory state, which could contribute to the development of autoimmunity. In this regard, Defert et al. (2012) demonstrated in CGD animal models that NOX2-deficient mice respond to intradermal injection with β-glucans showing high levels of proinflammatory cytokines (TNFα, IL-6, and IL1β) in the skin lesions. These cytokines were mainly secreted by macrophages and DCs [84]. It is known that DCs are critical actors in immune response, both, regulating the delicate balance between inflammation and tolerance and acting as linkers between innate and adaptive immunity [123–125]. Thus, there is a particular subset of NO and TNFα producing DCs (CD11b$^+$ CD11c^{int}-TIP DCs) which are derived from Ly6C^{Hi} monocytes and migrate to inflamed tissues [126,127]. On the other hand, Si et al. (2016) showed that DCs-derived NO controls the balance between the differentiation of effectors DCs and regulatory DCs. Thus, these authors reported that mice deficient in the NO-producing enzyme (iNOS) have an increased number of effectors DCs (IL-12, TNFα, and IL-6 producing), but a normal number of regulatory DCs (IL-10 producing) [123]. Therefore, NO would be acting as an inhibitor agent in the differentiation of effectors DCs. In this regard, the suppressive activity on NFκB pathways and inflammasome activation demonstrated that this molecule may contribute, at least in part, to the observed effects on DC differentiation [123]. These results demonstrate that DCs through NO plays a central role in the regulation of the immune response and in the avoidance of hyperinflammation states observed in CGD.

It is known that when apoptotic neutrophils cannot be phagocytosed by macrophages in an infectious focus, they can suffer necrosis and release their content into the environment, causing more inflammation and favoring autoimmunity [128]. Macrophages can recognize apoptotic neutrophils through the lipid phosphatidylserine (PS) and regulate the immune response by secreting TGFβ to control inflammation. There is evidence suggesting that ROS can induce apoptosis in neutrophils [129] and that both patients and mice with CGD have decreased/delayed exposure to PS. Therefore, it is hypothesized that the failed intake of apoptotic bodies present in granulomas could contribute to immunization with self-antigens and the development of autoimmunity [128,129].

Cahact et al. (2018) showed that both patients and mice with CGD present an alteration in the proportion of IgG isotypes, which was associated with an increased production of IFNγ and interpreted as a possible cause of the higher IgG2c production observed in B cells [130]. On the other hand, there are results showing that the defect in the NADPH oxidase enzyme could alter the repertoire of peptides presented by the MHCII molecule in B cells. These findings suggest that NADPH oxidase plays a critical role in the development of autoimmunity in CGD patients [117]. Therefore, the increased cytokines by DC and the participation of B cells could be the master key in the integration between increased T cell activation, antibody production, and development of autoimmunity related to CGD.

7. Therapeutic Considerations

Identification of the pathogenic variant(s) in one of the six genes that encode or permit assembly of the phagocyte NADPH oxidase subunits establishes the diagnosis of CGD. Pathogenic variants in CYBA, CYBC1, NCF1, NCF2, and NCF4 cause autosomal recessive CGD; pathogenic variants in CYBB cause X-linked CGD [131]. The phenotypic diagnosis of CGD is made by using the 1,2,3-dihydrorhodamine (DHR) test which evaluates the functionality of neutrophils by flow cytometry. The optimal therapeutic management of CGD is based on the antimicrobial prophylaxis, aggressive treatment of infectious and inflammatory complications, and in some cases, stem hematopoietic cell transplant [20] (Table 2). Currently, combination strategies that typically involve prophylactic antibacterial agents, antifungal agents, and immunomodulation via interferon-gamma (IFN-γ) are used [132]. In this regard, IFN-γ mediated therapy has been proposed to offer prophylactic benefits [133] promoting NO production. This, in turn may prevent bacterial-induced inflammation by depleting inflammasome activity [134]. Although there are discrepancies about whether or not IFN-γ therapy increases serum NO levels in CGD patients [77], many authors have found that prolonged IFN-γ treatment enhances the generation of NO through the activity of TNF-α [135]. It has been proposed that the increase in NO generation during the phagocytosis process generated by treatment with IFN-γ or Trimetropin-Sulfomethoxazole (used to treat bacterial infections) collaborates to achieve a more efficient respiratory burst [79,135] highlighting the aspect of NO as a molecular aggressor [136]. This role of NO is of particular importance in the immune response against *Mycobacterium tuberculosis* [137], one of the most frequent infectious agents in CGD patients [138]. In addition, IFN-γ treatment has been shown to enhance clearance of apoptotic bodies through a NO-dependent process in a CGD model of murine macrophages [128]. However, IFN-γ therapy has certain side effects such as fever, fatigue, myalgia, rash, erythema, and pain. The cost-benefit balance for the therapeutic use of IFN-γ is favorable, especially for patients with the X-linked variant and with a history of invasive aspergillosis. Despite the benefits, IFN-γ drug therapy does not prevent granuloma formation and does not appear to improve symptoms of chronic inflammation [139]. On the other hand, working with cells from CGD patients and murine models, it has been shown that the blockade of the IL-1β receptor restores autophagy and inhibits the activity of the inflammasome, generating beneficial effects such as the attenuation of inflammation, resistance to invasive aspergillosis, and improvement of symptoms typical of colitis [140]. Treatment with Anakinra, an IL-1β antagonist, showed pharmacological efficacy in the treatment of colitis in CGD patients. Rapamycin, an mTOR inhibitor and autophagy restorer, is capable of reducing the release of pro-inflammatory cytokines. Thus, it has been suggested that combination therapy with Anakinra and Rapamycin can be used to treat the inflammatory complications present in CGD patients [139].

Table 2. Clinical management of CGD.

Manifestations Treatment	Prevention of Primary Manifestations	Cure	Pregnancy Management
New azole drugs for fungal infections. Long courses of antibacterials. Abscesses may require percutaneous drainage or excisional surgery. Combination of antimicrobials and corticosteroids for inflammatory response	Antibacterials and antifungals combined with immunomodulatory therapy (IFN-γ).	Allogeneic hematopoietic stem cell transplantation (HSCT)	Trimethoprim, a folic acid antagonist, is discontinued during pregnancy. Sulfamethoxazole is typically administered. Data regarding the teratogenicity of itraconazole are limited.

8. Conclusions

Nitric oxide (NO) is a widespread gaseous mediator that acts through the activation of soluble guanylate cyclase or by inducing nitrosylation on different protein targets. Three isoforms of Nitric Oxide Synthase are the source of this signaling molecule, which acts as a neuromodulator, immunomodulatory, and regulator of cardiovascular tone in health and disease. In an immune context, NO originated by iNOS together with ROS generated by NADPH oxidase act as molecular aggressors. iNOS and NADPH oxidase have certain similarities. They are part of the effector mechanisms of phagocytes and both derived species have regulatory properties that shape the immune response with the transcription factor NF-kB. Different studies have evaluated whether the NO or the ROS of NADPH oxidase have a predominant role over the action of the other; however, to date, the results are inconclusive. Even though the expression of one of the enzymes is not dependent on the presence of the other, they are subjected to mutual influence. In this regard, in Chronic Granulomatous Disease (deficient NADPH oxidase), there is an unbalanced production of NO in response to inducing stimuli, such as IFN-γ. There are few but convincing works that demonstrate the participation of NO in the pathogenesis of CGD. Thus, the production of NO in phagocytes compensates for the ROS deficit in CGD patients treated with IFN-γ, increasing the quality of their respiratory burst and even improving other aspects of phagocytic function such as the clearance of apoptotic bodies. On the other hand, NO plays a pathological role in mediating the generation of granulomas in the presence of ubiquitous microbial components of a polysaccharide nature, one of the hallmark signs of CGD. In this regard, these patients present a series of less recognized features such as chronic inflammation, mucosal hypersensitivity reactions, autoimmune manifestations, and neurological symptoms. Given the pleiotropic effects of NO and its multiple functions, together with the critical regulatory functions of NADPH oxidase, it is likely that an unbalanced activity between both enzymes and their products plays a predominant role in the pathophysiology of these less conventional symptoms. Finally, it is known that one of the main pharmacological effects of IFN-γ is the increase in NO production, which acts as an executing arm of IFN-γ, mediating its beneficial and adverse effects in CGD patients.

Thus, though the IFN-γ-induced NO production does not improve the number and size of granulomas, it seems that it promotes their formation. All in all, this review has addressed the pathophysiological aspects of NO and signaling ROS in CGD and highlighted the importance of a comprehensive knowledge of these mediators for the development of more rational therapies and the improvement of those already available.

Author Contributions: Conceptualization, R.C.D., J.A.G., J.E.S. and M.S.D.G.; investigation, R.C.D., J.A.G. and J.E.S.; resources, R.C.D. and M.S.D.G.; writing—original draft preparation, R.C.D., J.A.G., and J.E.S.; writing—review and editing, R.C.D., J.A.G., J.E.S. and M.S.D.G.; supervision, R.C.D. and M.S.D.G. All authors have read and agreed to the published version of the manuscript.

Funding: This work was supported by grants from the National Agency for Promotion of Science and Technology, [PICT-2020-1868] and from the National Research Council Scientific and Technical (CONICET), [P-UE 013, IMIBIO-SL, CONICET].

Institutional Review Board Statement: Not applicable.

Informed Consent Statement: Not applicable.

Data Availability Statement: Not applicable.

Acknowledgments: We are grateful to Gabinete de Asesoramiento en Escritura Científica en Inglés (GAECI) staff for writing assistance.

Conflicts of Interest: The authors declare no conflict of interest.

References

1. Stuehr, D.J.; Santolini, J.; Wang, Z.-Q.; Wei, C.-C.; Adak, S. Update on Mechanism and Catalytic Regulation in the NO Synthases. *J. Biol. Chem.* **2004**, *279*, 36167–36170. [CrossRef] [PubMed]
2. Medeiros, K.A.A.L.; Almeida-Souza, T.H.; Silva, R.S.; Santos, H.F.; Santos, E.V.; Gois, A.M.; Leal, P.C.; Santos, J.R. Involvement of Nitric Oxide in the Neurobiology of Fear-like Behavior. *Nitric Oxide* **2022**, *124*, 24–31. [CrossRef] [PubMed]
3. Igrunkova, A.; Fayzullin, A.; Churbanov, S.; Shevchenko, P.; Serejnikova, N.; Chepelova, N.; Pahomov, D.; Blinova, E.; Mikaelyan, K.; Zaborova, V.; et al. Spray with Nitric Oxide Donor Accelerates Wound Healing: Potential Off-The-Shelf Solution for Therapy? *Drug Des. Dev. Ther.* **2022**, *16*, 349–362. [CrossRef] [PubMed]
4. Forstermann, U.; Kleinert, H. Nitric Oxide Synthase: Expression and Expressional Control of the Three Isoforms. *Naunyn-Schmiedebergs Arch. Pharmacol.* **1995**, *352*, 351–364. [CrossRef]
5. Lacza, Z.; Pankotai, E.; Csordás, A.; Gero, D.; Kiss, L.; Horváth, E.M.; Kollai, M.; Busija, D.W.; Szabó, C. Mitochondrial NO and Reactive Nitrogen Species Production: Does MtNOS Exist? *Nitric Oxide* **2006**, *14*, 162–168. [CrossRef]
6. Man, M.-Q.; Wakefield, J.S.; Mauro, T.M.; Elias, P.M. Regulatory Role of Nitric Oxide in Cutaneous Inflammation. *Inflammation* **2022**, *45*, 949–964. [CrossRef]
7. Jung, P.; Ha, E.; Zhang, M.; Fall, C.; Hwang, M.; Taylor, E.; Stetkevich, S.; Bhanot, A.; Wilson, C.G.; Figueroa, J.D.; et al. Neuroprotective Role of Nitric Oxide Inhalation and Nitrite in a Neonatal Rat Model of Hypoxic-Ischemic Injury. *PLoS ONE* **2022**, *17*, e0268282. [CrossRef]
8. Kumar, R.; Coggan, A.R.; Ferreira, L.F. Nitric Oxide and Skeletal Muscle Contractile Function. *Nitric Oxide* **2022**, *122–123*, 54–61. [CrossRef]
9. Rajendran, R.; Chathambath, A.; Al-Sehemi, A.G.; Pannipara, M.; Unnikrishnan, M.K.; Aleya, L.; Raghavan, R.P.; Mathew, B. Critical Role of Nitric Oxide in Impeding COVID-19 Transmission and Prevention: A Promising Possibility. *Environ. Sci. Pollut. Res.* **2022**, *29*, 38657–38672. [CrossRef]
10. Lee, C.H.; Kim, H.J.; Lee, Y.-S.; Kang, G.M.; Lim, H.S.; Lee, S.; Song, D.K.; Kwon, O.; Hwang, I.; Son, M.; et al. Hypothalamic Macrophage Inducible Nitric Oxide Synthase Mediates Obesity-Associated Hypothalamic Inflammation. *Cell Rep.* **2018**, *25*, 934–946.e5. [CrossRef]
11. Amini-Khoei, H.; Nasiri Boroujeni, S.; Maghsoudi, F.; Rahimi-Madiseh, M.; Bijad, E.; Moradi, M.; Lorigooini, Z. Possible Involvement of L-Arginine-Nitric Oxide Pathway in the Antidepressant Activity of Auraptene in Mice. *Behav. Brain Funct.* **2022**, *18*, 4. [CrossRef] [PubMed]
12. Noroozi, N.; Shayan, M.; Maleki, A.; Eslami, F.; Rahimi, N.; Zakeri, R.; Abdolmaleki, Z.; Dehpour, A.R. Protective Effects of Dapsone on Scopolamine-Induced Memory Impairment in Mice: Involvement of Nitric Oxide Pathway. *Dement. Geriatr. Cogn. Disord. Extra* **2022**, *12*, 43–50. [CrossRef] [PubMed]
13. Ren, P.; Xiao, B.; Wang, L.-P.; Li, Y.-S.; Jin, H.; Jin, Q.-H. Nitric Oxide Impairs Spatial Learning and Memory in a Rat Model of Alzheimer's Disease via Disturbance of Glutamate Response in the Hippocampal Dentate Gyrus during Spatial Learning. *Behav. Brain Res.* **2022**, *422*, 113750. [CrossRef]
14. Massion, P.B.; Feron, O.; Dessy, C.; Balligand, J.-L. Nitric Oxide and Cardiac Function. *Circ. Res.* **2003**, *93*, 388–398. [CrossRef] [PubMed]

15. Chen, X.; Niroomand, F.; Liu, Z.; Zankl, A.; Katus, H.A.; Jahn, L.; Tiefenbacher, C.P. Expression of nitric oxide related enzymes in coronary heart disease. *Basic Res. Cardiol.* **2006**, *101*, 346–353. [CrossRef] [PubMed]
16. Büttner, P.; Werner, S.; Baskal, S.; Tsikas, D.; Adams, V.; Lurz, P.; Besler, C.; Knauth, S.; Bahls, M.; Schwedhelm, E.; et al. Arginine metabolism and nitric oxide turnover in the ZSF1 animal model for heart failure with preserved ejection fraction. *Sci. Rep.* **2021**, *11*, 20684. [CrossRef]
17. Zhu, D.; Hou, J.; Qian, M.; Jin, D.; Hao, T.; Pan, Y.; Wang, H.; Wu, S.; Liu, S.; Wang, F.; et al. Nitrate-Functionalized Patch Confers Cardioprotection and Improves Heart Repair after Myocardial Infarction via Local Nitric Oxide Delivery. *Nat. Commun.* **2021**, *12*, 4501. [CrossRef]
18. Tsuji, S.; Iharada, A.; Taniuchi, S.; Hasui, M.; Kaneko, K. Increased Production of Nitric Oxide by Phagocytic Stimulated Neutrophils in Patients with Chronic Granulomatous Disease. *J. Pediatr. Hematol. Oncol.* **2012**, *34*, 500–502. [CrossRef]
19. Maydanaa, M.; Cabanillasb, D.; Regairazb, L.; Bastonsa, S.; Uriartea, V.; García, M.; Sosa, M.F.; Vinuesaa, M.; del Palacioc, P.; Morales, J. Enfermedad granulomatosa crónica: Infecciones múltiples como forma de presentación. Caso clínico pediátrico. *Arch. Argent. Pediatr.* **2018**, *116*, e744–e748.
20. Anjani, G.; Vignesh, P.; Joshi, V.; Shandilya, J.K.; Bhattarai, D.; Sharma, J.; Rawat, A. Recent Advances in Chronic Granulomatous Disease. *Genes Dis.* **2020**, *7*, 84–92. [CrossRef]
21. Wientjes, F.B.; Segal, A.W. NADPH Oxidase and the Respiratory Burst. *Semin. Cell Biol.* **1995**, *6*, 357–365. [CrossRef]
22. Vermot, A.; Petit-Härtlein, I.; Smith, S.M.E.; Fieschi, F. NADPH Oxidases (NOX): An Overview from Discovery, Molecular Mechanisms to Physiology and Pathology. *Antioxidants* **2021**, *10*, 890. [CrossRef]
23. Medzhitov, R.; Janeway, C.A. Innate Immunity: Impact on the Adaptive Immune Response. *Curr. Opin. Immunol.* **1997**, *9*, 4–9. [CrossRef]
24. Rich, R.R. *Clinical Immunology: Principles and Practice*, 4th ed.; Elsevier: Amsterdam, The Netherlands, 2019; pp. 35–46.
25. Weckel, A.; Guilbert, T.; Lambert, C.; Plainvert, C.; Goffinet, F.; Poyart, C.; Méhats, C.; Fouet, A. Streptococcuspyogenes Infects Human Endometrium by Limiting the Innate Immune Response. *J. Clin. Investig.* **2021**, *131*, e130746. [CrossRef] [PubMed]
26. Rajeeve, K.; Das, S.; Prusty, B.K.; Rudel, T. Chlamydia Trachomatis Paralyses Neutrophils to Evade the Host Innate Immune Response. *Nat. Microbiol.* **2018**, *3*, 824–835. [CrossRef] [PubMed]
27. Carty, M.; Guy, C.; Bowie, A.G. Detection of Viral Infections by Innate Immunity. *Biochem. Pharmacol.* **2021**, *183*, 114316. [CrossRef]
28. Salazar, F.; Brown, G.D. Antifungal Innate Immunity: A Perspective from the Last 10 Years. *J. Innate Immun.* **2018**, *10*, 373–397. [CrossRef]
29. Karaś, M.A.; Turska-Szewczuk, A.; Janczarek, M.; Szuster-Ciesielska, A. Glycoconjugates of Gram-Negative Bacteria and Parasitic Protozoa – Are They Similar in Orchestrating the Innate Immune Response? *Innate Immun.* **2019**, *25*, 73–96. [CrossRef]
30. Motran, C.C.; Silvane, L.; Chiapello, L.S.; Theumer, M.G.; Ambrosio, L.F.; Volpini, X.; Celias, D.P.; Cervi, L. Helminth Infections: Recognition and Modulation of the Immune Response by Innate Immune Cells. *Front. Immunol.* **2018**, *9*, 664. [CrossRef]
31. Constant, D.A.; Nice, T.J.; Rauch, I. Innate Immune Sensing by Epithelial Barriers. *Curr. Opin. Immunol.* **2021**, *73*, 1–8. [CrossRef]
32. Eriksson, O.; Mohlin, C.; Nilsson, B.; Ekdahl, K.N. The Human Platelet as an Innate Immune Cell: Interactions between Activated Platelets and the Complement System. *Front. Immunol.* **2019**, *10*, 1590. [CrossRef] [PubMed]
33. Medzhitov, R.; Janeway, C. Innate Immunity. *N. Engl. J. Med.* **2000**, *343*, 338–344. [CrossRef] [PubMed]
34. Penberthy, K.K.; Lysiak, J.J.; Ravichandran, K.S. Rethinking Phagocytes: Clues from the Retina and Testes. *Trends Cell Biol.* **2018**, *28*, 317–327. [CrossRef] [PubMed]
35. Beutler, B. Innate Immunity: An Overview. *Mol. Immunol.* **2004**, *40*, 845–859. [CrossRef]
36. Tarr, A.W.; Urbanowicz, R.A.; Ball, J.K. The Role of Humoral Innate Immunity in Hepatitis c Virus Infection. *Viruses* **2012**, *4*, 1–27. [CrossRef]
37. Dini, L.; Lentini, A.; Diez, G.D.; Rocha, M.; Falasca, L.; Serafino, L.; Vidal-Vanaclocha, F. Phagocytosis of Apoptotic Bodies by Liver Endothelial Cells. *J. Cell Sci.* **1995**, *108*, 967–973. [CrossRef]
38. Allen, L.-A.H.; Aderem, A. Mechanisms of Phagocytosis. *Curr. Opin. Immunol.* **1996**, *8*, 36–40. [CrossRef]
39. Mitrović, M.; Arapović, J.; Traven, L.; Krmpotić, A.; Jonjić, S. Innate Immunity Regulates Adaptive Immune Response: Lessons Learned from Studying the Interplay between NK and CD8+ T Cells during MCMV Infection. *Med. Microbiol. Immunol.* **2012**, *201*, 487–495. [CrossRef]
40. Mayordomo, A.C.; Silva, J.E.; Gorlino, C.V.; Arias, J.L.; Berón, W.; Di Genaro, M.S. IL-12/23p40 Overproduction by Dendritic Cells Leads to an Increased Th1 and Th17 Polarization in a Model of Yersinia Enterocolitica-Induced Reactive Arthritis in TNFRp55-/- Mice. *PLoS ONE* **2018**, *13*, e0193573. [CrossRef]
41. Goldblatt, D.; Thrasher, A.J. Chronic granulomatous disease. *Clin. Exp. Immunol.* **2000**, *122*, 11–19. [CrossRef]
42. Akar-Ghibril, N. Defects of the Innate Immune System and Related Immune Deficiencies. *Clin. Rev. Allergy Immunol.* **2021**, *63*, 36–54. [CrossRef]
43. Bogdan, C.; Röllinghoff, M.; Diefenbach, A. The Role of Nitric Oxide in Innate Immunity. *Immunol. Rev.* **2000**, *173*, 17–26. [CrossRef]
44. Frances, R. Bacterial DNA Activates Cell Mediated Immune Response and Nitric Oxide Overproduction in Peritoneal Macrophages from Patients with Cirrhosis and Ascites. *Gut* **2004**, *53*, 860–864. [CrossRef] [PubMed]
45. Davicino, R.C.; Eliçabe, R.J.; Di Genaro, M.S.; Rabinovich, G.A. Coupling Pathogen Recognition to Innate Immunity through Glycan-Dependent Mechanisms. *Int. Immunopharmacol.* **2011**, *11*, 1457–1463. [CrossRef]
46. Eliçabe, R.J.; Arias, J.L.; Rabinovich, G.A.; Di Genaro, M.S. TNFRp55 Modulates IL-6 and Nitric Oxide Responses Following Yersinia Lipopolysaccharide Stimulation in Peritoneal Macrophages. *Immunobiology* **2011**, *216*, 1322–1330. [CrossRef]
47. Zhang, T.; Ma, C.; Zhang, Z.; Zhang, H.; Hu, H. NF-κB signaling in inflammation and cancer. *Med. Comm.* **2021**, *16*, 618–653. [CrossRef]

48. Abramson, S.B.; Amin, A.R.; Clancy, R.M.; Attur, M. The Role of Nitric Oxide in Tissue Destruction. *Best Pract. Res. Clin. Rheumatol.* **2001**, *15*, 831–845. [CrossRef] [PubMed]
49. Gopallawa, I.; Freund, J.R.; Lee, R.J. Bitter Taste Receptors Stimulate Phagocytosis in Human Macrophages through Calcium, Nitric Oxide, and Cyclic-GMP Signaling. *Cell. Mol. Life Sci.* **2020**, *78*, 271–286. [CrossRef]
50. Tsai, W.C.; Strieter, R.M.; Zisman, D.A.; Wilkowski, J.M.; Bucknell, K.A.; Chen, G.H.; Standiford, T.J. Nitric Oxide Is Required for Effective Innate Immunity against Klebsiella Pneumoniae. *Infect. Immun.* **1997**, *65*, 1870–1875. [CrossRef] [PubMed]
51. Ribeiro, C.V.; Rocha, B.F.B.; Oliveira, E.; Teixeira-Carvalho, A.; Martins-Filho, O.A.; Murta, S.M.F.; Peruhype-Magalhães, V. Leishmania Infantum Induces High Phagocytic Capacity and Intracellular Nitric Oxide Production by Human Proinflammatory Monocyte. *Memórias Do Inst. Oswaldo Cruz* **2020**, *115*, e190408. [CrossRef] [PubMed]
52. Jofre, B.L.; Eliçabe, R.J.; Silva, J.E.; Pérez Sáez, J.M.; Paez, M.D.; Callegari, E.; Mariño, K.V.; Di Genaro, M.S.; Rabinovich, G.A.; Davicino, R.C. Galectin-1 Cooperates with Yersinia Outer Protein (Yop) P to Thwart Protective Immunity by Repressing Nitric Oxide Production. *Biomolecules* **2021**, *11*, 1636. [CrossRef]
53. Cabral, F.V.; Pelegrino, M.T.; Seabra, A.B.; Ribeiro, M.S. Nitric-Oxide Releasing Chitosan Nanoparticles towards Effective Treatment of Cutaneous Leishmaniasis. *Nitric Oxide* **2021**, *113–114*, 31–38. [CrossRef] [PubMed]
54. García-Ortiz, A.; Serrador, J.M. Nitric Oxide Signaling in T Cell-Mediated Immunity. *Trends Mol. Med.* **2018**, *24*, 412–427. [CrossRef] [PubMed]
55. Wei, X.; Charles, I.G.; Smith, A.; Ure, J.; Feng, G.; Huang, F.; Xu, D.; Mullers, W.; Moncada, S.; Liew, F.Y. Altered Immune Responses in Mice Lacking Inducible Nitric Oxide Synthase. *Nature* **1995**, *375*, 408–411. [CrossRef] [PubMed]
56. Taylor-Robinson, A.W.; Liew, F.Y.; Severn, A.; Xu, D.; McSorley, S.J.; Garside, P.; Padron, J.; Phillips, R.S. Regulation of the Immune Response by Nitric Oxide Differentially Produced by T Helper Type 1 and T Helper Type 2 Cells. *Eur. J. Immunol.* **1994**, *24*, 980–984. [CrossRef]
57. Yang, J.; Zhang, R.; Lu, G.; Shen, Y.; Peng, L.; Zhu, C.; Cui, M.; Wang, W.; Arnaboldi, P.; Tang, M.; et al. T Cell–Derived Inducible Nitric Oxide Synthase Switches off TH17 Cell Differentiation. *J. Exp. Med.* **2013**, *210*, 1447–1462. [CrossRef]
58. Cartwright, A.N.R.; Suo, S.; Badrinath, S.; Kumar, S.; Melms, J.; Luoma, A.; Bagati, A.; Saadatpour, A.; Izar, B.; Yuan, G.-C.; et al. Immunosuppressive Myeloid Cells Induce Nitric Oxide–Dependent DNA Damage and P53 Pathway Activation in CD8+ T Cells. *Cancer Immunol. Res.* **2021**, *9*, 470–485. [CrossRef]
59. Thwe, P.M.; Amiel, E. The Role of Nitric Oxide in Metabolic Regulation of Dendritic Cell Immune Function. *Cancer Lett.* **2018**, *412*, 236–242. [CrossRef]
60. Palmieri, E.M.; McGinity, C.; Wink, D.A.; McVicar, D.W. Nitric Oxide in Macrophage Immunometabolism: Hiding in Plain Sight. *Metabolites* **2020**, *10*, 429. [CrossRef]
61. Monteiro, H.P.; Rodrigues, E.G.; Amorim Reis, A.K.C.; Longo, L.S.; Ogata, F.T.; Moretti, A.I.S.; da Costa, P.E.; Teodoro, A.C.S.; Toledo, M.S.; Stern, A. Nitric Oxide and Interactions with Reactive Oxygen Species in the Development of Melanoma, Breast, and Colon Cancer: A Redox Signaling Perspective. *Nitric Oxide* **2019**, *89*, 1–13. [CrossRef]
62. Mijatović, S.; Savić-Radojević, A.; Plješa-Ercegovac, M.; Simić, T.; Nicoletti, F.; Maksimović-Ivanić, D. The Double-Faced Role of Nitric Oxide and Reactive Oxygen Species in Solid Tumors. *Antioxidants* **2020**, *9*, 374. [CrossRef] [PubMed]
63. Matziouridou, C.; Rocha, S.D.C.; Haabeth, O.A.; Rudi, K.; Carlsen, H.; Kielland, A. INOS- and NOX1-Dependent ROS Production Maintains Bacterial Homeostasis in the Ileum of Mice. *Mucosal Immunol.* **2017**, *11*, 774–784. [CrossRef] [PubMed]
64. Li, J.; Baud, O.; Vartanian, T.; Volpe, J.J.; Rosenberg, P.A. Peroxynitrite Generated by Inducible Nitric Oxide Synthase and NADPH Oxidase Mediates Microglial Toxicity to Oligodendrocytes. *Proc. Natl. Acad. Sci. USA* **2005**, *102*, 9936–9941. [CrossRef] [PubMed]
65. Breitbach, K.; Klocke, S.; Tschernig, T.; van Rooijen, N.; Baumann, U.; Steinmetz, I. Role of Inducible Nitric Oxide Synthase and NADPH Oxidase in Early Control of Burkholderia Pseudomallei Infection in Mice. *Infect. Immun.* **2006**, *74*, 6300–6309. [CrossRef] [PubMed]
66. Kaul, N.; Forman, H.J. Activation of NFκB by the Respiratory Burst of Macrophages. *Free Radic. Biol. Med.* **1996**, *21*, 401–405. [CrossRef]
67. Liu, J.; Iwata, K.; Zhu, K.; Matsumoto, M.; Matsumoto, K.; Asaoka, N.; Zhang, X.; Ibi, M.; Katsuyama, M.; Tsutsui, M.; et al. NOX1/NADPH Oxidase in Bone Marrow-Derived Cells Modulates Intestinal Barrier Function. *Free Radic. Biol. Med.* **2020**, *147*, 90–101. [CrossRef]
68. Lanone, S.; Bloc, S.; Foresti, R.; Almolki, A.; Taillé, C.; Callebert, J.; Conti, M.; Goven, D.; Aubier, M.; Dureuil, B.; et al. Bilirubin Decreases NOS2 Expression via Inhibition of NAD(P)H Oxidase: Implications for Protection against Endotoxic Shock in Rats. *FASEB J.* **2005**, *19*, 1890–1892. [CrossRef]
69. Wu, F.; Tyml, K.; Wilson, J.X. INOS Expression Requires NADPH Oxidase-Dependent Redox Signaling in Microvascular Endothelial Cells. *J. Cell. Physiol.* **2008**, *217*, 207–214. [CrossRef]
70. Jang, A.; Choi, G.; Kim, Y.; Lee, G.; Hyun, K. Neuroprotective Properties of Ethanolic Extract of Citrus Unshiu Markovich Peel through NADPH Oxidase 2 Inhibition in Chemotherapy-Induced Neuropathic Pain Animal Model. *Phytother. Res.* **2021**, *35*, 6918–6931. [CrossRef]
71. Kumar, A.; Singh, K.P.; Bali, P.; Anwar, S.; Kaul, A.; Singh, O.P.; Gupta, B.K.; Kumari, N.; Alam, M.N.; Raziuddin, M.; et al. INOS Polymorphism Modulates INOS/NO Expression via Impaired Antioxidant and ROS Content in P. Vivax and P. Falciparum Infection. *Redox Biol.* **2018**, *15*, 192–206. [CrossRef]
72. Hou, L.; Zhang, L.; Hong, J.-S.; Zhang, D.; Zhao, J.; Wang, Q. NADPH Oxidase and Neurodegenerative Diseases: Mechanisms and Therapy. *Antioxid. Redox Signal.* **2020**, *33*, 374–393. [CrossRef] [PubMed]

73. Aviello, G.; Knaus, U.G. NADPH Oxidases and ROS Signaling in the Gastrointestinal Tract. *Mucosal Immunol.* **2018**, *11*, 1011–1023. [CrossRef] [PubMed]
74. Breitenbach, M.; Rinnerthaler, M.; Weber, M.; Breitenbach-Koller, H.; Karl, T.; Cullen, P.; Basu, S.; Haskova, D.; Hasek, J. The Defense and Signaling Role of NADPH Oxidases in Eukaryotic Cells. *Wien. Med. Wochenschr.* **2018**, *168*, 286–299. [CrossRef] [PubMed]
75. Thomas, D.C. How the Phagocyte NADPH Oxidase Regulates Innate Immunity. *Free Radic. Biol. Med.* **2018**, *125*, 44–52. [CrossRef]
76. Heropolitanska-Pliszka, E.; Berk, K.; Maciejczyk, M.; Sawicka-Powierza, J.; Bernatowska, E.; Wolska-Kusnierz, B.; Pac, M.; Dabrowska-Leonik, N.; Piatosa, B.; Lewandowicz-Uszynska, A.; et al. Systemic Redox Imbalance in Patients with Chronic Granulomatous Disease. *J. Clin. Med.* **2020**, *9*, 1397. [CrossRef]
77. Condino-Neto, A.; Muscara, M.; Grumach, A.; Carneiro-Sampaio, M.; Nucci, G. Neutrophils and Mononuclear Cells from Patients with Chronic Granulomatous Disease Release Nitric Oxide. *Br. J. Clin. Pharmacol.* **1993**, *35*, 485–490. [CrossRef]
78. Clark, S.R.; Coffey, M.J.; Maclean, R.M.; Collins, P.W.; Lewis, M.J.; Cross, A.R.; O'Donnell, V.B. Characterization of Nitric Oxide Consumption Pathways by Normal, Chronic Granulomatous Disease and Myeloperoxidase-Deficient Human Neutrophils. *J. Immunol.* **2002**, *169*, 5889–5896. [CrossRef]
79. Tsuji, S.; Taniuchi, S.; Hasui, M.; Yamamoto, A.; Kobayashi, Y. Increased Nitric Oxide Production by Neutrophils from Patients with Chronic Granulomatous Disease on Trimethoprim–Sulfamethoxazole. *Nitric Oxide* **2002**, *7*, 283–288. [CrossRef]
80. Blancas-Galicia, L.; Santos-Chávez, E.; Deswarte, C.; Mignac, Q.; Medina-Vera, I.; León-Lara, X.; Roynard, M.; Scheffler-Mendoza, S.C.; Rioja-Valencia, R.; Alvirde-Ayala, A.; et al. Genetic, Immunological, and Clinical Features of the First Mexican Cohort of Patients with Chronic Granulomatous Disease. *J. Clin. Immunol.* **2020**, *40*, 475–493. [CrossRef]
81. Williams, G.T.; Williams, W.J. Granulomatous Inflammation—A Review. *J. Clin. Pathol.* **1983**, *36*, 723–733. [CrossRef]
82. Lewis, C.J.; Cobb, B.A. Adaptive Immune Defects against Glycoantigens in Chronic Granulomatous Disease via Dysregulated Nitric Oxide Production. *Eur. J. Immunol.* **2011**, *41*, 2562–2572. [CrossRef] [PubMed]
83. Mantegazza, A.R.; Savina, A.; Vermeulen, M.; Pérez, L.; Geffner, J.; Hermine, O.; Rosenzweig, S.D.; Faure, F.; Amigorena, S. NADPH Oxidase Controls Phagosomal PH and Antigen Cross-Presentation in Human Dendritic Cells. *Blood* **2008**, *112*, 4712–4722. [CrossRef] [PubMed]
84. Deffert, C.; Carnesecchi, S.; Yuan, H.; Rougemont, A.-L.; Kelkka, T.; Holmdahl, R.; Krause, K.-H.; Schäppi, M.G. Hyperinflammation of Chronic Granulomatous Disease Is Abolished by NOX2 Reconstitution in Macrophages and Dendritic Cells. *J. Pathol.* **2012**, *228*, 341–350. [CrossRef] [PubMed]
85. Meissner, F.; Seger, R.A.; Moshous, D.; Fischer, A.; Reichenbach, J.; Zychlinsky, A. Inflammasome Activation in NADPH Oxidase Defective Mononuclear Phagocytes from Patients with Chronic Granulomatous Disease. *Blood* **2010**, *116*, 1570–1573. [CrossRef] [PubMed]
86. Poole, R.K. *Nitric Oxide and Other Small Signalling Molecules*, 1st ed.; Oxford Academic Press: London, UK; Elsevier: Alpharetta, GA, USA, 2018; pp. 62–115.
87. Shi, C.-S.; Shenderov, K.; Huang, N.-N.; Kabat, J.; Abu-Asab, M.; Fitzgerald, K.A.; Sher, A.; Kehrl, J.H. Activation of Autophagy by Inflammatory Signals Limits IL-1β Production by Targeting Ubiquitinated Inflammasomes for Destruction. *Nat. Immunol.* **2012**, *13*, 255–263. [CrossRef] [PubMed]
88. Saitoh, T.; Akira, S. Regulation of inflammasomes by autophagy. *J. Allergy Clin. Immunol.* **2016**, *138*, 28–36. [CrossRef]
89. Sarkar, S.; Korolchuk, V.I.; Renna, M.; Imarisio, S.; Fleming, A.; Williams, A.; Garcia-Arencibia, M.; Rose, C.; Luo, S.; Underwood, B.R.; et al. Complex Inhibitory Effects of Nitric Oxide on Autophagy. *Mol. Cell* **2011**, *43*, 19–32. [CrossRef]
90. Schwenkenbecher, P.; Neyazi, A.; Donnerstag, F.; Ringshausen, F.C.; Jacobs, R.; Stoll, M.; Kirschner, P.; Länger, F.P.; Valizada, E.; Gingele, S.; et al. Chronic Granulomatous Disease First Diagnosed in Adulthood Presenting with Spinal Cord Infection. *Front. Immunol.* **2018**, *9*, 1258. [CrossRef]
91. Hadfield, M.G.; Ghatak, N.R.; Laine, F.J.; Myer, E.C.; Massie, F.S.; Kramer, W.M. Brain Lesions in Chronic Granulomatous Disease. *Acta Neuropathol.* **1991**, *81*, 467–470. [CrossRef]
92. Prabhat, N.; Chakravarty, K.; Pattnaik, S.N.; Takkar, A.; Ray, S.; Lal, V. Systemic Lupus Erythematosus with Autoimmune Neurological Manifestations in a Carrier of Chronic Granulomatous Disease—A Rare Presentation. *J. Neuroimmunol.* **2020**, *343*, 577229. [CrossRef]
93. Mori, H.; Mishina, M. Structure and Function of the NMDA Receptor Channel. *Neuropharmacology* **1995**, *34*, 1219–1237. [CrossRef]
94. Pao, M.; Wiggs, E.A.; Anastacio, M.M.; Hyun, J.; DeCarlo, E.S.; Miller, J.T.; Anderson, V.L.; Malech, H.L.; Gallin, J.I.; Holland, S.M. Cognitive Function in Patients with Chronic Granulomatous Disease: A Preliminary Report. *Psychosomatics* **2004**, *45*, 230–234. [CrossRef] [PubMed]
95. Kishida, K.T.; Hoeffer, C.A.; Hu, D.; Pao, M.; Holland, S.M.; Klann, E. Synaptic Plasticity Deficits and Mild Memory Impairments in Mouse Models of Chronic Granulomatous Disease. *Mol. Cell. Biol.* **2006**, *26*, 5908–5920. [CrossRef] [PubMed]
96. Garthwaite, J.; Garthwaite, G.; Palmer, R.M.J.; Moncada, S. NMDA Receptor Activation Induces Nitric Oxide Synthesis from Arginine in Rat Brain Slices. *Eur. J. Pharmacol. Mol. Pharmacol.* **1989**, *172*, 413–416. [CrossRef]
97. Olthof, B.M.J.; Gartside, S.E.; Rees, A. Puncta of Neuronal Nitric Oxide Synthase (NNOS) Mediate NMDA Receptor Signaling in the Auditory Midbrain. *J. Neurosci.* **2018**, *39*, 876–887. [CrossRef]
98. Faria, M.P.; Laverde, C.F.; Nunes-de-Souza, R.L. Anxiogenesis Induced by Social Defeat in Male Mice: Role of Nitric Oxide, NMDA, and CRF1 Receptors in the Medial Prefrontal Cortex and BNST. *Neuropharmacology* **2020**, *166*, 107973. [CrossRef]
99. Weitzdoerfer, R.; Hoeger, H.; Engidawork, E.; Engelmann, M.; Singewald, N.; Lubec, G.; Lubec, B. Neuronal Nitric Oxide Synthase Knock-out Mice Show Impaired Cognitive Performance. *Nitric Oxide* **2004**, *10*, 130–140. [CrossRef]

100. Paul, V.; Ekambaram, P. Involvement of nitric oxide in learning & memory processes. *Indian J. Med. Res.* **2011**, *133*, 471–478.
101. Yeo, I.J.; Yun, J.; Son, D.J.; Han, S.-B.; Hong, J.T. Antifungal Drug Miconazole Ameliorated Memory Deficits in a Mouse Model of LPS-Induced Memory Loss through Targeting INOS. *Cell Death Dis.* **2020**, *11*, 623. [CrossRef]
102. Wang, B.; Han, S. Inhibition of Inducible Nitric Oxide Synthase Attenuates Deficits in Synaptic Plasticity and Brain Functions Following Traumatic Brain Injury. *Cerebellum* **2018**, *17*, 477–484. [CrossRef]
103. Contestabile, A. Roles of NMDA Receptor Activity and Nitric Oxide Production in Brain Development. *Brain Res. Rev.* **2000**, *32*, 476–509. [CrossRef]
104. Szydlowska, K.; Tymianski, M. Calcium, Ischemia and Excitotoxicity. *Cell Calcium* **2010**, *47*, 122–129. [CrossRef] [PubMed]
105. Lam, T.I.; Brennan-Minnella, A.M.; Won, S.J.; Shen, Y.; Hefner, C.; Shi, Y.; Sun, D.; Swanson, R.A. Intracellular PH Reduction Prevents Excitotoxic and Ischemic Neuronal Death by Inhibiting NADPH Oxidase. *Proc. Natl. Acad. Sci. USA* **2013**, *110*, E4362–E4368. [CrossRef] [PubMed]
106. Wang, Y.; Golledge, J. Neuronal Nitric Oxide Synthase and Sympathetic Nerve Activity in Neurovascular and Metabolic Systems. *Curr. Neurovascular Res.* **2013**, *10*, 81–89. [CrossRef] [PubMed]
107. Liu, H.; Liu, J.; Li, H.; Peng, Y.; Zhao, S. Mimicking Hypersensitivity Pneumonitis as an Uncommon Initial Presentation of Chronic Granulomatous Disease in Children. *Orphanet J. Rare Dis.* **2017**, *12*, 169. [CrossRef]
108. Liu, H.; Yang, H.; Li, H.; Liu, J.; Zhao, S. Hypersensitive Pneumonitis: An Initial Presentation of Chronic Granulomatous Disease in a Child. *J. Clin. Immunol.* **2018**, *38*, 155–158. [CrossRef]
109. Esenboga, S.; Emiralioglu, N.; Cagdas, D.; Erman, B.; De Boer, M.; Oguz, B.; Kiper, N.; Tezcan, İ. Diagnosis of Interstitial Lung Disease Caused by Possible Hypersensitivity Pneumonitis in a Child: Think CGD. *J. Clin. Immunol.* **2017**, *37*, 269–272. [CrossRef]
110. Chandra, D.; Cherian, S.V. Hypersensitivity Pneumonitis. In *StatPearls [Internet]*; StatPearls Publishing: Treasure Island, FL, USA, 2022.
111. Shirai, T.; Ikeda, M.; Morita, S.; Asada, K.; Suda, T.; Chida, K. Elevated Alveolar Nitric Oxide Concentration after Environmental Challenge in Hypersensitivity Pneumonitis. *Respirology* **2010**, *15*, 721–722. [CrossRef]
112. Girard, M.; Cormier, Y. Hypersensitivity pneumonitis. *Curr. Opin. Allergy Clin. Immunol.* **2010**, *10*, 99–103. [CrossRef] [PubMed]
113. Boughton-Smith, N.K.; Evans, S.M.; Whittle, B.J.R.; Moncada, S.; Hawkey, C.J.; Cole, A.T.; Balsitis, M. Nitric Oxide Synthase Activity in Ulcerative Colitis and Crohn's Disease. *Lancet* **1993**, *342*, 338.e2. [CrossRef]
114. Cross, R.K.; Wilson, K.T. Nitric Oxide in Inflammatory Bowel Disease. *Inflamm. Bowel Dis.* **2003**, *9*, 179–189. [CrossRef] [PubMed]
115. Marciano, B.E.; Rosenzweig, S.D.; Kleiner, D.E.; Anderson, V.L.; Darnell, D.N.; Anaya-O'Brien, S.; Hilligoss, D.M.; Malech, H.L.; Gallin, J.I.; Holland, S.M. Gastrointestinal Involvement in Chronic Granulomatous Disease. *Pediatrics* **2004**, *114*, 462–468. [CrossRef] [PubMed]
116. Angelino, G.; De Angelis, P.; Faraci, S.; Rea, F.; Romeo, E.F.; Torroni, F.; Tambucci, R.; Claps, A.; Francalanci, P.; Chiriaco, M.; et al. Inflammatory Bowel Disease in Chronic Granulomatous Disease: An Emerging Problem over a Twenty Years' Experience. *Pediatric Allergy Immunol.* **2017**, *28*, 801–809. [CrossRef]
117. Kalra, N.; Ghaffari, G. The Association between Autoimmune Disorders and Chronic Granulomatous Disease. *Pediatric Allergy Immunol. Pulmonol.* **2014**, *27*, 147–150. [CrossRef]
118. Yu, H.-H.; Yang, Y.-H.; Chiang, B.-L. Chronic Granulomatous Disease: A Comprehensive Review. *Clin. Rev. Allergy Immunol.* **2020**, *61*, 101–113. [CrossRef] [PubMed]
119. Rawat, A.; Bhattad, S.; Singh, S. Chronic Granulomatous Disease. *Indian J. Pediatr.* **2016**, *83*, 345–353. [CrossRef]
120. Chávez, M.D.; Tse, H.M. Targeting Mitochondrial-Derived Reactive Oxygen Species in T Cell-Mediated Autoimmune Diseases. *Front. Immunol.* **2021**, *12*, 3972. [CrossRef]
121. Kraaij, M.D.; Savage, N.D.L.; van der Kooij, S.W.; Koekkoek, K.; Wang, J.; van den Berg, J.M.; Ottenhoff, T.H.M.; Kuijpers, T.W.; Holmdahl, R.; van Kooten, C.; et al. Induction of Regulatory T Cells by Macrophages Is Dependent on Production of Reactive Oxygen Species. *Proc. Natl. Acad. Sci. USA* **2010**, *107*, 17686–17691. [CrossRef]
122. Hatzioannou, A.; Boumpas, A.; Papadopoulou, M.; Papafragkos, I.; Varveri, A.; Alissafi, T.; Verginis, P. Regulatory T Cells in Autoimmunity and Cancer: A Duplicitous Lifestyle. *Front. Immunol.* **2021**, *12*, 731947. [CrossRef]
123. Si, C.; Zhang, R.; Wu, T.; Lu, G.; Hu, Y.; Zhang, H.; Xu, F.; Wei, P.; Chen, K.; Tang, H.; et al. Dendritic Cell-Derived Nitric Oxide Inhibits the Differentiation of Effector Dendritic Cells. *Oncotarget* **2016**, *7*, 74834–74845. [CrossRef]
124. Martin-Gayo, E.; Yu, X.G. Role of Dendritic Cells in Natural Immune Control of HIV-1 Infection. *Front. Immunol.* **2019**, *10*, 1306. [CrossRef] [PubMed]
125. Stagg, A.J. Intestinal Dendritic Cells in Health and Gut Inflammation. *Front. Immunol.* **2018**, *9*, 2883. [CrossRef] [PubMed]
126. Hey, Y.-Y.; Tan, J.K.H.; O'Neill, H.C. Redefining Myeloid Cell Subsets in Murine Spleen. *Front. Immunol.* **2016**, *6*, 652. [CrossRef] [PubMed]
127. Sundquist, M.; Wick, M.J. Salmonella Induces Death of CD8 + Dendritic Cells but Not CD11cintCD11b+ Inflammatory Cells in Vivo via MyD88 and TNFR1. *J. Leukoc. Biol.* **2008**, *85*, 225–234. [CrossRef]
128. Fernandez-Boyanapalli, R.; McPhillips, K.A.; Frasch, S.C.; Janssen, W.J.; Dinauer, M.C.; Riches, D.W.H.; Henson, P.M.; Byrne, A.; Bratton, D.L. Impaired Phagocytosis of Apoptotic Cells by Macrophages in Chronic Granulomatous Disease Is Reversed by IFN-γ in a Nitric Oxide-Dependent Manner. *J. Immunol.* **2010**, *185*, 4030–4041. [CrossRef]
129. Roxo-Junior, P.; Simão, H.M.L. Chronic Granulomatous Disease: Why an Inflammatory Disease? *Braz. J. Med. Biol. Res.* **2014**, *47*, 924–928. [CrossRef]

130. Cachat, J.; Deffert, C.; Alessandrini, M.; Roux-Lombard, P.; Le Gouellec, A.; Stasia, M.-J.; Hugues, S.; Krause, K.-H. Altered Humoral Immune Responses and IgG Subtypes in NOX2-Deficient Mice and Patients: A Key Role for NOX2 in Antigen-Presenting Cells. *Front. Immunol.* **2018**, *9*, 1555. [CrossRef]
131. Leiding, J.W.; Holland, S.M. Chronic Granulomatous Disease. In *GeneReviews® [Internet]*; Adam, M.P., Everman, D.B., Mirzaa, G.M., Pagon, R.A., Wallace, S.E., Eds.; Updated 2022; University of Washington: Seattle, WA, USA, 2012; pp. 1993–2022. Available online: https://www.ncbi.nlm.nih.gov/books/NBK99496/ (accessed on 29 July 2022).
132. Slack, M.A.; Thomsen, I.P. Prevention of Infectious Complications in Patients with Chronic Granulomatous Disease. *J. Pediatric Infect. Dis. Soc.* **2018**, *7*, S25–S30. [CrossRef]
133. Assari, T. Chronic Granulomatous Disease; Fundamental Stages in Our Understanding of CGD. *Med. Immunol.* **2006**, *5*, 4. [CrossRef]
134. Lacey, C.A.; Chambers, C.A.; Mitchell, W.J.; Skyberg, J.A. IFN-γ-Dependent Nitric Oxide Suppresses Brucella -Induced Arthritis by Inhibition of Inflammasome Activation. *J. Leukoc. Biol.* **2019**, *106*, 27–34. [CrossRef]
135. Naderi beni, F.; Fattahi, F.; Mirshafiey, A.; Ansari, M.; Mohsenzadegan, M.; Movahedi, M.; Pourpak, Z.; Moin, M. Increased Production of Nitric Oxide by Neutrophils from Patients with Chronic Granulomatous Disease on Interferon-Gamma Treatment. *Int. Immunopharmacol.* **2012**, *12*, 689–693. [CrossRef] [PubMed]
136. Nagarkoti, S.; Sadaf, S.; Awasthi, D.; Chandra, T.; Jagavelu, K.; Kumar, S.; Dikshit, M. L-Arginine and Tetrahydrobiopterin Supported Nitric Oxide Production Is Crucial for the Microbicidal Activity of Neutrophils. *Free Radic. Res.* **2019**, *53*, 281–292. [CrossRef] [PubMed]
137. McNeill, E.; Stylianou, E.; Crabtree, M.J.; Harrington-Kandt, R.; Kolb, A.-L.; Diotallevi, M.; Hale, A.B.; Bettencourt, P.; Tanner, R.; O'Shea, M.K.; et al. Regulation of Mycobacterial Infection by Macrophage Gch1 and Tetrahydrobiopterin. *Nat. Commun.* **2018**, *9*, 5409. [CrossRef] [PubMed]
138. Gao, L.; Yin, Q.; Tong, Y.; Gui, J.; Liu, X.; Feng, X.; Yin, J.; Liu, J.; Guo, Y.; Yao, Y.; et al. Clinical and Genetic Characteristics of Chinese Pediatric Patients with Chronic Granulomatous Disease. *Pediatric Allergy Immunol.* **2019**, *30*, 378–386. [CrossRef]
139. Gennery, A.R. Progress in Treating Chronic Granulomatous Disease. *Br. J. Haematol.* **2020**, *192*, 251–264. [CrossRef] [PubMed]
140. de Luca, A.; Smeekens, S.P.; Casagrande, A.; Iannitti, R.; Conway, K.L.; Gresnigt, M.S.; Begun, J.; Plantinga, T.S.; Joosten, L.A.B.; van der Meer, J.W.M.; et al. IL-1 Receptor Blockade Restores Autophagy and Reduces Inflammation in Chronic Granulomatous Disease in Mice and in Humans. *Proc. Natl. Acad. Sci. USA* **2014**, *111*, 3526–3531. [CrossRef]

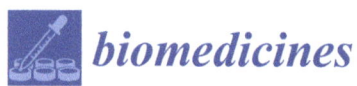

Review

Enhancement of Nitric Oxide Bioavailability by Modulation of Cutaneous Nitric Oxide Stores

Christoph V. Suschek [1], Dennis Feibel [1], Maria von Kohout [2,3] and Christian Opländer [3,*]

1. Department for Orthopedics and Trauma Surgery, Medical Faculty, Heinrich-Heine-University Dusseldorf, 40225 Düsseldorf, Germany
2. Plastic Surgery, Hand Surgery, Burn Center, Cologne-Merheim Hospital, 51109 Cologne, Germany
3. Institute for Research in Operative Medicine (IFOM), University Witten/Herdecke, 51109 Cologne, Germany
* Correspondence: christian.oplaender@uni-wh.de; Tel.: +49-221-989-57-13

Abstract: The generation of nitric oxide (NO) in the skin plays a critical role in wound healing and the response to several stimuli, such as UV exposure, heat, infection, and inflammation. Furthermore, in the human body, NO is involved in vascular homeostasis and the regulation of blood pressure. Physiologically, a family of enzymes termed nitric oxide synthases (NOS) generates NO. In addition, there are many methods of non-enzymatic/NOS-independent NO generation, e.g., the reduction of NO derivates (NODs) such as nitrite, nitrate, and nitrosylated proteins under certain conditions. The skin is the largest and heaviest human organ and contains a comparatively high concentration of these NODs; therefore, it represents a promising target for many therapeutic strategies for NO-dependent pathological conditions. In this review, we give an overview of how the cutaneous NOD stores can be targeted and modulated, leading to a further accumulation of NO-related compounds and/or the local and systemic release of bioactive NO, and eventually, NO-related physiological effects with a potential therapeutical use for diseases such as hypertension, disturbed microcirculation, impaired wound healing, and skin infections.

Keywords: UVA; nitrite; cold atmospheric plasma; nitric oxide donor; skin; wound healing; microcirculation

1. Nitric Oxide

Chemically, nitric oxide (NO) is an inorganic gas and can be dissolved in water up to concentrations of 2 mM [1]. In organisms, NO formation is catalyzed by the NO synthases (NOS), which synthesize NO directly from NADPH and L-arginine [2,3]. NO is a biological signal and effector molecule and has a large number of physiological as well as pathophysiological functions in an organism, which depend on concentration, the release profile, and the biological environment, among other things. As the smallest bioactive molecule produced by mammalian cells with lipophilic properties, NO is highly diffusible and can easily cross tissues and cell membranes [1,4].

NO controls pivotal physiological functions such as neurotransmission and vascular tone by activation of the soluble guanylyl cyclase [5,6], known to be the primary physiological effector for NO, and also by modulating gene transcription and mRNA translation [7,8].

2. Enzymatic Nitric Oxide Generation by Nitric Oxide Synthases

No only has a half-life of five seconds, which is why it has to be constantly regenerated. In humans, three isoforms of NO synthase, which are encoded by different genes, are known. These include the two constitutively expressed NOS isoenzymes, which are referred to as nNOS and eNOS, because of their initial discovery in neuronal cells and endothelial cells [9]. However, the expressions of the nNOS and the eNOS are not limited to the two cell types. The eNOS is expressed in many other cell types such as fibroblasts, osteoblasts, or hepatocytes, and the expression of the nNOS is not limited to neurons and is also expressed

in skin keratinocytes, among other cells. It is characteristic of the constitutively expressed NO synthases that after agonist activation, in a pulsatile manner, generate small amounts of NO in the pM–nM range over a relatively short period of time [2,9]. For example, the NO generated by eNOS in the endothelial cell lining, the inside of vessels, indirectly causes relaxation of smooth vascular muscle by increasing intracellular cyclic guanosine monophosphate (cGMP) levels, leading to vasodilation and, thus, a reduction in cardiac afterload and blood pressure. This reaction helped to understand how a whole group of drugs worked, including amyl nitrite, nitroprusside, and nitroglycerin: these drugs lead to a direct or indirect release of NO in the body [10–13].

The NO detected in the brain is predominantly the product of the nNOS in neurons. There it takes over the function of a neurotransmitter, whereby it also increases the synthesis of cGMP, among other things. It is also assumed that NO, due to its rapid diffusion, can modulate relatively large areas of the CNS [6,13].

The third NOS is an inducible isoform, the iNOS. After activation by pro-inflammatory mediators (cytokines) and/or bacterial components such as lipopolysaccharides (LPS), iNOS expression is induced, leading to a longer-lasting production of NO in comparatively high physiological concentrations in the µM range [13,14]. For example, the NO generated in high amounts by the iNOS in macrophages or the microglial cells after corresponding activation have fewer signal transductive effects and serve to protect the organism against bacteria, viruses, and helminths due to the radical and toxic character of NO. However, an excessive and, above all, insufficiently regulated high production rate of NO by iNOS can also have side effects such as tissue damage and, for example, profound vasodilatation leading to a dangerous drop in blood pressure, which is observed in the vasculature during septic shock [15,16].

While the role of eNOS- or nNOS-generated NO in human health as a physiological signaling and effector molecule in lower concentrations is not in doubt, many researchers assume that NO at an elevated concentration must have a predominantly negative to pathogenic effect.

In this context, NO-related diseases can be differentiated by either a lack or excess of NO. For example, NO in the brain regulates many physiological processes that can have an effect on cognitive function and behavior. Moreover, NO promotes angiogenesis and controls brain blood flow, and maintains cell immunity and the survival of neurons. However, an overproduction may result in neurodegeneration [17]. In addition, it was suggested that NO generation may be a major inherited factor of insulin sensitivity and that a diet-induced oxidative scavenging of NO is the first hit toward insulin resistance [18]. In the vasculature, NO from eNOS and nNOS that is also present around arterioles controls the vascular tone and blood flow. Moreover, a steady NO production is essential for leukocyte adhesion and platelet aggregation. Aberrations in vascular NO production can result in endothelial dysfunction, which is associated with several cardiovascular disorders, such as hypertension and angiogenesis-associated disorders (for review see [19]). Here, higher levels of NO generated by iNOS induced by chronic or acute inflammatory processes promote atherosclerosis directly or by the generation of NO metabolites such as peroxynitrite [20].

Thus, improving or protecting constitutive nitric oxide production in the vasculature may avoid the development of vascular diseases, whereas the inhibition of excessive NO by iNOS could also represent a therapeutic target [21].

3. Nitric Oxide and Skin

In the skin, too, NO-related diseases are caused by either a lack or excess of NO. In low concentrations, NO is a signaling molecule with regulatory and homeostatic functions, such as melanogenesis, vasodilation, and protection against environmental challenges [22]. The eNOS activity of endothelial cells in the skin vessels generates small pulses of NO, resulting in a basal level of vascular smooth muscle relaxation [23]. Thus, the inhibition of eNOS impairs local skin circulation, demonstrating the involvement of NO in maintaining resting cutaneous blood flow [24]. A local NO deficiency in skin contributes to vasospasms, which take part in the vasoconstrictive processes of Raynaud's disease [23].

NO can control pathogen growth in skin infections caused by epidermotropic viruses and many different species of bacteria, protozoa, helminths, and fungi that are often susceptible to NO. For example, NO at high concentrations produced by macrophages via iNOS is able to eliminate intracellular pathogens such as the *Leishmania* species and *Mycobacterium leprae*. It was presumed that this type of NO-induced antimicrobial efficacy would be restricted to macrophages. However, it has become obvious that many cell types, in tissues with immunological barrier functions in particular, use the iNOS-derived NO for defense, contributing to innate immunity [25–27].

The dark side of a high-output NO generation by iNOS may be seen in the pathogenesis of immune-mediated inflammatory skin diseases such as cutaneous lupus erythematosus, psoriasis, and possibly allergic skin lesions [28–30].

NO is a key molecule in dermal wound healing and tissue regeneration and here, too, the NO concentration can determine its function [31]. In primary cell cultures of human keratinocytes, low NO concentrations increased cell proliferation, whereas differentiation was blocked. Using higher NO concentrations, keratinocyte proliferation was inhibited and keratinocyte differentiation was induced. Analogous experiments with human dermal fibroblasts showed a decrease in proliferation correlated with increasing NO concentrations [32]. Independently of any MMP and TIMP action, NO exerts direct regulating properties on collagen metabolism [33,34]; thus, the inhibition of enzymatic NO synthesis causes a significant decrease in collagen synthesis and a delayed wound contraction in rats. In contrast, in vivo transfection of healthy rats with iNOS-cDNA resulted in enhanced collagen accumulation in cutaneous wounds due to increased NO generation [35].

4. Nitric Oxide and Nitric Oxide Derivates

Nitric oxide, as a free radical, reacts or binds with a wide range of biomolecules in humans such as proteins at heme, sulfhydryl sites, and cysteine residues, thereby regulating crucial cell functions. Many different bioactive NO-related compounds are generated in the process, such as S-nitrosylated proteins (RSNO), N-nitrosamine, and metal nitrosyls (RNNO), whereas the sum of RSNOs and RNNOs is called RNXOs. A major part of NO is known to be oxidized to nitrite (NO_2^-) and nitrate (NO_3^-) [36].

The biological catalysts of NO oxidation in an organism are not fully elucidated. Oxyhemoglobin and oxymyoglobin as catalysts are restricted to muscle tissues and blood lumen. Intracellularly, possible catalysts are heme-containing peroxidases (e.g., myeloperoxidase, eosinophil peroxidase, lactoperoxidase), which exert intrinsic NO oxidase activity resulting in the formation of nitrite but not nitrate [37,38]. Such NO oxidation activities are suggested to serve as a catalytic sink for NO in areas of inflammatory processes [37].

The reaction products of NO—(nitrite, nitrate, and RXNO) we call nitric oxide derivates (NODs), but they have many other names, for example NO-related species, NO metabolites, NO-related compounds, or NO derivatives, dependent on the authors. Some of these NODs, in particular nitrite and RSNO, are known to exert NO bioactivity under certain conditions, for example hypoxia, acidosis, or UVA exposure, and contribute to the global NO bioavailability [39,40].

Nitrite has been used for millennia to preserve meat (for review, see [41]). Here, the reduction of nitrite to NO, possibly via S-nitrosothiol formation [42], forms iron-nitrosyl, which gives cured meat a distinctive red color and protection against oxidation and bacterial contamination (for review, see [43]).

Thus, nitrite in the body either stems from NO synthases using L-arginine as a substrate, from dietary intake, or from reduction of dietary nitrate by commensal bacteria. The main sources of nitrate and nitrite in our diet are green vegetables, such as lettuce and spinach, and root vegetables, water, and cured meat. In the USA and many European countries, the estimated dietary intake range of nitrate is from 31 to 185 mg/day and of nitrite from 0.7 to 8.7 mg/day [44]. It is known that in vivo nitrite and secondary amines can react to produce carcinogenic nitrosamines. Therefore, stringent regulations were enforced to lower nitrate as well as nitrite concentrations in food and water. However, urinary excretion in human volunteers is about 1 mmol nitrate per day when nitrate intake is strictly excluded, and, therefore, in the same range of urinary nitrate levels provided by food [45]. Thus, it is assumed that the amount of nitrate synthesized by NO synthases is comparable to the amount of nitrate ingested with diet (for review, see [46]). The impact of dietary nitrite/nitrate intake on human health is a matter of scientific controversy. On the one hand, inorganic nitrates and nitrites are frequently used to avoid bacterial growth in processed meats, the high consumption of which is linked with a greater risk of cancer of the upper gastrointestinal tract [47]. On the other hand, reviews do not show an association between dietary nitrate consumption and cancer risk [48,49]. The predictions that dietary intake of nitrate and/or nitrite may increase the risk of gastric cancer, extrapolated from animal studies, have not been substantiated epidemiologically [44,50]. On the contrary, several studies have observed the beneficial effects of dietary nitrate supplementation on, for example, blood pressure and endothelial function, demonstrating that NO homeostasis can be restored by nitrite and/or nitrate independent from enzymatic NO sources and may represent a further system for endogenous NO production [51–53].

However, it is known that nitrite is capable of causing severe methemoglobinemia with a high mortality following the intake of sodium nitrite, which is often misused for self-poisoning [54]. However, nitrite, when administered in a clinical setting for specific diseases, reveals health benefits because most of the published reports identify NO production as the mechanism of action for nitrite applications [52].

The beneficial effects of a higher dietary nitrate intake seem to be related to an increase in NO generation, via the reduction to nitrite by oral commensal bacteria and then nitrite further reduction to NO [55,56]. In this nitrate–nitrite–NO pathway, nitrate is absorbed from the stomach and proximal small intestine into the blood stream, whereas a part of it is actively absorbed by the salivary glands resulting in a nitrate accumulation in the saliva. After excretion, the nitrate in salvia is rapidly reduced to nitrite by commensal oral facultative anaerobic bacteria located in the mouth (sublingual), swallowed, and then absorbed in the gut. Here, it enters the systemic circulation or is partly reduced further to NO under the acidic conditions in the stomach, from where it, in turn, enters the circulation, where it is oxidized to nitrite and nitrate [55,57]. As an overall effect, a higher nitrate consumption increases the general levels of available nitrite/NO in blood, body fluids, and in tissues [58]. Vegetarians are at reduced risk of developing hypertension and other cardiovascular diseases. Therefore, it can be speculated that the high nitrate/nitrite content of many consumed vegetables may possibly contribute to these beneficial cardioprotective effects [41,59], in addition to the often-cited antioxidant effects of vegetables.

There are many pathways in the body involving hemoglobin, myoglobin, xanthine oxidoreductase, or the further reduction of nitrite to bioactive NO, which is particularly enhanced during acidosis and hypoxia. Therefore, it is thought that these mechanisms represent a back-up system to ensure NO generation when oxygen-dependent NOS are compromised [51,55].

In the next sections, we present the NOD stores in the human body and introduce the non-enzymatic pathways, which generate NO from nitrite, affecting skin physiology in particular and many secondary systemic parameters.

5. NOD Content of Tissues and Skin

As products of enzymatic NO synthesis, nitrite and nitrate are widely distributed in the human body. However, their distribution varies, so that their concentrations in different body fluids can differ significantly [60]. In body fluids such as urine and saliva, nitrate concentrations are found in up to triple-digit micromolar concentrations, whereas in blood plasma, gastric juice, or milk only single- to double-digit micromolar nitrate concentrations are found. Nitrite levels in the human body are generally lower than nitrate levels. Without a bacterial urinary tract infection, no nitrite is found in the urine under physiological conditions, while concentrations of up to 200 µM and higher are observed in the saliva. The concentrations in blood plasma and milk are also very low and often below the detection limit. In the stomach, the nitrite concentrations in the gastric juice can be very variable and can be significantly increased in people with gastric diseases, with up to 200 µM present [61]. Weller et al. were also able to detect relevant amounts of nitrate and nitrite in human sweat [62]. Since it is easier to take body fluids and measure them quickly, there are fewer studies that have examined the concentrations of nitrite and nitrate in different tissues. A study of Nyakayiru et al. showed that, in humans, the content of skeletal muscle nitrate is clearly higher than in blood plasma. However, in this study, the nitrite concentration in skeletal muscle remained below the detection limit [63].

In human skin homogenizates (epidermis + dermis) we showed that the concentration of nitrate was around 6-fold, of nitrite 25-fold, and of RSNO/RNNO up to 40-fold higher than in blood plasma [64]. These results are consistent with another study by Mowbray et al. using another experimental set-up. Interestingly, they found that most of the nitrate and nitrite is found in the epidermis and cornea, and only a small portion of it in the underlying dermis [65]. In addition, they further described a strong inter-individual variation in the concentration of NO-related products in the blood plasma, saliva, sweat, superficial vascular dermis, and epidermis. They also demonstrated that the concentration of NODs found in the blood plasma strongly correlated with the NOD concentration in the superficial dermis or sweat. It was suggested that the majority of nitrite found in tissues may have originated from exogenous dietary intake of nitrite and nitrate instead of from endogenous sources, which may cause great inter-individual variation in tissue nitrite levels, depending on individual nitrate and nitrite intake [41]. In contrast, nitrite blood plasma concentrations are more stable, suggesting the existence of regulatory mechanisms in the blood [66].

In conclusion, normal human skin of healthy volunteers can contain NODs such as nitrite and RSNO in many-fold higher concentrations than in blood plasma. Why and how NODs accumulate in the skin although there is fast renal elimination is a matter of much speculation. There are studies that provide direct evidence that the existing dermal NODs are jointly responsible for NOS-independent NO generation and can thus exert local and systemic NO-specific effects, which we introduce in the following sections.

6. NO Generation by Decomposition of Dermal Nitric Oxide Derivates

6.1. Acid-Induced Nitrite Decomposition of Nitrite in Sweat

There are many possible ways to generate NO in skin and on the skin surface besides the NOS-dependent NO synthesis. Analogously oral bacteria and also the skin commensal bacteria can synthesize the nitrate reductase enzyme, which reduces nitrate of sweat to nitrite. Owing to the acidic nature of sweat, nitrite is reduced further to NO, which in turn can evaporate in ambient air and also easily cross the epidermal barrier, thus entering the skin tissue and reaching skin cells, and also possibly the superficial blood vessels and the blood circulation [62]. In addition, it was postulated that ammonia-oxidizing bacteria may contribute to superficial dermal nitrite concentration via oxidation of ammonia to nitrite [67]. In previous studies, we found that NO generation by acidification of low concentrations of nitrite (10 µM) depends on the pH value and can be enhanced in the presence of antioxidants such as vitamin C (see Equations (1)–(4))

$$NO_2^- + H^+ \rightleftarrows HNO_2 \quad (1)$$

$$2\,HNO_2 \rightleftarrows N_2O_3 + H_2O \quad (2)$$

$$N_2O_3 \rightleftarrows NO + NO_2^\bullet \quad (3)$$

$$HNO_2 + Asc \rightarrow 2\,NO + DHAsc + 2\,H_2O \quad (4)$$

This enhancement is more pronounced under lower pH values (pH 2–4), whereas under normal skin pH values the presence of vitamin C does not play a big role. However, the antioxidant-assisted NO generation can be boosted manifold by copper ions at the pH value of 5.5 and under normoxia conditions [68]. Technically, when using higher nitrite concentrations, the underlying mechanism of antioxidant/copper-assisted NO generation at normal skin pH values can be used as an NO donor system with therapeutic potential, e.g., for increasing dermal microcirculation in critically perfused flaps in plastic surgery [69,70].

There are reports confirming the presence of relevant amounts of water-soluble vitamins, e.g., vitamin C in sweat [71]. Interestingly, these concentrations are in the same range as found in blood plasma [72]. In addition, copper can be found in sweat and, although there was no correlation between serum copper and sweat copper, there were hints that a high dietary intake of copper resulted in larger excreted amounts of copper in sweat [73].

In conclusion, besides nitrate/nitrite concentration of sweat, bacterial nitrate reductase activity, and the sweat pH value, it is very probable that further individual factors (such as the presence of copper ions and antioxidants) have a strong impact on acid-induced nitrite decomposition in sweat and consequent NO generation, making in vivo investigations more difficult.

6.2. UV-Induced Photolysis of NOD Stores in Skin

As early as 1961 the term photorelaxation was introduced by Nobel Prize winner R.F. Furchgott to describe the relaxation of rings of rabbit aorta under light (<450 nm) and UV radiation [74], potentiated in the presence of nitrite [75]. Nitrite can undergo photodecomposition induced by UVA irradiation, resulting eventually in the generation of bioactive NO [76]. Therefore, it is obvious that dermal nitrite can be targeted by UVA, as demonstrated by a study by Paunel et al. Here, UVA exposure of skin specimens causes an enzyme-independent high-output NO generation above the skin surface and within the skin, which not only correlates with the nitrite and RSNO concentrations in the skin but also with concentrations of free and protein-bound thiols, which may serve as antioxidants. Further experiments show that the UVA/nitrite-induced biological effects on keratinocyte differentiation and proliferation could be enhanced in the presence of antioxidants such as vitamin C and glutathione (GSH) [64]. In additional studies, we found that the NO formation from UVA-induced decomposition could be enhanced manifold by antioxidants such as Trolox (water-soluble vitamin E derivate), GSH, and vitamin C [77].

In healthy volunteers, an increase in RXNO and nitrite concentration in the blood plasma could be observed at an interval of 15 to 45 min after a whole-body UVA irradiation, indicating a possible UVA-induced mobilization of nitrite-derived NO from skin tissue into the blood plasma [78]. These effects were accompanied by and correlated with a significant drop in systemic blood pressure, raising the question whether UVA could be good for the heart [79,80]. These results were supported by Mowbray et al., showing in healthy volunteers, via microdialysis, a likewise increase in NO-related products by UVA irradiation [65]. In addition, a study by Liu et al. using confocal fluorescence microscopy and an NO imaging probe on human skin samples revealed that UVA-induced NO release occurs in a dose-dependent manner, with the majority of the light-sensitive NO pool in the upper epidermis, independent of NOS activity. In addition, here, UVA lowered blood pressure independent of NOS [81].

It can be assumed that UVA also has an effect on photolabile NODs such as nitrite and other RXNO in sweat, which in turn is produced more under warm and sunny conditions. Our in vitro experiments (data not published, see Supplementary Materials) show that buffers (pH 5.5) containing low concentrations of nitrite release NO upon UVA exposure. As shown in Figure 1B,C, this NO release can be boosted by the addition of an antioxidant, e.g., vitamin C. We observed in vivo that under UVA exposure, the increase in NO evaporation from human skin increased manifold. However, the addition of topical vitamin C could only slightly enhance the NO amount, indicating that the process of UVA-induced decomposition on the skin surface and upper skin layers was already using naturally occurring antioxidants (sweat) in sufficient concentrations (see Figure 1D,E). However, washing of the skin prior to UVA exposure halved the NO yield. In a parallel study, using the same experimental set-up, we showed that heat generation was not primarily responsible for the increase in skin NO release, but the used wavelengths for irradiation (Section 6.3) [82].

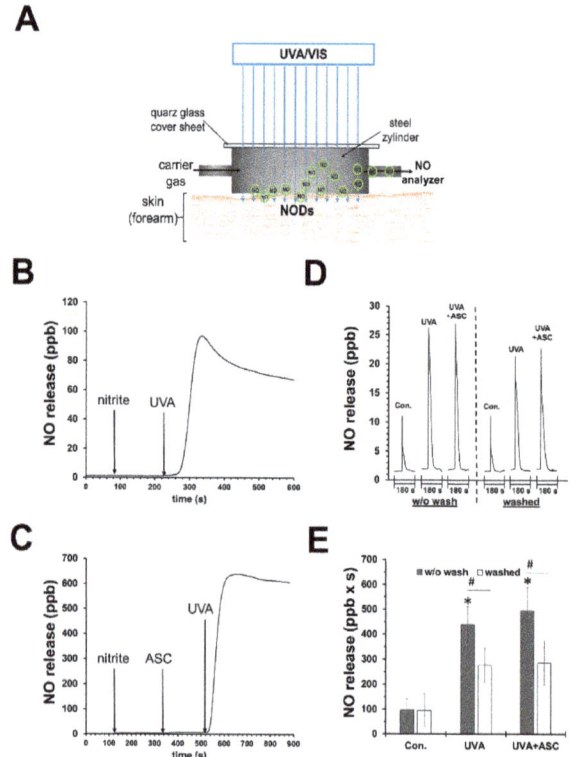

Figure 1. UVA can induce nitric oxide release by photodecomposition of nitrite. (A) Experimental set-up to measure nitric oxide (NO) emanation from human skin. (B) NO release from an UVA-irradiated (70 mW/cm^2) reaction chamber with saline buffer (PBS; pH 7.4; 20 mL) containing nitrite (10 µM) and (C) in addition sodium ascorbate (1 mM). There was not any significant release of NO without nitrite (not shown). (D) Representative registration of NO release from skin of one volunteer after 180 s UVA exposure (18 mW/cm^2) using the experimental set-up pictured in (A). Mean values ± SD of integrated NO peaks ($n = 4$) are shown in (E); * $p < 0.05$ as compared to the controls and # $p < 0.05$ as compared to respective values obtained from unwashed arms.

Investigating the NO release action spectrum in human skin, Pelegrino et al. observed that NO can be generated by UVA and also UVB irradiation, which both could trigger the dermal NOD store, mainly composed of nitrite, nitrate, and RSNOs [83].

It is possible that NO released by photolabile NOD, in particular nitrite, may serve as a protection against UV challenge. In human skin cells, even supra-physiological high concentrations of NO protected cells from oxidative stress and UVA-induced apoptosis. However, in other cell systems, the number of apoptotic events, even at physiological concentrations of NO, increased [84]. Nevertheless, skin fibroblasts depleted from intracellular nitrite showed a higher UVA susceptibility and died at lower doses than control fibroblasts or fibroblast cultures supplemented with physiological nitrite concentrations found in the skin [85].

Thus, it seems that skin-derived nitrite and other NODs may play an important role in human skin physiology, as it is postulated for NO itself. However, further experiments showed that nitrite at higher supra-physiological concentrations enhanced UVA-induced cell deaths in skin fibroblasts, probably due to the generation of toxic NO_2 radicals produced simultaneously by UVA-induced nitrite decomposition [86]. Here, the addition of the antioxidant ascorbate could reverse the UVA/nitrite-induced toxic effects, whereas GSH and Trolox enhanced them. Although NO formation via photodecomposition of nitrite may serve as an effective antioxidant and protector in skin, the simultaneous generation of toxic side products may have adverse and harmful effects.

Thus, besides the nitrite concentration, here the individual antioxidative capacity of a cell type and the microenvironment during UVA exposure are also crucial for the outcome and should be considered when dealing with UV/A-induced skin effects such as sunburn, erythema, and premature skin ageing.

In conclusion, analogous to acid-induced nitrite decomposition, the UV-induced photolysis of NODs depends on the wavelength, irradiance, and dose; individual factors such as nitrate/nitrite/antioxidant concentrations and pH of the skin, skin surface, and sweat; as well as skin hygiene, skin type, and others. In addition, possible interactions with light/radiation of other wavelengths (visible light/IR) should not be forgotten, as they are part of the natural sunlight and can have a direct impact on NO release and NOD stores (see the following section).

6.3. VIS/IR-Induced Photolysis of NOD Stores in Skin

Apart from UVA radiation, we demonstrated that blue light at shorter wavelengths is also able to mobilize NO from photolabile NODs in the skin. We found a significant increase in the intradermal levels of free NO caused by blue light irradiation in human skin specimens. Furthermore, blue light induced an emanation of NO from the skin area in healthy volunteers, whereas other wavelengths in the green, red, and infrared spectrum did not have significant effects [82].

In a randomized crossover study conducted by Stern et al., 14 healthy male volunteers were irradiated by monochromatic blue using a full-body blue light device, and the circulating nitric oxide species (nitrite/RXNO) in blood plasma were measured. The results showed that 30 min after the end of irradiation, the levels of nitric oxide species increased in circulation. In particular, the levels of RXNOs were significantly elevated by 30–50% [87].

There are reports that IR and red light may have an impact on NO stores in the skin or NO release, possibly via photolysis [88]. However, further investigation showed that enzymatic pathways were dominant in the induction of NO release found in ex vivo human skin homogenates [89]. In experiments using human keratinocytes, an increase in NOS-dependent NO production was observed after infrared low-level laser stimulation [90]. Since the observed increase in NO production was very quick, the authors postulated that the existing NOS activity may be enhanced instead of a de novo NOS protein synthesis, indicating that IR may stabilize NOS, cofactors, and enhance substrate binding ability, possibly by heating.

7. Modulation of Dermal NOD Content and Possible Effects

7.1. NO Donors

Since NO is important for wound healing and shows antibacterial efficacy in many studies, different types of NO donors such as RSNOs (S-nitrosocysteine, S-nitrosoalbumin S-nitrosoglutathione), N-diazeniumdiolates (NONOates), metal nitrosyls, and others were used [91,92]. There are many reports that state exogenous NO donors represent a promising method to promote wound healing by enhancing cell proliferation, collagen deposition, and angiogenic activities improving granulation tissue formation [93].

Acidified nitrite creams were also used, as NO donor systems showed good therapeutic effects on wound healing in mice. However, the outcome was better when cream was applied in the first 4 days after wounding [94]. In a prospective study (8 patients, 15 infected wounds), the possibility of MRSA eradication was also demonstrated (9 of 15 wounds) using the same cream formula [95].

A possible clinical application of NO donors is to improve dermal microcirculation and tissue perfusion, which are often pathologic in patients with hypertension, obesity, and diabetes mellitus, but also often critical after skin flap surgery [96,97]. Many studies have proven the effectiveness of NO donors to improve flap survival in experimental models [98]. In humans, we showed that topically applied NO (acidified nitrite/ascorbate) significantly increased vasodilatation and blood flow. These beneficial effects were also observed in a patient with a critically perfuse flap preventing further surgery [70].

Nevertheless, in spite of these beneficial results of using NO donors, they are not very common in clinical practice. In cells, NO can cause cell death, induce DNA damage, and disturb mitochondrial functions. High concentrations of NO are toxic, as seen in inflammatory responses where a high-level activity of iNOS results in high NO concentration associated with the destruction of cells and tissues [99–101].

Therefore, one major problem involves the therapeutic windows and possible adverse side effects, as reported in some studies [102,103]. Here, a repeated topical application of acidified nitrite exerted pro-inflammatory effects in the skin, and a dose-related increase in itching, pain, and edema were observed in patients with anogenital warts. A study by Mowbray et al. suggested that the observed potent inflammation by acidified nitrite produced by a combination of nitrite and ascorbic acid was secondary to the release of additional mediators (e.g., ascorbyl radicals), whereas using a chemically inert pure NO donor (NO zeolite) providing the same NO release exerted only minimal inflammation [104].

Nonetheless, we demonstrated in vitro using an acidified nitrite/ascorbate/copper system and gas permeable cell culture well bottoms that the NO release profile was crucial for the outcome. Here, directly after mixing and application of liniments, the obtained initial high peaks of NO amounts in the first 200 s correlated better to cell toxicity than the total amount of applied NO in 600 s [69]. Evaluating potential damage effects on human skin in further studies (see Supplementary Materials), we observed an increase in apoptotic events in epidermis and dermis in freshly donated human skin after topical application of slightly acidified nitrite/ascorbate liniments with different nitrite concentrations (see Figure 2). Here, higher nitrite concentrations led to higher NO penetration through the epidermis (Figure 2B). We observed that the rate of apoptosis in the epidermis correlated with the generated NO amount in the liniment (see Figure 2C,E). Furthermore, within the dermis, the number of apoptotic events was seen to generally increase for all tested NO-releasing liniments, but neither showed a good correlation to NO doses nor to the penetrated NO amounts (see Figure 2C,D,F). These results indicate that different cell populations and possible fibroblast subpopulation in the dermis may show different NO sensitivity, which could be interesting for therapeutic approaches to hyperproliferative fibrotic conditions, for example, excessive scaring after burns.

Most studies relating to the use of NO donors for skin pathologies only investigated the direct NO effects on bacteria, dermal microcirculation, and skin cells. However, less studied is the fate of topically applied NO. Apart from the direct local effects, the application of any NO donor should increase the amount of more stable NODs in the treated area via NO reduction and other chemical reactions, e.g., S-nitrosylation. These NODs may accumulate locally and remain in the treated tissue and/or may be distributed systemically. By using 15N-labeleld nitrite we observed that topical application of NO (acidified nitrite/ascorbate) on skin samples and the skin of healthy volunteers led to a transepidermal translocation of NO into the underlying tissue, resulting in a significant increase in nitrite and RSNO in the skin and blood [70]. Depending on the size of the treated skin area (torso), a significant systemic increase in the NOD (nitrite and RXNO) was also found in blood plasma, accompanied by an increased systemic vasodilatation and blood flow as well as a reduced blood pressure [105].

In summary, apart from direct effects on wound healing, bacterial contamination, microcirculation, blood pressure, and others, the topical application of NO donors represent an approach to directly increase circulatory NO bioavailability, and also indirectly by increasing the local and systemic NOD stores, which in turn may have longer lasting effects on, for example, skin physiology/bacterial colonization and circulation parameters.

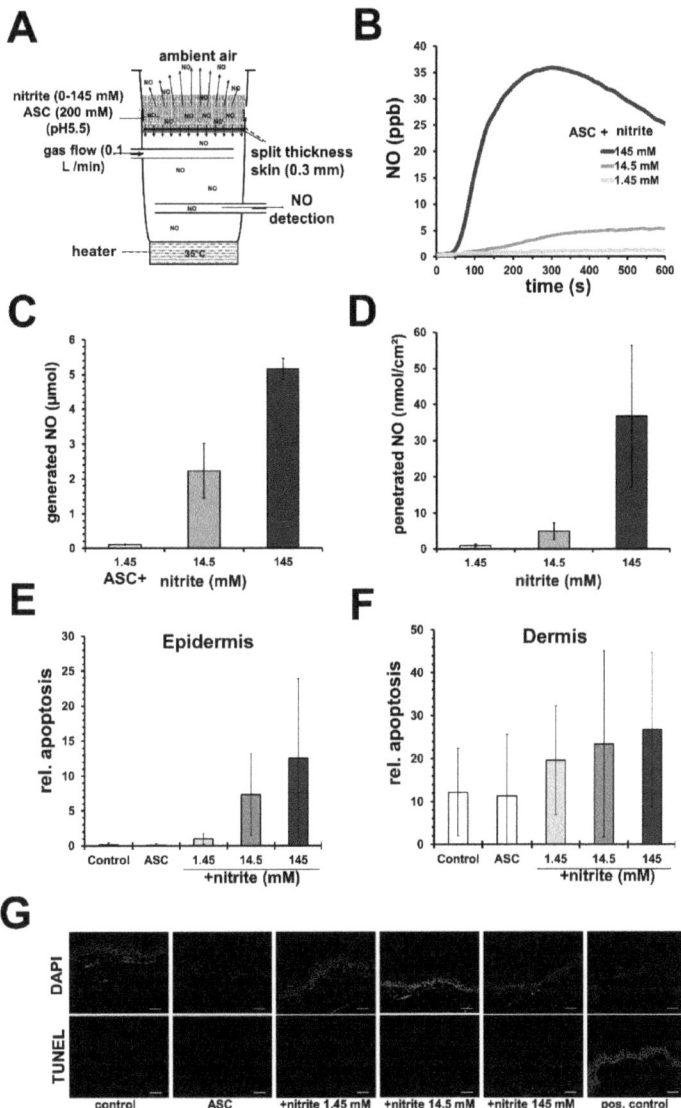

Figure 2. Nitric oxide–releasing solutions can induce apoptosis in human skin. (**A**) Experimental set-up to measure nitric oxide (NO) penetration through human split skin. (**B**) Exemplary registration of measured NO below skin with sodium ascorbate (ASC; 100 mM)-containing acetate buffer (pH 5.5) and nitrite in concentration as indicated. (**C**) Shows the amount of generated NO from 1 mL of the nitrite solution (described in (**B**) in 600 s). (**D**) By integration the amounts of penetrated NO were calculated. Shown are the mean values + SD of 3 independent experiments using different skin specimens. (**E**) Different nitrite/ascorbate buffers were applied on vital human skin samples and apoptosis was detected 24 h later by TUNEL assay. Shown are the mean values ± SD (n = 3) of relative apoptosis, the counted number of TUNEL-positive cells in relation to the total number (DAPI-stained) of cells found in the epidermis or (**F**) dermis. (**G**) Exemplary fluorescence microscope images obtained from skin samples treated as indicated (white bar = 100 µm).

7.2. Cold Atmospheric Plasma

Physical plasma is referred to as the fourth state of matter alongside solid, liquid, and gas and has become increasingly interesting in medical research in recent years. Plasma can be generated at room temperature under normal atmosphere (cold atmospheric plasma; CAP); thus, it can also be applied to sensitive surfaces such as human skin and tissue. By supplying energy, for example, by applying a strong electric field, ions, atoms, and especially electrons of a gas are set in motion. Through impact ionization, electrons are accelerated and catapulted out of their orbits and react with other molecules/atoms generating, among other things, radical nitrogen and oxygen species. Within CAP, other components such as UV rays (UVA, UVB, UVC), ions, neutral atoms, and heat are generated, determining the effects of the CAP [106]. There are many types of CAP sources using different approaches to CAP generation. Direct CAP sources use the surface to be treated as a counter electrode, and the active particles are generated directly on this surface. The energy-generating first electrode is covered with ceramic, so that an attenuated discharge occurs, which discharges homogeneously in the form of many small lightning strikes on an uneven surface. It is important that the distance electrode/surface is uniform and not more than 1–2 mm. A device using this kind of CAP generation is called a "dielectric barrier discharge" or DBD for short, and the ambient air is used as the gas to be ionized.

Indirect plasmas are generated at two identically constructed electrodes and then transported with a carrier gas (e.g., helium or argon) to the surface to be treated [107]. The plasma becomes visible as a narrow gas jet. The treated surface is not in an electric field, which means that mainly uncharged particles are transported [108].

CAP becomes complex through the various factors that influence its composition and, thus, its effects on cells and tissues/body fluids. Among other things, it is characterized by its particle composition, temperature, type of generation, spatial distribution, and strength of the electric field. These factors can be individually designed and, thus, optimized to suit the field of application.

CAP has been thought to be used for disinfection and sterilization of surfaces, such as infected wounds, and may have potential besides its antibacterial efficacy to promote wound healing [109–111]. However, we found that CAP treatment using a commercially available and clinically approved plasmajet obtained good results on dry surfaces but did not lead to the desired significant reduction in the bacterial burden in a wet wound milieu or in biofilms [112].

Investigating a direct CAP source/DBD (see Supplementary Materials), we found that topical CAP treatment induces NOD accumulation in the treated skin area, as shown in Figure 3A–C, accompanied by an acidification of the skin surface (down to pH 2) and NO-like effects, such as increasing dermal microcirculation without significant toxic effects to skin or skin cells (Figure 3D) [113].

Similar results were obtained using a commercially available and clinically approved PlasmaDerm device based on DBD, showing increased cutaneous capillary blood flow at the radial forearm of healthy volunteers after CAP treatment [114].

In summary, apart from the supposed antibacterial and wound healing effects, the topical application of CAP and the use of direct CAP sources, in particular, may represent an alternative approach to increasing dermal and perhaps systemic NOD stores and NO bioavailability (for overview see Figure 4).

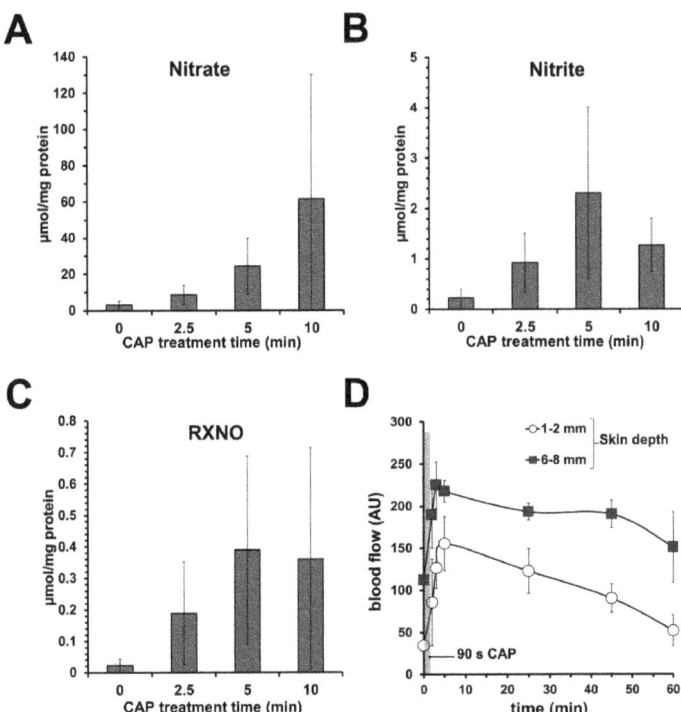

Figure 3. Topical application of cold atmospheric plasma (CAP) increases dermal microcirculation and the amount of nitric oxide derivates (NODs) in skin. Using a dielectric barrier device as CAP source, topical CAP treatment of human skin samples led to an increase in (A) nitrate, (B) nitrite, and (C) nitrosylated compounds (RXNOs) found in the respective skin homogenizates. Shown are the mean values ± SD of 6 independent experiments (treated skin surface 0.64 cm^2). (D) Hairless areas of forearm were treated with CAP (90 s) and blood flow was measured in different skin depths as indicated by a microlight guide spectrophotometer (O2C) device. Given are blood flow mean values ± SD of volunteers (n = 4) showing a CAP-induced increase in dermal blood flow in the treated area.

Showing similar effects as acidified nitrite/NO donors, CAP may also exert beneficial and detrimental effects, depending on the treatment regimen and dose. Although there are many reports of CAP/DBD-induced cell death, we found in our experiments that CAP/DBD did not induce apoptosis in human donor skin but sometimes a slight inflammatory response [113].

7.3. Nitrate-Rich Diet

Assuming that permanently higher NOD blood plasma levels are also reflected in higher NOD concentrations in tissues, oral intake of NOD such as nitrate and nitrite should not only increase plasma levels but also replenish dermal NOD stores.

Since Mowbray et al. demonstrated that NOD concentration in blood plasma is correlated with NOD concentration in superficial dermis or sweat [65], it is probable that this assumption is right and that the dermal NOD stores can be filled by a regular nitrate-rich diet, preferably with high contents of vitamins and antioxidants by eating vegetables, such as spinach and red beetroot. Moreover, because certain bacteria are essential for the enterosalivary nitrate–nitrite–nitric oxide pathway, disturbing the oral bacterial fauna by, for example, antiseptic mouthwash, may have strong negative impact on NO bioavailability and NOD levels mediated by oral nitrate uptake [115].

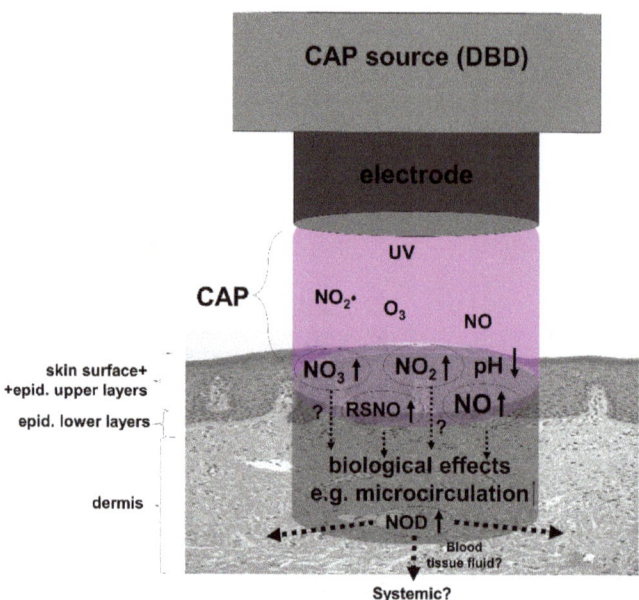

Figure 4. The use of cold atmospheric plasma (CAP) to enrich skin with nitric oxide derivates (NOD). Shown is a simplified assumption of possible reactions of CAP during treatment of skin. A dielectric barrier discharge (DBD) device as CAP source operated under ambient air generates, i.e., water-soluble nitrogen dioxide ($NO_2\bullet$), which in turn hydrolyzes to nitric acid (HNO_3) and nitrous acid (HNO_2) on skin leading to an acidification of the skin surface. Thus, the skin surface, sweat, and the upper skin layers can be loaded with the anions nitrate (NO_3) and nitrite (NO_2), which may partially decompose under the induced acidic conditions and UV irradiation generated in CAP to nitric oxide (NO) that can penetrate deeper through the epidermal barrier and/or leading to the formation of S-nitrosylated proteins (RSNO), both capable of increasing local dermal microcirculation.

To what extent the dermal NOD content can be influenced by nutrition and the possible physiological consequences this may have has not yet been sufficiently investigated and needs further research. However, increasing dermal NOD stores via nutrition and support of the oral bacteria seem feasible and delicious approaches.

7.4. UV/VIS Modulation of Dermal NOD

UV radiation and visible light—blue light in particular—are able to target photolabile NOD in the skin, resulting in NO release. This kind of NO mobilization also leads to possibly long-lasting changes in the dermal NOD stores. Paunel et al. described how UVA irradiation of skin induced an increase in the dermal RSNO content, which can be enhanced by incubation with nitrite [64]. On the other hand, a depletion of photolabile NOD can be expected by UV/VIS, which can be an interesting pathway in photo-induced premature skin ageing. To our knowledge, no study has been conducted in this direction yet. However, in a combination, for example, with a topical neutral nitrite application, UV/VIS may be used to mobilize NO from more superficial NODs (nitrite) into deeper skin layers, where it is possible to be stored as bioactive RSNOs and nitrite, increasing the level of NOD stores in skin. On the other hand, NO donors (acidified nitrite/ascorbate) increased the NOD levels in skin, which in turn may result in a higher NO release upon UVA or VIS. Personal observations indicate that the increased NOD levels in the skin induced by NO donors can remain for days, as was found out by chance when we investigated the skin NO release upon UV irradiation. Here, the irradiation of one forearm of a volunteer, which was in contact with an acidified nitrite/ascorbate cream three days before, led to a manifold stronger (~10×) NO release than the other (uncreamed) arm.

Thus, elevated dermal NOD levels obtained also, for example, by a nitrite/nitrate-rich diet or inflammation, should be affected by UV/VIS, possibly leading to more dermal/circulatory RSNO/RXNO concentrations with consequent NO-induced effects on blood pressure and microcirculation [87].

In order to avoid any misunderstandings, of course, it is appropriate at this point to point out the potential dangers of UV exposure. UV radiation can be a harmful and carcinogenic environmental medium, and frequent UV exposure with higher radiation doses that can lead to erythema or even sunburn should be avoided at all costs [116].

However, it is also undisputed that sunlight, as the most important physical environmental factor in human evolution, has a positive influence on many human physiological processes and that insufficient sun exposure has become a real public health problem [117]. The positive aspects of moderate UVR exposure on numerous areas of human physiology relate not only to the UV-mediated synthesis of the vitamin D required throughout the organism, but also, as has recently been recognized, to the release of NO by photodecomposition of cutaneous NO precursors, such as the photolabile NO derivatives nitrite and RSNO [79,118,119]. In the current literature, a positive effect is attributed to both UVR-dependent factors on a wide variety of physiological processes, with the positive effect on the cardiovascular system being particularly emphasized [118]. Against this background, it makes perfect sense to point out that a system of increased cutaneous NOD concentration, either through food or exogenous application, as well as moderate UVR exposure, represents a cardiovascular supportive measure [120].

Furthermore, although epidemiological, mechanistic, and study data provide solid evidence that sunlight is a risk factor for skin cancer, the prevalence of cardiovascular and cerebrovascular death is about 100 times higher than that of skin cancer. Interventions that result in small changes in the incidence of cardiovascular disease therefore have even greater public health benefits than large changes in skin cancer. Epidemiological and mechanistic data now suggest that sunlight has cardiovascular benefits. A priority of photobiology research should now be the development of advice that balances the established carcinogenic effects of ultraviolet radiation with the possible or probable benefits of the same UV radiation on cardiovascular health and all-cause mortality [118,121].

8. Summary and Conclusions

There is a strong line of evidence to show that an increase in NO bioavailability has beneficial effects on health. In this context, bioactive NODs such as nitrite and S-nitrosylated proteins are jointly responsible for NOS-independent NO generation and may act as an NO store or back-up system when oxygen-dependent NO synthesis is compromised. Human skin can store and contain comparatively high concentrations of these NODs. The modulation of these stores, as shown in Figure 5 (e.g., by nitrate-rich diet, NO donor, CAP), and/or the induction of dermal NO release by NOD decomposition (e.g., by UVA/blue light) may represent promising therapeutic strategies against local pathological conditions such as disturbed microcirculation, skin infections, and impaired wound healing, and also against systemic conditions such as hypertension, arteriosclerosis, and diabetes.

However, it seems that many other factors, in particular the levels of antioxidants, have a strong impact on NO release. Moreover, further studies are necessary concerning NOD stores and possible premature skin ageing and/or skin cancerogenesis.

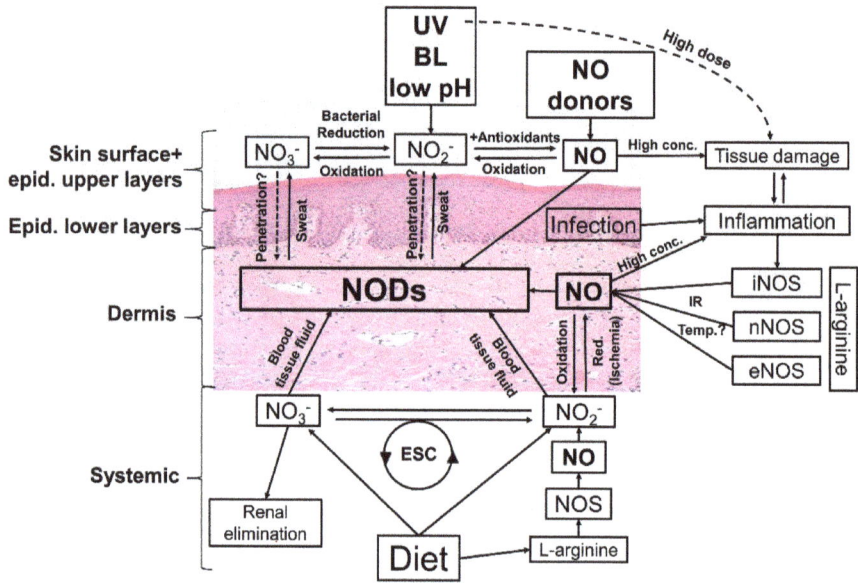

Figure 5. Possible ways to modulate the nitric oxide derivates (NODs) in the human skin. Targeting the skin there are many ways to affect the amounts and composition of NODs in skin tissues. Topical application of nitric oxide (NO) donors and nitrate (NO_3), nitrite (NO_2) +/− acidification can increase the NOD concentrations in skin layers and eventually in underlying tissues and circulation. Irradiation with UV/UVA, or blue light (BL)-photolabile NODs found in skin, in particular nitrite, generates NO, which in turn penetrates deeper in the skin and may directly enter the circulatory system and/or react to bioactive NODs, exerting vasodilatory effects and lowering the blood pressure. By tissue damage, infection, and inflammation, the inducible NO synthase (iNOS) is activated, producing high amounts of NO via reduction of L-arginine. The generated NO reacts in the skin with biomolecules (e.g., proteins) or is oxidized to nitrite/nitrate, leading to an increase in NOD content in the skin. It seems possible to enhance the activity of iNOS and also the constitutively expressed eNOS and/or nNOS via higher temperature/infrared radiation (IR). By oral intake of nitrate/nitrite it is possible to increase, with help of the enterosalivary circle (ESC), the general amount of NODs in the human body and theoretically also the NODs in the skin. A major part of nitrate is excreted via the urine, which opens up further possibilities for influencing blood and therefore tissue concentrations of nitrate and perhaps further NODs.

Supplementary Materials: The following supporting information can be downloaded at: https://www.mdpi.com/article/10.3390/biomedicines10092124/s1, Methods S1 [64,82,113,122–125].

Author Contributions: Conceptualization, C.O. and C.V.S.; methodology, C.O. and C.V.S.; investigation, C.O., M.v.K. and D.F.; resources, C.O.; data curation, C.O. and C.V.S.; writing—original draft preparation, C.O. and C.V.S.; writing—review and editing, D.F. and M.v.K.; visualization, C.O.; supervision, C.O.; project administration, C.O.; funding acquisition, C.O. All authors have read and agreed to the published version of the manuscript.

Funding: This research was funded by GERMAN RESEARCH FOUNDATION DFG, grant number OP 207/11-1, and by the internal grant program (project IFF 2022-18) of the Faculty of Health at Witten/Herdecke University, Germany.

Institutional Review Board Statement: The use of human material was approved by the local ethics committees of the Medical Faculty of the RWTH University Aachen (Votum No. EK163/07) and the Medical Faculty of the Heinrich-Heine-University Düsseldorf (Study No. 3634). All experiments were conducted in compliance with the Declaration of Helsinki Principles.

Informed Consent Statement: Informed consent was obtained from all subjects involved in the study.

Data Availability Statement: The data that support the findings of this study are available from the corresponding author upon reasonable request.

Conflicts of Interest: The authors declare no conflict of interest.

References

1. Lancaster, J.R., Jr. A tutorial on the diffusibility and reactivity of free nitric oxide. *Nitric Oxide* **1997**, *1*, 18–30. [CrossRef] [PubMed]
2. Knowles, R.G.; Moncada, S. Nitric oxide synthases in mammals. *Biochem. J.* **1994**, *298*, 249–258. [CrossRef]
3. Marsden, P.; Heng, H.; Scherer, S.; Stewart, R.; Hall, A.; Shi, X.; Tsui, L.; Schappert, K. Structure and chromosomal localization of the human constitutive endothelial nitric oxide synthase gene. *J. Biol. Chem.* **1993**, *268*, 17478–17488. [CrossRef]
4. Cary, S.P.; Winger, J.A.; Derbyshire, E.R.; Marletta, M.A. Nitric oxide signaling: No longer simply on or off. *Trends Biochem. Sci.* **2006**, *31*, 231–239. [CrossRef] [PubMed]
5. Snyder, S.H. Nitric Oxide: First in a New Class of Neurotransmitters. *Science* **1992**, *257*, 494–496. [CrossRef]
6. Förstermann, U.; Closs, E.I.; Pollock, J.S.; Nakane, M.; Schwarz, P.; Gath, I.; Kleinert, H. Nitric oxide synthase isozymes. Characterization, purification, molecular cloning, and functions. *Hypertension* **1994**, *23*, 1121–1131. [CrossRef] [PubMed]
7. Peunova, N.; Enikolopov, G. Amplification of calcium-induced gene transcription by nitric oxide in neuronal cells. *Nature* **1993**, *364*, 450–453. [CrossRef]
8. Weiss, G.; Goossen, B.; Doppler, W.; Fuchs, D.; Pantopoulos, K.; Werner-Felmayer, G.; Wachter, H.; Hentze, M.W. Translational regulation via iron-responsive elements by the nitric ox-ide/NO-synthase pathway. *Embo J.* **1993**, *12*, 3651–3657. [CrossRef]
9. Mayer, B.; John, M.; Bohme, E. Purification of a Ca^{2+}/calmodulin-dependent nitric oxide synthase from porcine cerebellum. Cofactor-role of tetrahydrobiopterin. *FEBS Lett.* **1990**, *277*, 215–219. [CrossRef]
10. De Tejada, I.S.; Goldstein, I.; Azadzoi, K.; Krane, R.J.; Cohen, R.A. Impaired Neurogenic and Endothelium-Mediated Relaxation of Penile Smooth Muscle from Diabetic Men with Impotence. *N. Engl. J. Med.* **1989**, *320*, 1025–1030. [CrossRef]
11. Ignarro, L.J.; Bush, P.A.; Buga, G.M.; Wood, K.S.; Fukuto, J.M.; Rajfer, J. Nitric oxide and cyclic GMP formation upon electrical field stimulation cause relaxation of corpus cavernosum smooth muscle. *Biochem. Biophys. Res. Commun.* **1990**, *170*, 843–850. [CrossRef]
12. Schlossmann, J.; Feil, R.; Hofmann, F. Signaling through NO and cGMP-dependent protein kinases. *Ann Med.* **2003**, *35*, 21–27. [CrossRef] [PubMed]
13. Moncada, S.; Higgs, E.A. Endogenous nitric oxide: Physiology, pathology and clinical relevance. *Eur. J. Clin. Investig.* **1991**, *21*, 361–374. [CrossRef]
14. Nathan, C.; Xie, Q.-W. Nitric oxide synthases: Roles, tolls, and controls. *Cell* **1994**, *78*, 915–918. [CrossRef]
15. Granger, D.L.; Hibbs, J.B.; Perfect, J.R.; Durack, D.T. Metabolic fate of L-arginine in relation to microbiostatic capability of murine macrophages. *J. Clin. Investig.* **1990**, *85*, 264–273. [CrossRef]
16. Moncada, S.; Higgs, A. The L-arginine-nitric oxide pathway. *N. Engl. J. Med.* **1993**, *329*, 2002–2012.
17. Moncada, S.; Bolanos, J.P. Nitric oxide, cell bioenergetics and neurodegeneration. *J. Neurochem.* **2006**, *97*, 1676–1689. [CrossRef]
18. Blouet, C.; Mariotti, F.; Mathe, V.; Tome, D.; Huneau, J.-F. Nitric Oxide Bioavailability and Not Production Is First Altered During the Onset of Insulin Resistance in Sucrose-Fed Rats. *Exp. Biol. Med.* **2007**, *232*, 1458–1464. [CrossRef]
19. Chen, K.; Pittman, R.N.; Popel, A. Nitric Oxide in the Vasculature: Where Does It Come from and Where Does It Go? A Quantitative Perspective. *Antioxid. Redox Signal.* **2008**, *10*, 1185–1198. [CrossRef]
20. Moncada, S.; Higgs, E.A. The discovery of nitric oxide and its role in vascular biology. *J. Cereb. Blood Flow Metab.* **2006**, *147*, S193–S201. [CrossRef]
21. Luiking, Y.C.; Engelen, M.P.; Deutz, N.E. Regulation of nitric oxide production in health and disease. *Curr. Opin. Clin. Nutr. Metab. Care* **2010**, *13*, 97–104. [CrossRef]
22. Cals-Grierson, M.-M.; Ormerod, A.D. Nitric oxide function in the skin. *Nitric Oxide* **2004**, *10*, 179–193. [CrossRef]
23. Änggård, E. Nitric oxide: Mediator, murderer, and medicine. *Lancet* **1994**, *343*, 1199–1206. [CrossRef]
24. Goldsmith, P.C.; Leslie, T.A.; Hayes, N.A.; Levell, N.J.; Dowd, P.M.; Foreman, J.C. Inhibitors of Nitric Oxide Synthase in Human Skin. *J. Investig. Dermatol.* **1996**, *106*, 113–118. [CrossRef]
25. Bruch-Gerharz, D.; Ruzicka, T.; Kolb Bachofen, V. Nitric oxide and its implications in skin homeostasis and dis-ease—A review. *Arch. Dermatol. Res.* **1998**, *290*, 643–651. [CrossRef]
26. Liew, F.Y.; Cox, F.E.G. Nonspecific defense mechanism: The role of nitric oxide. *Immunol. Today* **1991**, *12*, A17–A21. [CrossRef]
27. Stenger, S.; Donhauser, N.; Thüring, H.; Röllinghoff, M.; Bogdan, C. Reactivation of latent leishmaniasis by inhibition of inducible nitric oxide synthase. *J. Exp. Med.* **1996**, *183*, 1501–1514. [CrossRef]
28. Kolb-Bachofen, V.; Fehsel, K.; Michel, G.; Ruzicka, T. Epidermal keratinocyte expression of inducible nitric oxide synthase in skin lesions of psoriasis vulgaris. *Lancet* **1994**, *344*, 139. [CrossRef]
29. Bécherel, P.-A.; Le Goff, L.; Ktorza, S.; Chosidow, O.; Francès, C.; Issaly, F.; Mencia-Huerta, J.-M.; Debre, P.; Mossalayi, M.D.; Arock, M. CD23-Mediated Nitric Oxide Synthase Pathway Induction in Human Keratinocytes Is Inhibited by Retinoic Acid Derivatives. *J. Investig. Dermatol.* **1996**, *106*, 1182–1186. [CrossRef]

30. Kuhn, A.; Fehsel, K.; Lehmann, P.; Krutmann, J.; Ruzicka, T.; Kolb-Bachofen, V. Aberrant Timing in Epidermal Expression of Inducible Nitric Oxide Synthase After UV Irradiation in Cutaneous Lupus Erythematosus. *J. Investig. Dermatol.* **1998**, *111*, 149–153. [CrossRef]
31. Frank, S.; Kämpfer, H.; Wetzler, C.; Pfeilschifter, J. Nitric oxide drives skin repair: Novel functions of an established mediator. *Kidney Int.* **2002**, *61*, 882–888. [CrossRef]
32. Krischel, V.; Bruch-Gerharz, D.; Suschek, C.; Kröncke, K.-D.; Ruzicka, T.; Kolb-Bachofen, V. Biphasic Effect of Exogenous Nitric Oxide on Proliferation and Differentiation in Skin Derived Keratinocytes but Not Fibroblasts. *J. Investig. Dermatol.* **1998**, *111*, 286–291. [CrossRef]
33. Ishii, Y.; Ogura, T.; Tatemichi, M.; Fujisawa, H.; Otsuka, F.; Esumi, H. Induction of matrix metalloproteinase gene transcription by nitric oxide and mechanisms of MMP-1 gene induction in human melanoma cell lines. *Int. J. Cancer* **2002**, *103*, 161–168. [CrossRef]
34. Witte, M.B.; Thornton, F.J.; Efron, D.T.; Barbul, A. Enhancement of Fibroblast Collagen Synthesis by Nitric Oxide. *Nitric Oxide* **2000**, *4*, 572–582. [CrossRef]
35. Thornton, F.J.; Schäffer, M.R.; Witte, M.B.; Moldawer, L.L.; MacKay, S.L.; Abouhamze, A.; Tannahill, C.L.; Barbul, A. Enhanced Collagen Accumulation Following Direct Transfection of the Inducible Nitric Oxide Synthase Gene in Cutaneous Wounds. *Biochem. Biophys. Res. Commun.* **1998**, *246*, 654–659. [CrossRef]
36. Umbrello, M.; Dyson, A.; Pinto, B.B.; Fernandez, B.O.; Simon, V.; Feelisch, M.; Singer, M. Short-term hypoxic vasodilationin vivois mediated by bioactive nitric oxide metabolites, rather than free nitric oxide derived from haemoglobin-mediated nitrite reduction. *J. Physiol.* **2014**, *592*, 1061–1075. [CrossRef]
37. Abu-Soud, H.M.; Hazen, S.L. Nitric Oxide Is a Physiological Substrate for Mammalian Peroxidases. *J. Biol. Chem.* **2000**, *275*, 37524–37532. [CrossRef]
38. Eiserich, J.P.; Baldus, S.; Brennan, M.-L.; Hoffman, S.L.; Zhang, C.; Tousson, A.; Castro, L.; Lusis, A.J.; Nauseef, W.M.; White, C.R.; et al. Myeloperoxidase, a Leukocyte-Derived Vascular NO Oxidase. *Science* **2002**, *296*, 2391–2394. [CrossRef]
39. Suschek, C.V.; Opländer, C.; van Faassen, E.E. Non-enzymatic NO production in human skin: Effect of UVA on cutaneous NO stores. *Nitric Oxide* **2010**, *22*, 120–135. [CrossRef]
40. DeMartino, A.W.; Kim-Shapiro, D.B.; Patel, R.P.; Gladwin, M.T. Nitrite and nitrate chemical biology and signalling. *J. Cereb. Blood Flow Metab.* **2018**, *176*, 228–245. [CrossRef]
41. Gladwin, M.T.; Schechter, A.N.; Kim-Shapiro, D.B.; Patel, R.; Hogg, N.; Shiva, S.; Cannon, R.O.; Kelm, M.; Wink, D.A.; Espey, M.G.; et al. The emerging biology of the nitrite anion. *Nat. Chem. Biol.* **2005**, *1*, 308–314. [CrossRef]
42. Mirna, A.; Hofmann, K. Über den Verbleib von Nitrit in Fleischwaren. 1. Umsetzung von Nitrit mit Sulfhydryl-Verbindungen. *Fleischwirtschaft* **1969**, *49*, 1362–1366.
43. Cammack, R.; Joannou, C.; Cui, X.-Y.; Martinez, C.T.; Maraj, S.R.; Hughes, M.N. Nitrite and nitrosyl compounds in food preservation. *Biochim. Biophys. Acta* **1999**, *1411*, 475–488. [CrossRef]
44. Gangolli, S.D.; Brandt, P.A.V.D.; Feron, V.J.; Janzowsky, C.; Koeman, J.H.; Speijers, G.J.; Spiegelhalder, B.; Walker, R.; Wishnok, J.S. Nitrate, nitrite and N-nitroso compounds. *Eur. J. Pharmacol. Environ. Toxicol. Pharmacol.* **1994**, *292*, 1–38. [CrossRef]
45. Wishnok, J.S.; Tannenbaum, S.R.; Tamir, S. Endogenous formation of nitrate. Health aspects of nitrate and its metabolites (particularly nitrite). In Proceedings of the International Workshop, Bilthoven, The Netherlands, 1994; Council of Europe Press: Bilthoven, The Netherlands, 1995; pp. 151–179.
46. Walker, R. The metabolism of dietary nitrites and nitrates. *Biochem. Soc. Trans.* **1996**, *24*, 780–785. [CrossRef]
47. Lin, J. Nitrosamines as potential environmental carcinogens in man. *Clin. Biochem.* **1990**, *23*, 67–71. [CrossRef]
48. Lidder, S.; Webb, A.J. Vascular Effects of Dietary Nitrate (as Found in Green Leafy Vegetables and Beetroot) via the Nitrate-Nitrite-Nitric Oxide Pathway. *Br. J. Clin. Pharmacol.* **2013**, *75*, 677–696. [CrossRef] [PubMed]
49. Babateen, A.M.; Fornelli, G.; Donini, L.; Mathers, J.C.; Siervo, M. Assessment of dietary nitrate intake in humans: A systematic review. *Am. J. Clin. Nutr.* **2018**, *108*, 878–888. [CrossRef]
50. Wylie, L.J.; Kelly, J.; Bailey, S.J.; Blackwell, J.R.; Skiba, P.F.; Winyard, P.G.; Jeukendrup, A.E.; Vanhatalo, A.; Jones, A.M. Beetroot juice and exercise: Pharmacodynamic and dose-response relationships. *J. Appl. Physiol.* **2013**, *115*, 325–336. [CrossRef]
51. Siervo, M.; Scialò, F.; Shannon, O.M.; Stephan, B.C.; Ashor, A.W. Does dietary nitrate say NO to cardiovascular ageing? Current evidence and implications for research. *Proc. Nutr. Soc.* **2018**, *77*, 112–123. [CrossRef]
52. Bryan, N.S. Dietary Nitrite: From menace to marvel. *Funct. Foods Health Dis.* **2016**, *6*, 691. [CrossRef]
53. Lundberg, J.O.; Carlstrom, M.; Larsen, F.J.; Weitzberg, E. Roles of dietary inorganic nitrate in cardiovascular health and disease. *Cardiovasc. Res.* **2010**, *89*, 525–532. [CrossRef]
54. Matin, A.M.; Boie, E.T.; Moore, G.P. Survival after self-poisoning with sodium nitrite: A case report. *J. Am. Coll. Emerg. Physicians Open* **2022**, *3*, 12702. [CrossRef]
55. Lundberg, J.O.; Weitzberg, E.; Gladwin, M.T. The nitrate–nitrite–nitric oxide pathway in physiology and therapeutics. *Nat. Rev. Drug Discov.* **2008**, *7*, 156–167. [CrossRef] [PubMed]
56. McNally, B.; Griffin, J.L.; Roberts, L.D. Dietary inorganic nitrate: From villain to hero in metabolic disease? *Mol. Nutr. Food Res.* **2015**, *60*, 67–78. [CrossRef]
57. Duncan, C.; Dougall, H.; Johnston, P.R.; Green, S.; Brogan, R.; Leifert, C.; Smith, L.; Golden, M.H.N.; Benjamin, N. Chemical generation of nitric oxide in the mouth from the enterosalivary circulation of dietary nitrate. *Nat. Med.* **1995**, *1*, 546–551. [CrossRef] [PubMed]

58. Henrohn, D.; Björkstrand, K.; Lundberg, J.O.; Granstam, S.-O.; Baron, T.; Ingimarsdóttir, I.J.; Hedenström, H.; Malinovschi, A.; Wernroth, M.-L.; Jansson, M.; et al. Effects of Oral Supplementation with Nitrate-Rich Beetroot Juice in Patients with Pulmonary Arterial Hypertension—Results From BEET-PAH, an Exploratory Randomized, Double-Blind, Placebo-Controlled, Crossover Study. *J. Card. Fail.* **2018**, *24*, 640–653. [CrossRef] [PubMed]
59. Lundberg, J.O.; Govoni, M. Inorganic nitrate is a possible source for systemic generation of nitric oxide. *Free Radic. Biol. Med.* **2004**, *37*, 395–400. [CrossRef]
60. Archer, D.L. Evidence that Ingested Nitrate and Nitrite Are Beneficial to Health. *J. Food Prot.* **2002**, *65*, 872–875. [CrossRef]
61. Green, L.C.; Wagner, D.A.; Glogowski, J.; Skipper, P.L.; Wishnok, J.S.; Tannenbaum, S.R. Analysis of nitrate, nitrite, and [15N] nitrate in biological fluids. *Anal. Biochem.* **1982**, *126*, 131–138. [CrossRef]
62. Weller, R.; Pattullo, S.; Smith, L.; Golden, M.; Ormerod, A.; Benjamin, N. Nitric Oxide Is Generated on the Skin Surface by Reduction of Sweat Nitrate. *J. Investig. Dermatol.* **1996**, *107*, 327–331. [CrossRef] [PubMed]
63. Nyakayiru, J.; Kouw, I.; Cermak, N.M.; Senden, J.M.; van Loon, L.J.; Verdijk, L.B. Sodium nitrate ingestion increases skeletal muscle nitrate content in humans. *J. Appl. Physiol.* **2017**, *123*, 637–644. [CrossRef] [PubMed]
64. Paunel, A.N.; Dejam, A.; Thelen, S.; Kirsch, M.; Horstjann, M.; Gharini, P.; Mürtz, M.; Kelm, M.; de Groot, H.; Kolb-Bachofen, V.; et al. Enzyme-independent nitric oxide formation during UVA challenge of human skin: Characterization, molecular sources, and mechanisms. *Free Radic. Biol. Med.* **2005**, *38*, 606–615. [CrossRef] [PubMed]
65. Mowbray, M.; McLintock, S.; Weerakoon, R.; Lomatschinsky, N.; Jones, S.; Rossi, A.G.; Weller, R. Enzyme-Independent NO Stores in Human Skin: Quantification and Influence of UV Radiation. *J. Investig. Dermatol.* **2009**, *129*, 834–842. [CrossRef] [PubMed]
66. Bryan, N.S.; Fernandez, B.; Bauer, S.M.; Garcia-Saura, M.F.; Milsom, A.B.; Rassaf, T.; Maloney, R.E.; Bharti, A.; Rodriguez, J.; Feelisch, M. Nitrite is a signaling molecule and regulator of gene expression in mammalian tissues. *Nat. Chem. Biol.* **2005**, *1*, 290–297. [CrossRef]
67. Whitlock, D.R.; Feelisch, M. Soil bacteria, nitrite and the skin. In *The Hygiene Hypothesis and Darwinian Medicine*; Rook, G.A.W., Ed.; Progress in Inflammation Research: Birkhäuser, Basel, 2009; pp. 103–115.
68. Opländer, C.; Rösner, J.; Gombert, A.; Brodski, A.; Suvorava, T.; Grotheer, V.; van Faassen, E.E.; Kröncke, K.-D.; Kojda, G.; Windolf, J.; et al. Redox-mediated mechanisms and biological responses of copper-catalyzed reduction of the nitrite ion in vitro. *Nitric Oxide* **2013**, *35*, 152–164. [CrossRef]
69. Opländer, C.; Müller, T.; Baschin, M.; Bozkurt, A.; Grieb, G.; Windolf, J.; Pallua, N.; Suschek, C.V. Characterization of novel nitrite-based nitric oxide generating delivery systems for topical dermal application. *Nitric Oxide* **2012**, *28*, 24–32. [CrossRef]
70. Opländer, C.; Römer, A.; Paunel-Görgülü, A.; Fritsch, T.; Van Faassen, E.E.; Mürtz, M.; Bozkurt, A.; Grieb, G.; Fuchs, P.; Pallua, N.; et al. Dermal Application of Nitric Oxide In Vivo: Kinetics, Biological Responses, and Therapeutic Potential in Humans. *Clin. Pharmacol. Ther.* **2012**, *91*, 1074–1082. [CrossRef]
71. Peng, Y.; Cui, X.; Liu, Y.; Li, Y.; Liu, J.; Cheng, B. Systematic Review Focusing on the Excretion and Protection Roles of Sweat in the Skin. *Dermatology* **2014**, *228*, 115–120. [CrossRef]
72. Hagel, A.F.; Albrecht, H.; Dauth, W.; Hagel, W.; Vitali, F.; Ganzleben, I.; Schultis, H.W.; Konturek, P.C.; Stein, J.; Neurath, M.F.; et al. Plasma concentrations of ascorbic acid in a cross section of the German population. *J. Int. Med. Res.* **2017**, *46*, 168–174. [CrossRef]
73. Stauber, J.; Florence, T. A comparative study of copper, lead, cadmium and zinc in human sweat and blood. *Sci. Total Environ.* **1988**, *74*, 235–247. [CrossRef]
74. Furchgott, R.F.; Ehrreich, S.J.; Greenblatt, E. The Photoactivated Relaxation of Smooth Muscle of Rabbit Aorta. *J. Gen. Physiol.* **1961**, *44*, 499. [CrossRef] [PubMed]
75. Matsunaga, K.; Furchgott, R.F. Interactions of light and sodium nitrite in producing relaxation of rabbit aorta. *J. Pharmacol. Exp. Ther.* **1989**, *248*, 687–695.
76. Strehlow, H.; Wagner, I. Flash Photolysis in Aqueous Nitrite Solutions. *Z. Für Phys. Chem.* **1982**, *132*, 151–160. [CrossRef]
77. Opländer, C.; Suschek, C.V. The Role of Photolabile Dermal Nitric Oxide Derivates in Ultraviolet Radiation (UVR)-Induced Cell Death. *Int. J. Mol. Sci.* **2012**, *14*, 191–204. [CrossRef]
78. Opländer, C.; Volkmar, C.M.; Paunel-Görgülü, A.; Van Faassen, E.E.; Heiss, C.; Kelm, M.; Halmer, D.; Mürtz, M.; Pallua, N.; Suschek, C.V. Whole Body UVA Irradiation Lowers Systemic Blood Pressure by Release of Nitric Oxide From Intracutaneous Photolabile Nitric Oxide Derivates. *Circ. Res.* **2009**, *105*, 1031–1040. [CrossRef]
79. Feelisch, M.; Kolb-Bachofen, V.; Liu, D.; Lundberg, J.O.; Revelo, L.P.; Suschek, C.V.; Weller, R.B. Is sunlight good for our heart? *Eur. Heart J.* **2010**, *31*, 1041–1045. [CrossRef]
80. Weller, R. Sunlight Has Cardiovascular Benefits Independently of Vitamin D. *Blood Purif.* **2016**, *41*, 130–134. [CrossRef]
81. Liu, D.; Fernandez, B.O.; Hamilton, A.; Lang, N.N.; Gallagher, J.M.; Newby, D.E.; Feelisch, M.; Weller, R.B. UVA Irradiation of Human Skin Vasodilates Arterial Vasculature and Lowers Blood Pressure Independently of Nitric Oxide Synthase. *J. Investig. Dermatol.* **2014**, *134*, 1839–1846. [CrossRef]
82. Opländer, C.; Deck, A.; Volkmar, C.M.; Kirsch, M.; Liebmann, J.; Born, M.; van Abeelen, F.; van Faassen, E.E.; Kröncke, K.-D.; Windolf, J.; et al. Mechanism and biological relevance of blue-light (420–453 nm)-induced nonenzymatic nitric oxide generation from photolabile nitric oxide derivates in human skin in vitro and in vivo. *Free Radic. Biol. Med.* **2013**, *65*, 1363–1377. [CrossRef]
83. Pelegrino, M.T.; Paganotti, A.; Seabra, A.B.; Weller, R.B. Photochemistry of nitric oxide and S-nitrosothiols in human skin. *Histochem. Cell Biol.* **2020**, *153*, 431–441. [CrossRef]

84. Suschek, C.V.; Schroeder, P.; Aust, O.; Sies, H.; Mahotka, C.; Horstjann, M.; Ganser, H.; Mürtz, M.; Hering, P.; Schnorr, O.; et al. The presence of nitrite during UVA irradiation protects from apoptosis. *FASEB J.* **2003**, *17*, 2342–2344. [CrossRef] [PubMed]
85. Oplander, C.; Wetzel, W.; Cortese, M.M.; Pallua, N.; Suschek, C.V. Evidence for a physiological role of intracellularly occurring pho-tolabile nitrogen oxides in human skin fibroblasts. *Free. Radic. Biol. Med.* **2008**, *44*, 1752–1761. [CrossRef] [PubMed]
86. Opländer, C.; Cortese, M.M.; Korth, H.-G.; Kirsch, M.; Mahotka, C.; Wetzel, W.; Pallua, N.; Suschek, C.V. The impact of nitrite and antioxidants on ultraviolet-A-induced cell death of human skin fibroblasts. *Free Radic. Biol. Med.* **2007**, *43*, 818–829. [CrossRef]
87. Stern, M.; Broja, M.; Sansone, R.; Gröne, M.; Skene, S.; Liebmann, J.; Suschek, C.V.; Born, M.; Kelm, M.; Heiss, C. Blue light exposure decreases systolic blood pressure, arterial stiffness, and improves endothelial function in humans. *Eur. J. Prev. Cardiol.* **2018**, *25*, 1875–1883. [CrossRef] [PubMed]
88. Barolet, A.C.; Barolet, D.; Cormack, G.; Auclair, M.; Lachance, G. In vivo quantification of nitric oxide (NO) release from intact human skin following exposure to photobiomodulation wavelengths in the visible and near infrared spectrum. In Proceedings of the Mechanisms of Photobiomodulation Therapy XIV, San Francisco, CA, USA, 2–3 February 2019. [CrossRef]
89. Barolet, A. *Photobiomodulation in the Near Infrared and Red Spectra Induces Nitric Oxide Release in Ex-Vivo Human Skin Homogenate via Enzymatic Pathways*; McGill University: Montreal, QC, Canada, 2021.
90. Rizzi, M.; Migliario, M.; Tonello, S.; Rocchetti, V.; Renò, F. Photobiomodulation induces in vitro re-epithelialization via nitric oxide production. *Lasers Med. Sci.* **2018**, *33*, 1003–1008. [CrossRef]
91. Zhou, X.; Zhang, J.; Feng, G.; Shen, J.; Kong, D.; Zhao, Q. Nitric Oxide-Releasing Biomaterials for Biomedical Applications. *Curr. Med. Chem.* **2016**, *23*, 2579–2601. [CrossRef]
92. Ahmed, R.; Augustine, R.; Chaudhry, M.; Akhtar, U.A.; Zahid, A.A.; Tariq, M.; Falahati, M.; Ahmad, I.S.; Hasan, A. Nitric oxide-releasing biomaterials for promoting wound healing in impaired diabetic wounds: State of the art and recent trends. *Biomed. Pharmacother.* **2022**, *149*, 112707. [CrossRef]
93. Zhang, Y.; Tang, K.; Chen, B.; Zhou, S.; Li, N.; Liu, C.; Yang, J.; Lin, R.; Zhang, T.; He, W. A polyethylenimine-based diazeniumdiolate nitric oxide donor accelerates wound healing. *Biomater. Sci.* **2019**, *7*, 1607–1616. [CrossRef]
94. Weller, R.; Finnen, M.J. The effects of topical treatment with acidified nitrite on wound healing in normal and diabetic mice. *Nitric Oxide* **2006**, *15*, 395–399. [CrossRef]
95. Ormerod, A.D.; Shah, A.A.; Li, H.; Benjamin, N.B.; Ferguson, G.P.; Leifert, C. An observational prospective study of topical acidified nitrite for killing methicillin-resistant Staphylococcus aureus (MRSA) in contaminated wounds. *BMC Res. Notes* **2011**, *4*, 458. [CrossRef] [PubMed]
96. Levy, B.I.; Schiffrin, E.; Mourad, J.-J.; Agostini, D.; Vicaut, E.; Safar, M.E.; Struijker-Boudier, H.A. Impaired Tissue Perfusion. *Circulation* **2008**, *118*, 968–976. [CrossRef] [PubMed]
97. Lin, J.; Jia, C.; Wang, Y.; Jiang, S.; Jia, Z.; Chen, N.; Sheng, S.; Li, S.; Jiang, L.; Xu, H.; et al. Therapeutic potential of pravastatin for random skin flaps necrosis: Involvement of promoting angiogenesis and inhibiting apoptosis and oxidative stress. *Drug Des. Dev. Ther.* **2019**, *13*, 1461–1472. [CrossRef]
98. Engel, H.; Sauerbier, M.; Germann, G.; Küntscher, M.V. Dose-Dependent Effects of a Nitric Oxide Donor in a Rat Flap Model. *Ann. Plast. Surg.* **2007**, *58*, 456–460. [CrossRef] [PubMed]
99. Kroncke, K.D.; Fehsel, K.; Kolb-Bachofen, V. Nitric oxide: Cytotoxicity versus cytoprotection–how, why, when, and where? *Nitric Oxide* **1997**, *1*, 107–120. [CrossRef]
100. Kroncke, K.D.; Suschek, C.V.; Kolb-Bachofen, V. Implications of inducible nitric oxide synthase expression and en-zyme activity. *Antioxid. Redox Signal.* **2000**, *2*, 585–605. [CrossRef]
101. Bolanos, J.; Almeida, A.; Stewart, V.; Peuchen, S.; Land, J.M.; Clark, J.B.; Heales, S.J.R. Nitric Oxide-Mediated Mitochondrial Damage in the Brain: Mechanisms and Implications for Neurodegenerative Diseases. *J. Neurochem.* **2002**, *68*, 2227–2240. [CrossRef]
102. Ormerod, A.D.; Vader, P.C.V.V.; Majewski, S.; Vanscheidt, W.; Benjamin, N.; Van Der Meijden, W. Evaluation of the Efficacy, Safety, and Tolerability of 3 Dose Regimens of Topical Sodium Nitrite with Citric Acid in Patients with Anogenital Warts. *JAMA Dermatol.* **2015**, *151*, 854–861. [CrossRef]
103. Ormerod, A.; White, M.; Shah, S.; Benjamin, N. Molluscum contagiosum effectively treated with a topical acidified nitrite, nitric oxide liberating cream. *Br. J. Dermatol.* **1999**, *141*, 1051–1053. [CrossRef]
104. Mowbray, M.; Tan, X.; Wheatley, P.S.; Morris, R.E.; Weller, R.B. Topically Applied Nitric Oxide Induces T-Lymphocyte Infiltration in Human Skin, but Minimal Inflammation. *J. Investig. Dermatol.* **2008**, *128*, 352–360. [CrossRef]
105. Opländer, C.; Volkmar, C.M.; Paunel-Görgülü, A.; Fritsch, T.; van Faassen, E.E.; Mürtz, M.; Grieb, G.; Bozkurt, A.; Hemmrich, K.; Windolf, J.; et al. Dermal application of nitric oxide releasing acidified nitrite-containing liniments significantly reduces blood pressure in humans. *Nitric Oxide* **2012**, *26*, 132–140. [CrossRef] [PubMed]
106. Nosenko, T.; Shimizu, T.; Morfill, G.E. Designing plasmas for chronic wound disinfection. *New J. Phys.* **2009**, *11*, 115013. [CrossRef]
107. Shimizu, T.; Steffes, B.; Pompl, R.; Jamitzky, F.; Bunk, W.; Ramrath, K.; Georgi, M.; Stolz, W.; Schmidt, H.-U.; Urayama, T.; et al. Characterization of Microwave Plasma Torch for Decontamination. *Plasma Process. Polym.* **2008**, *5*, 577–582. [CrossRef]
108. Mann, M.S.; Tiede, R.; Gavenis, K.; Daeschlein, G.; Bussiahn, R.; Weltmann, K.-D.; Emmert, S.; Von Woedtke, T.; Ahmed, R. Introduction to DIN-specification 91315 based on the characterization of the plasma jet kINPen® MED. *Clin. Plasma Med.* **2016**, *4*, 35–45. [CrossRef]

109. Lademann, J.M.; Richter, H.; Alborova, A.; Humme, D.; Patzelt, A.; Kramer, A.; Weltmann, K.-D.; Hartmann, B.; Ottomann, C.; Fluhr, J.W.; et al. Risk assessment of the application of a plasma jet in dermatology. *J. Biomed. Opt.* **2009**, *14*, 054025. [CrossRef] [PubMed]
110. Von Woedtke, T.; Kramer, A.; Weltmann, K.-D. Plasma Sterilization: What are the Conditions to Meet this Claim? *Plasma Process. Polym.* **2008**, *5*, 534–539. [CrossRef]
111. Blackert, S.; Haertel, B.; Wende, K.; von Woedtke, T.; Lindequist, U. Influence of non-thermal atmospheric pressure plasma on cellular structures and processes in human keratinocytes (HaCaT). *J. Dermatol. Sci.* **2013**, *70*, 173–181. [CrossRef]
112. Plattfaut, I.; Besser, M.; Severing, A.-L.; Stürmer, E.K.; Opländer, C. Plasma medicine and wound management: Evaluation of the antibacterial efficacy of a medically certified cold atmospheric argon plasma jet. *Int. J. Antimicrob. Agents* **2021**, *57*, 106319. [CrossRef]
113. Heuer, K.; Hoffmanns, M.A.; Demir, E.; Baldus, S.; Volkmar, C.M.; Röhle, M.; Fuchs, P.C.; Awakowicz, P.; Suschek, C.V.; Opländer, C. The topical use of non-thermal dielectric barrier discharge (DBD): Nitric oxide related effects on human skin. *Nitric Oxide* **2015**, *44*, 52–60. [CrossRef]
114. Kisch, T.; Helmke, A.; Schleusser, S.; Song, J.; Liodaki, E.; Stang, F.H.; Mailaender, P.; Kraemer, R. Improvement of cutaneous microcirculation by cold atmospheric plasma (CAP): Results of a controlled, prospective cohort study. *Microvasc. Res.* **2015**, *104*, 55–62. [CrossRef]
115. Blot, S. Antiseptic mouthwash, the nitrate–nitrite–nitric oxide pathway, and hospital mortality: A hypothesis generating review. *Intensive Care Med.* **2020**, *47*, 28–38. [CrossRef] [PubMed]
116. Levine, J.A.; Sorace, M.; Spencer, J.; Siegel, D.M. The indoor UV tanning industry: A review of skin cancer risk, health benefit claims, and regulation. *J. Am. Acad. Dermatol.* **2005**, *53*, 1038–1044. [CrossRef] [PubMed]
117. Alfredsson, L.; Armstrong, B.K.; Butterfield, D.A.; Chowdhury, R.; De Gruijl, F.R.; Feelisch, M.; Garland, C.F.; Hart, P.H.; Hoel, D.G.; Jacobsen, R.; et al. Insufficient Sun Exposure Has Become a Real Public Health Problem. *Int. J. Environ. Res. Public Health* **2020**, *17*, 5014. [CrossRef] [PubMed]
118. Weller, R.B. The health benefits of UV radiation exposure through vitamin D production or non-vitamin D pathways. Blood pressure and cardiovascular disease. *Photochem. Photobiol. Sci.* **2016**, *16*, 374–380. [CrossRef]
119. Hoel, D.G.; De Gruijl, F.R. Sun Exposure Public Health Directives. *Int. J. Environ. Res. Public Health* **2018**, *15*, 2794. [CrossRef]
120. Johnson, R.S.; Titze, J.; Weller, R. Cutaneous control of blood pressure. *Curr. Opin. Nephrol. Hypertens.* **2016**, *25*, 11–15. [CrossRef]
121. Wright, F.; Weller, R.B. Risks and benefits of UV radiation in older people: More of a friend than a foe? *Maturitas* **2015**, *81*, 425–431. [CrossRef]
122. Suschek, C.V.; Paunel, A.; Kolb-Bachofen, V. Nonenzymatic Nitric Oxide Formation during Uva Irradiation of Human Skin: Experimental Setups and Ways to Measure. *Methods Enzymol.* **2005**, *396*, 568–578.
123. Ben-Sasson, S.A.; Sherman, Y.; Gavrieli, Y. Identification of Dying Cells–in Situ Staining. *Methods Cell Biol.* **1995**, *46*, 29–39.
124. Feelisch, M.; Rassaf, T.; Mnaimneh, S.; Singh, N.; Bryan, N.S.; Jourd'Heuil, D.; Kelm, M. Concomitant S-, N-, and Heme-Nitros(Yl)Ation in Biological Tissues and Fluids: Implications for the Fate of No in Vivo. *FASEB J.* **2002**, *16*, 1775–1785. [CrossRef]
125. Beckert, S.; Witte, M.B.; Konigsrainer, A.; Coerper, S. The Impact of the Micro-Lightguide O2c for the Quantification of Tissue Ischemia in Diabetic Foot Ulcers. *Diabetes Care* **2004**, *27*, 2863–2867. [CrossRef] [PubMed]

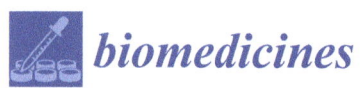

Review

Endothelial Nitric Oxide Synthase in the Perivascular Adipose Tissue

Andy W. C. Man, Yawen Zhou, Ning Xia and Huige Li *

Department of Pharmacology, Johannes Gutenberg University Medical Center, 55131 Mainz, Germany; wingcman@uni-mainz.de (A.W.C.M.); yawezhou@uni-mainz.de (Y.Z.); xianing@uni-mainz.de (N.X.)
* Correspondence: huigeli@uni-mainz.de

Abstract: Perivascular adipose tissue (PVAT) is a special type of ectopic fat depot that adheres to most vasculatures. PVAT has been shown to exert anticontractile effects on the blood vessels and confers protective effects against metabolic and cardiovascular diseases. PVAT plays a critical role in vascular homeostasis via secreting adipokine, hormones, and growth factors. Endothelial nitric oxide synthase (eNOS; also known as NOS3 or NOSIII) is well-known for its role in the generation of vasoprotective nitric oxide (NO). eNOS is primarily expressed, but not exclusively, in endothelial cells, while recent studies have identified its expression in both adipocytes and endothelial cells of PVAT. PVAT eNOS is an important player in the protective role of PVAT. Different studies have demonstrated that, under obesity-linked metabolic diseases, PVAT eNOS may be even more important than endothelium eNOS in obesity-induced vascular dysfunction, which may be attributed to certain PVAT eNOS-specific functions. In this review, we summarized the current understanding of eNOS expression in PVAT, its function under both physiological and pathological conditions and listed out a few pharmacological interventions of interest that target eNOS in PVAT.

Keywords: vascular function; obesity; nitric oxide; adiponectin; SIRT1

Citation: Man, A.W.C.; Zhou, Y.; Xia, N.; Li, H. Endothelial Nitric Oxide Synthase in the Perivascular Adipose Tissue. *Biomedicines* 2022, 10, 1754. https://doi.org/10.3390/biomedicines10071754

Academic Editors: Mats Eriksson and Anders O. Larsson

Received: 15 June 2022
Accepted: 18 July 2022
Published: 21 July 2022

Publisher's Note: MDPI stays neutral with regard to jurisdictional claims in published maps and institutional affiliations.

Copyright: © 2022 by the authors. Licensee MDPI, Basel, Switzerland. This article is an open access article distributed under the terms and conditions of the Creative Commons Attribution (CC BY) license (https://creativecommons.org/licenses/by/4.0/).

1. Introduction

Perivascular adipose tissue (PVAT) is a special type of ectopic fat depot that adheres to most large arteries and veins, small and resistance vessels, and microvessels of the musculoskeletal system [1]. The beneficial role of PVAT was first observed by Soltis and Cassis in the aorta of a Sprague–Dawley rat where that PVAT diminished agonists-induced vasocontraction in vitro [2]. Till now, PVAT has been shown to exert anticontractile effects in the blood vessels in both rodents and humans [3,4]. Similar to other adipose tissues, PVAT is an important endocrine tissue that secretes adipokines, hormones, growth factors, chemokine, reactive oxygen species (ROS), nitric oxide (NO), and hydrogen sulfide (H_2S) [1]. As PVAT has a very close proximity to the vasculature, PVAT has been recognized as an active player in vascular physiology and pathology, and studies of PVAT in maintaining vascular homeostasis have been focused on in recent decades. Endothelial nitric oxide synthase (eNOS; also known as NOS3 or NOSIII) is an enzyme named after the cell type (endothelial cell) in which it was first identified. eNOS is well-known for its role in the generation of vasoprotective NO. To date, numerous studies using global eNOS-deficient mice have demonstrated the antihypertensive, antithrombotic, and anti-atherosclerotic effects of eNOS, which were mainly attributed to NO derived from the endothelium. Indeed, eNOS expression has been identified in both endothelial cells and adipocytes in PVAT and both contribute to the production of vascular NO and modulate vascular pathophysiology [5,6]. Although there are reviews discussing several aspects of PVAT, the functions of eNOS in PVAT have not been fully described. This review will address the current understanding of PVAT eNOS and propose possible roles of eNOS in PVAT for future directions.

2. What Is Special about PVAT?

There are three layers in the vascular wall of blood vessels, namely tunica intima, tunica media, and tunica adventitia. The inner layer, tunica intima, consists of a single layer of flattened, polygonal endothelial cells supported by a basal lamina of connective tissues. Tunica media is the middle layer that mainly consists of vascular smooth muscle cells (VSMCs), especially in arteries. Tunica adventitia is the strongest layer that contains connective tissues and elastic fibers [7]. Different from other adipose tissues, PVAT can be found outside the adventitia of the systemic blood vessels, including arteries and veins, small and resistance vessels, and microvessels in skeletal muscles. PVAT is absent in microvasculature and the cerebral vasculature [8,9]. There are no laminar structures or barriers between PVAT and the adventitia layer of blood vessels.

PVAT is a highly heterogenous tissue. In addition to stem cells, immune cells, and nerves, both white and brown adipocytes can be found in PVAT. White adipocytes mainly act as energy storage in the form of triglyceride [10], while brown adipocytes are more metabolically active and associated with thermogenesis [11]. There are regional phenotypic and functional differences among the PVAT in different locations of the vascular system [8,9]. Depending on its location on the vascular bed, PVAT can be white adipose tissue (WAT)-like (such as mesenteric PVAT), brown adipose tissue (BAT)-like (such as thoracic aortic PVAT) or mixed (such as abdominal aortic PVAT). Vascularization and innervation of these PVATs, as well as their adipokine profiles also highly vary [8,9,12–14], which could explain the local functional differences of PVATs. However, the morphology of PVAT in other species are currently less characterized than that in murine models.

Studies have shown evidence that as an anatomically separated adipose tissue, adipocytes from different PVATs may arise from unique progenitor cells, giving rise to its distinctive morphological and functional characteristics compared to other adipose tissues [15–17]. Nevertheless, the origins of adipocytes in the PVAT and the precise process of PVAT development are barely known. A recent study suggested that adipocytes in periaortic PVAT may partly originate from progenitors expressing smooth muscle protein 22-alpha (SM22α) [18]. Thoracic periaortic PVAT may present both SM22α+ and myogenic factor 5 (Myf5+) origins [19], whereas these progenitor cells are able to differentiate into uncoupling protein-1 (UCP-1) positive adipocytes in vitro [20]. A recent study has also shown that fibroblastic progenitor cells, but not VSMCs, are responsible for the adipogenesis of thoracic PVAT [21]. The origins of adipocytes in abdominal periaortic PVAT are less known. They may share, at least, similar developmental origins with SM22α+ and peroxisome proliferator-activated receptor gamma (PPARγ+) VSMCs, as the absence of PPARγ in the VSMCs resulted in a complete lack of abdominal periaortic PVAT development [22]. In the same study, Chang et al. also suggested that mesenteric PVAT may share a similar developmental origin with VSMCs, since the absence of PPARγ in VSMCs also resulted in a dramatic loss of mesenteric PVAT, while other adipose tissues were not affected [22]. Indeed, studies have also suggested that the developmental origins of mesenteric PVAT may be similar to the visceral adipose tissues [23,24]. Taken together, the lack of the discovery of unique cell markers makes the generation of PVAT-specific gene modified mouse models and the mechanistical study of PVAT function a challenging task.

3. What Is the Function of PVAT?

Since the first attention to the paracrine effects of PVAT on blood vessels [2], growing studies, from experimental animal models to clinical samples, have indicated that the cross-talk between PVAT and its connecting vessel plays a critical role in the physiological homeostasis and pathological changes of the cardiovascular system. The paracrine crosstalk between PVAT and its connecting vessel can actively regulate vascular inflammation and remodeling [23], while PVAT can also act as an endocrine organ to modulate multiple biological processes by releasing adipokines [25]. In 2002, using the physiological buffer in which PVAT from a healthy rat was incubated, Lohn et al. observed a direct relaxation in precontracted, isolated, PVAT-removed rat thoracic aorta [26]. They concluded the presence of transferable soluble substances from the PVAT that were released to the buffer and caused relaxation. It is currently known that PVAT is capable to synthesize and secrete substances via endocrine and paracrine mechanisms, including adipokines, growth factors, ROS, NO, and H_2S [1]. The previous literature already explored the function of PVAT in detail [1,25,27–30]. Here, we briefly summarized the area of PVAT-derived adipokine production and vascular function regulation, and some novel findings of exosomes/extracellular vesicles (Figure 1).

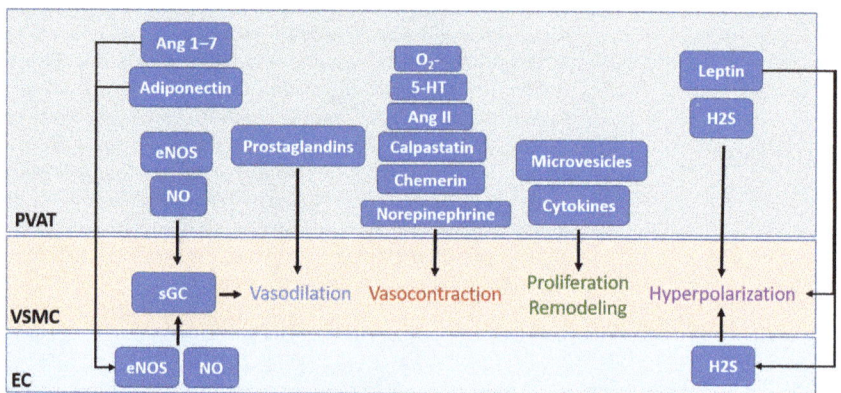

Figure 1. The crosstalk between PVAT and the vessel wall modulates vascular functions. PVAT releases vasoactive molecules, hormones, adipokines, and microvesicles. PVAT-derived relaxing factors (PVRFs) include leptin and adiponectin, hydrogen sulphide (H_2S), hydrogen peroxide (H_2O_2), prostaglandins, NO, and angiotensin (Ang) 1–7. PVAT-derived contracting factors (PVCFs) include chemerin, calpastatin, 5-hydroxytryptamine (5-HT), norepinephrine (NE), AngII, and ROS. These factors from PVAT may reach the endothelial layer of blood vessels by either direct diffusion or via vasa vasorum or small media conduit networks connecting the medial layer with the underlying adventitia and modulate vasodilation and vasocontraction. PVAT plays a critical role in vascular homeostasis via secreting adipokine, hormones, and growth factors to modulate the proliferation of VSMCs. Adipocytes from PVAT also secrete different types of extracellular vesicles, including exosomes and microvesicles, which have also been shown to trigger early vascular remodeling in vascular inflammation. Under pathological conditions, PVAT becomes dysfunctional, and the secretion of the PVAT-derived factor becomes imbalanced which could exert detrimental effects on vascular homeostasis and lead to vascular remodeling and arterial stiffening.

Similar to any other adipose tissues, PVAT plays a critical role in vascular homeostasis via secreting adipokine, hormones, and growth factors [31]. These PVAT-derived factors include both pro-inflammatory and anti-inflammatory vasoactive molecules that modulate vascular inflammation and oxidative stress, vascular tone, and VSMCs proliferation and migration [9,32]. In various models of metabolic and cardiovascular diseases, including obesity, hypertension, and diabetes, the loss of anticontractile function of PVAT was observed [33–35]. PVAT becomes dysfunctional and the secretion of the PVAT-derived factors becomes imbalanced which could exert detrimental effects on vascular homeostasis and lead to vascular remodeling and arterial stiffening [28,36–38].

It is currently known that PVAT exerts anticontractile function on the adherent blood vessel through secretion of various PVAT-derived relaxing factors (PVRFs), previously known as the adventitia-derived relaxing factors (ADRFs) [39]. Potential PVRFs include leptin and adiponectin [40], H_2S [41], hydrogen peroxide (H_2O_2) [42], prostaglandins [43,44], NO [45], and angiotensin (Ang) 1–7 [46]. In addition to PVRFs, recent studies have revealed that PVAT can secrete contracting factors (PVCFs) that modulate vasoconstriction [47–49]. Potential PVCFs include chemerin [50], calpastatin [51], 5-hydroxytryptamine (5-HT) [49], norepinephrine (NE) [52], AngII, and ROS [53]. Although the detailed mechanisms of how PVRFs and PVCFs exert their effects on the blood vessel remain unclear, it is hypothesized that PVAT modulates vascular functions through two distinct mechanisms: endothelium-dependent and endothelium-independent pathways [29,45]. These factors from PVAT may reach the endothelial layer of blood vessels by either direct diffusion or via vasa vasorum or small media conduit networks connecting the medial layer with the underlying adventitia [8,54,55] (Table 1). In addition, the same factors from PVAT can act as either PVRFs or PVCFs. For example, H_2S and prostanoids in PVAT have anticontractile effects under normal conditions, while they can induce contractile responses under disease conditions [56].

Table 1. List of focused PVAT-derived factors.

PVAT-Derived Factors	Effects	References
Adiponectin	Relaxation	[40]
Angiotensin (Ang) 1–7	Relaxation	[46]
Angiotensin II (Ang II)	Contraction	[14,56,57]
Calpastatin	Contraction	[51]
Chemerin	Contraction	[50,54]
Hydrogen peroxide (H_2O_2)	Relaxation	[42,55]
Hydrogen sulphide (H_2S)	Contraction	[41]
	Relaxation	[56,58]
Leptin	Relaxation	[57,59]
	Contraction	[51,60]
Nitric oxide (NO)	Relaxation	[45]
Norepinephrine (NE)	Contraction	[52]
Prostanoids		
-Prostaglandins	Contraction	[44,61]
-Prostacyclin	Relaxation	[22]
-Thromboxane	Contraction	[61]
Superoxide	Contraction	[53]
5-hydroxytryptamine (5-HT)	Contraction	[49]

A recent study has also shown that the anticontractile effects of PVAT can be attributed to its ability to uptake and metabolize vasoactive amines such as dopamine, NE, and 5-HT [62]. Monoamine oxidase A/B (MAO-A/B) catalyzes the oxidative deamination of vasoactive amines, while semicarbazide-sensitive amine oxidase (SSAO) catalyzes the generation of ammonia and H_2O_2. These two enzymes are present in PVAT, and the inhibition of these enzymes increased the NE-induced vasocontraction on vessel rings with PVAT [62]. PVAT can also prevent NE-induced vasocontraction, by taking up NE and preventing it from reaching the vessel wall [63].

In small arterioles, stepwise increase in blood pressure can induce vasoconstriction due to smooth muscle myogenic response, while this physiological function is absent in large arteries [64]. Until now, most of the in vitro pressure myograph studies about myogenic responses were performed in PVAT-denuded vessels. Therefore, there is an underlying question of whether PVAT may be involved in the regulation of myogenic responses. In resistance arteries with myogenic response, endothelial-derived hyperpolarization plays a more prominent role than NO in vasodilation [65]. Thus far, there has been no direct evidence on whether PVAT plays a role in myogenic response in vivo. Nevertheless, recent studies have shown the new function for PVAT in assisting stress-induced relaxation [66] and the presence of stretch sensitive, nonselective cation channel Piezo1 in PVAT [67]. These shed light on the possible function of PVAT in modulating myogenic responses.

Dysfunction of PVAT has also been linked to the development of atherosclerosis. Adipocytes and macrophages in PVAT can secrete various pro-inflammatory cytokines and adipokines including monocyte chemoattractant protein-1 (MCP-1), tumor necrosis factor alpha (TNF-α), leptin, adiponectin, omentin, etc. [68]. In obesity, inflammation in PVAT causes the phenotypic switch from anti-inflammatory to pro-inflammatory [69]. A recent study has also revealed that macrophage polarization in the PVAT is critically associated with coronary atherosclerosis [70]. M1 macrophages in the PVAT are positively correlated with a higher risk of coronary thrombosis and are correlated with plaque progression and destabilization. M2 macrophages in the PVAT are negatively correlated with increased arterial obstruction, calcification, necrosis, and decrease of the number of vasa vasorum in the adventitia layer [70]. Transplantation of PVAT from high-cholesterol diet-fed apolipoprotein E (ApoE) knockout mice to normal chow-fed ApoE-knockout mice resulted in a striking increase in atherosclerosis development [71]. These suggest that the inflammatory status of the PVAT is related to the progression of atherosclerosis.

Apart from the above secretory factors, adipocytes from PVAT also secrete different types of extracellular vesicles, including exosomes and microvesicles [72,73]. Exosomes are formed within the endosomal network and exocytosed by fusion with the plasma membrane, while microvesicles are directly formed from the plasma membrane. Extracellular vesicles are crucial regulators of vascular functions by transferring the enclosed biological messengers, including lipids, proteins, noncoding RNAs, and microRNAs (miRNAs) for intercellular communications [74]. Adipose tissues have been shown to produce circulating exosomal miRNAs, as a form of adipokine, to regulate gene expressions locally or distantly [75]. These miRNA-containing extracellular vesicles act as the agent for the crosstalk between adipose tissues and neighboring tissues, including endothelial cells, VSMCs, and macrophages [76–78]. In addition, the crosstalk between endothelial cells and adipocytes is modulated, at least partly, by the extracellular vesicles-mediated reciprocal trafficking of caveolin-1 (Cav-1) [79]. A recent study demonstrated that PVAT secretes encapsulated microRNAs, such as miR-221-3p, which can be taken up in neighboring VSMCs, and triggers an early vascular remodeling in vascular inflammation [72]. In another recent study, PVAT-derived exosomes were demonstrated to reduce macrophage foam cell formation through miR-382-5p- and bone morphogenetic protein 4 (BMP4)-PPARγ-mediated upregulation of cholesterol efflux transporters [76]. However, it is still unclear which cell types in PVAT generate these extracellular vesicles.

4. Current Proves of eNOS in PVAT

There are currently three isoforms of NO synthase (NOS), which is named by the cell types where they are first identified: neuronal NOS (nNOS or NOS1), inducible NOS (iNOS or NOS2), and eNOS (or NOS3) [77]. Vascular nNOS is expressed in perivascular nerve fibers and in the vascular wall, while the expression of iNOS is induced under conditions of inflammation and sepsis [77]. eNOS is primarily expressed, but not exclusively, in endothelial cells. All three isoforms of NO synthase catalyze the production of NO from L-arginine [80]. Under physiological conditions, eNOS is the main vascular source of NO, modulates vascular functions and confers protection against cardiovascular diseases.

In recent years, eNOS expression in other cell types has been demonstrated in vitro and in vivo. Indeed, eNOS expression has been found in dendrite cells [78], red blood cells [81], hepatocytes [80], as well as in adipocytes [6]. While the expression of iNOS in PVAT is only induced in pathological conditions [82], and the expression of nNOS in PVAT is controversial [83], the expression of eNOS in thoracic aortic PVAT has recently been demonstrated by various groups. Gene and protein expressions of eNOS in PVAT have been detected [6,84]. Using immunohistochemistry, eNOS can be stained in both adipocytes and endothelial cells of the capillaries and vasa vasorum in aortic PVAT [6,85]. Of the three isoforms of NOS, immunostaining of eNOS is the most abundant in PVAT of the saphenous vein, and eNOS activity is comparable in PVAT and the adherent vein [85]. In addition, in situ NO production in PVAT adipocytes can be directly detected by fluorescence imaging [13,86]. There is a high histological discrepancy of eNOS expression among the anatomical localizations of PVAT. Abdominal PVAT has been shown to have a lower eNOS expression compared with thoracic PVAT, while the eNOS expression remains the same along the vessel walls [13]. Indeed, unpublished data from our laboratory suggests a similar eNOS expression level of mesenteric PVAT and thoracic PVAT. Nevertheless, due to the highly heterogenous origins and compositions of different PVATs, detailed investigations of specific cell types that express eNOS in different PVATs is crucial.

5. What Are the Functions of eNOS in PVAT?

Unfortunately, due to the lack of PVAT-specific eNOS knockout animal models, the exact functions of eNOS in PVAT is relatively unclear. Most of the current knowledge about PVAT eNOS is based on evidence from studies using global eNOS knockout mice or mice with pathological conditions that leads to downregulation of PVAT eNOS. Here, we summarize current understanding of potential eNOS functions in PVAT under both basal and pathological conditions.

The first and most important function of eNOS in PVAT is, of course, to generate vasoactive NO. Previous studies with animal models have demonstrated that PVAT plays a crucial role in vascular NO production [1,6,29]. PVAT-derived NO can diffuse into the adjacent VSMC, stimulating soluble guanylate cyclase (sGC) and increasing the cyclic guanosine monophosphate (cGMP) level, which leads to the phosphorylation of large-conductance calcium-activated potassium channels in VSMC via protein kinase G, resulting in hyperpolarization and vascular relaxation [87,88]. In small arteries isolated from visceral fat of healthy individuals, basal vascular NO production is reduced after PVAT removal, which leads to an attenuated contractile response to L-NAME [89]. In PVAT-adhered, endothelium-denuded rat mesenteric arteries, inhibition of eNOS significantly enhances NE-induced contraction, indicating that eNOS in PVAT contributes to the vascular NO production, while the anticontractile effect of PVAT is, at least partly, independent of the endothelium [33,90]. In low-density lipoprotein receptor (Ldlr) knockout mice, the thoracic aortic PVAT shows significant upregulation of eNOS expression and NO production, which protects against impaired vasorelaxation to acetylcholine and insulin [84]. In a very recent clinical study, the authors demonstrated PVAT as a predominant source of NO in human vasculature in a no-touch saphenous vein grafts (NT-SVGs) coronary artery bypass model [91]. The study showed that PVAT, via NO production from eNOS, can induce vasorelaxation even in endothelium-denuded SVG. The above evidence suggests the protective role of PVAT eNOS in improving endothelial functions. Nevertheless, currently, there is a lack of detailed studies that are designed to compare the NO production and eNOS function among vascular components, such as the endothelium and PVAT.

In addition to direct modulation of vasodilation, PVAT-derived NO released toward the vascular lumen is a potent inhibitor of platelet aggregation and leukocyte adhesion [92]. PVAT has been shown to play a role in the inhibition of DNA synthesis, mitogenesis, and proliferation of VSMCs [93]. The inhibition of platelet aggregation and adhesion also protects VSMCs from exposure to platelet-derived growth factors. These confer the ability of PVAT to protect against the onset of atherogenesis and vascular remodeling in the adherent vessels. However, there is a lack of direct evidence of how PVAT eNOS and PVAT-derived NO act on atherogenesis and vascular remodeling.

Another important function of PVAT eNOS is to stimulate the expression of adiponectin, which is an important adipokine that contributes to vasodilation regulation, anti-inflammation, and inhibition of VSMCs proliferation and migration [36,94]. eNOS has been shown to regulate adiponectin synthesis in adipocytes by increasing mitochondrial biogenesis and enhancing mitochondrial function [95]. PVAT-derived adiponectin may regulate endothelial functions, partly by enhancing eNOS phosphorylation in the endothelium [96]. Indeed, the function of PVAT is determined by the browning and inflammation status. Mitochondrial biogenesis is involved in the browning of adipocytes [97]. Fitzgibbons et al. proposed that promoting the browning of PVAT might confer a protective effect to attenuate the development of vascular diseases [11]. PVAT eNOS may have a vital role in the mitochondrial biogenesis and browning of PVAT [98]. However, the detailed mechanisms underlying browning or thermogenesis of PVAT are barely known.

Apart from the functions of PVAT eNOS and NO mentioned above, NO is also known as an endogenously produced signaling molecule that regulates gene expression and cell phenotypes [99]. Currently, NO is known to regulate gene expression either by direct interaction with transcription factors or by post-translational modification of proteins. NO may mediate the transcriptional regulation of histone-modifying enzymes and modulate the activities and cellular localizations of transcription factors through the formation of S-nitrosothiols or iron nitrosyl complexes [100]. Additionally, NO may alter the cellular methylation, acetylation, phosphorylation, ubiquitylation, or sumoylation profiles of proteins and histones by modifying these enzymes [101]. Recent evidence has revealed the presence of S-nitrosylated (SNO) proteins in abdominal aortic PVAT [102]. For example, a reduced NO level results in the activation and cellular release of tissue transglutaminase (TG2), which is involved in vascular fibrosis and remodeling [103,104]. Normally, TG2 can be S-nitrosylated by NO, and is retained within the cytosolic compartment. Reduced bioavailability of NO leads to reduction of TG2 S-nitrosylation, which facilities its translocation to the extracellular compartment where it can induce crosslinking of extracellular matrix proteins and promote fibrosis [105]. Nevertheles, the complete nitrosylation profile of PVAT and vascular wall remains unclear. Identification of these SNO proteins could greatly enhance our understanding of the detailed function of PVAT eNOS and its derived NO.

A recent study has revealed the reciprocal regulation of eNOS and β-catenin [106]. eNOS and β-catenin are interactive partners. β-catenin is a membrane protein known to bind with eNOS to promote eNOS phosphorylation and activation, while this interaction facilitates the translocation of β-catenin to the nucleus and activates downstream gene transcription [106]. This suggests a potential role of eNOS as a 'carrier' protein to facilitate gene expression independent of NO production. In addition, another cobinding protein and negative regulator of eNOS, Cav-1, is expressed in both endothelial cells and adipocytes [107]. Cav-1 can regulate eNOS functions in PVAT [108], whereas eNOS-derived NO has been shown to promote caveolae trafficking [109]. These suggest that protein–protein interaction of eNOS may play a critical role in PVAT functions, such as the secretion of miRNA-encapsulated microvesicles.

6. PVAT eNOS under Pathological Conditions

Multiple studies with high-fat diet (HFD) and/or genetic manipulation models have reported the pathophysiological significance of PVAT eNOS in mediating vascular functions, inflammation, and other metabolic processes [6,29,110]. PVAT eNOS plays a crucial role in obesity-induced vascular dysfunction [1,28]. Indeed, endothelium-dependent, NO-mediated acetylcholine-induced vasodilation response has no significant changes in PVAT-removed aortas from HFD-fed mice compared with control mice, while vascular dysfunction of the thoracic aorta is only evident when PVAT is adhered [6,111]. Our group has also found evidence of PVAT eNOS dysfunction and eNOS uncoupling in HFD-induced obese mice [6]. Although an adaptive overproduction of NO from mesenteric PVAT was observed at the early phase of HFD-induced obesity in C57BL/6J mice [86], reduced eNOS expression was observed after long-time HFD feeding in the mesenteric PVAT of obese rats [33] and thoracic aortic PVAT of mice [112]. Either improving L-arginine availability [6] or restoring eNOS phosphorylation and acetylation [111] can ameliorate obese-linked vascular dysfunction. These suggest that obese-induced eNOS dysfunction in the PVAT can significantly reduce the vascular functions in the adherent vessels. In addition, basal NO production is reduced in small arteries from obese patients compared with nonobese controls, while this reduction in basal NO production is only evident in PVAT-adhered, but not in PVAT-removed arteries [89]. However, in HFD-fed ApoE knockout rat models of early atherosclerosis, Nakladel et al. demostrated an upregulation of eNOS in the inflammatory thoracic PVAT, which compensates severe endothelial dysfunction by contributing to NO production upon cholinergic stimulation [82]. Nevertheless, these results indicate that, under obesity-related metabolic diseases, PVAT eNOS may be even more important than endothelium eNOS in obesity-induced vascular dysfunction, which may be attributed to certain PVAT eNOS-specific functions [1,28,113].

The reduction of eNOS activity and PVAT function can be caused by the reduced L-arginine bioavailability and changes in post-translational modifications of eNOS in obese PVAT [28]. Deficiency in L-arginine is attributable to an upregulation of arginase in the

PVAT of obese mice [6]. The upregulation of arginase reduces L-arginine bioavailability for NO production and leads to eNOS uncoupling in PVAT [114], while uncoupled eNOS produces superoxide and increases oxidative stress in PVAT [6]. Indeed, acylation, acetylation, S-nitrosylation, glycosylation, glutathionylation, and phosphorylation of eNOS have been reported and involved in the dynamic control of its activity in response to different physiologic and pathophysiologic cues [115]. Reduction in eNOS phosphorylation at serine 1177 residue and inhibition of Akt, an upstream kinase of eNOS, were observed in the thoracic aortic PVAT of obese mice [6]. Another important post-translational modification of PVAT eNOS involved in obesity-induced vascular dysfunction is acetylation [35,115]. eNOS has been reported to be constitutively acetylated at Lys 497 and Lys 507 [115], which inhibits the activity of eNOS. Deacetylation of eNOS by SIRT1 increases the enzymatic activity of the eNOS [116]. In our previous study, we observed an upregulation of eNOS acetylation in the thoracic aortic PVAT of obese mice [111]. O-GlcNAcylation is another post-translational modification of eNOS that influences its stability, activity and subcellular localization [115]. O-GlcNAcylation of eNOS in PVAT is increased in high sugar diet-fed rats as well as in hyperglycemic human patients, suggesting that O-GlcNAcylation of eNOS may be involved in high sugar diet-induced oxidative stress in PVAT [117]. Other modifications of eNOS and the resulting changes in eNOS functions have not been reported or investigated in PVAT in pathological models.

One of the mechanisms leading to eNOS dysfunction in PVAT is the dysregulation of leptin, adiponectin, and chemerin. HFD-induced obesity enhances the leptin level in PVAT which leads to the reduction of eNOS activity and NO production [86]. The reduction in PVAT eNOS activity and NO production in obesity can be partially attributed to the reduced expression of adiponectin in PVAT [88]. Adiponectin and eNOS have a bidirectional regulation. The decreased adiponectin from PVAT may also reduce endothelial eNOS activity in obesity [110,113,118]. In obesity, chemerin from PVAT contributes to the positive amplification of sympathetic nerve stimulation and thereby increases vascular tone [119], while chemerin in the vessel wall decreases the expression of the rate-limiting enzyme for tetrahydrobiopterin (BH4) biosynthesis, GTP cyclohydrolase I (GTPCH1), decreases eNOS activation and NO production, and promotes ROS generation [120,121]. Nevertheless, the regulation of PVAT eNOS by chemerin has not been investigated.

On the other hand, both aging and obesity might affect PVAT in a comparable manner [10]. Aging has been shown to attenuate the anticontractile effect of aortic PVAT and reduce the browning phenotype of PVAT in rats [122]. Aging can also promote obesity-induced oxidative stress and inflammation in PVAT, which in turn exacerbates the secretion of inflammatory factors from PVAT, and affects vascular remodeling in obese mice [123]. In addition, ROS production in PVAT is progressively increased during aging, which subsequently contributes to aging-related vascular injuries [122,124]. eNOS uncoupling has been demonstrated in aged vessels [125]; however, the changes in expression and uncoupling of eNOS in aged PVAT is totally unknown. Future studies are needed to examine eNOS expression and function during aging in related to aging-induced vascular complications.

7. Pharmacological Targeting of PVAT eNOS

As mentioned above, under obesity-related metabolic diseases, PVAT eNOS may be even more important than endothelium eNOS in obesity-induced vascular dysfunction. Therefore, restoring the function of eNOS in obese PVAT may effectively improve and normalize vascular functions. As many studies have focused on the pharmacological interventions targeting PVAT eNOS in obesity, different targets that regulate eNOS in PVAT have been detailed [28,126,127]. Here, we briefly summarize a few of interest.

SIRT1 is known as a class III histone deacetylase which also deacetylates nonhistone proteins and cytosolic molecules such as eNOS. SIRT1 deacetylates eNOS at lysine 494 and 504 in the calmodulin-binding domain of eNOS, resulting in the activation of eNOS [116]. Adipose tissue-specific-SIRT1 knockout mice have increased obesity-induced brown-to-white transition in PVAT in vivo, leading to impaired vascular reactivity [128].

The deficiency of PVAT SIRT1 may reduce PVAT browning by promoting local superoxide production and reducing adipokines production [128], which could be attributed to the inactivation of eNOS due to the constitutive acetylation of eNOS. In a very recent study, we demonstrated that the PVAT SIRT1 activity is reduced in obese mice despite an enhanced SIRT1 expression [35]. This resulted from the downregulation of NAD^+-producing enzyme NAMPT, which leads to a reduced level of NAD^+ and $NAD^+/NADH$ ratio in PVAT. The reduced SIRT1 activity is associated with an enhanced acetylation of eNOS in the PVAT [35]. In addition, activation of SIRT1 promotes mitochondrial biogenesis via the peroxisome proliferator-activated receptor-gamma and coactivator 1 alpha (PGC-1α) mitochondrial pathway in adipose tissues [129]. Moreover, SIRT1 is reported to regulate adiponectin secretion in adipocytes [130]. Resveratrol, a SIRT1 activitor, has been shown to improve PVAT functions [131,132], but the change in PVAT eNOS activity has not been studied. Nevertheless, these suggest a tight interplay between PVAT SIRT1 and eNOS in controlling the browning and inflammation status of PVAT, which mediates vascular functions (Figure 2).

The serine/threonine protein kinase Akt mediates the activation of eNOS, leading to increased NO production. Inhibition of Akt or mutation of the Akt binding site on eNOS at serine 1177 attenuates the phosphorylation of eNOS and prevents eNOS activation [133]. The standardized Crataegus extract WS® 1442, with antioxidative properties, is known to enhance eNOS phosphorylation at the serine 1177 residue by stimulating Akt activity. Treatment with WS® 1442 can restore the vascular functions in the PVAT-adhered aorta of obese mice without any effect on body weight or fat mass [27].

AMP-activated protein kinase (AMPK) is an important regulator of energy metabolism homeostasis and can activate eNOS via phosphorylation [134,135]. The activation of the AMPK/eNOS pathway in PVAT is responsible for its anticontractile function. Treating PVAT with various AMPK activators 5-Aminoimidazole-4-carboxamide ribonucleotide (AICAR), salicylate, metformin, methotrexate, resveratrol, or diosgenin was reported to increase phosphorylation of PVAT eNOS and improve PVAT functions in different studies [131,132].

Exercise training was shown to increase eNOS expression and eNOS phosphorylation in both vascular wall and PVAT, which is associated with increased adiponectin expression in PVAT [136]. Aerobic exercise training has been shown to promote the anticontractile activities of PVAT by upregulating the expression of antioxidant enzymes and decreasing oxidative stress in PVAT [126]. Aerobic exercise training also stimulates angiogenesis, which improves blood flow and reduces hypoxia and macrophage infiltration in PVAT [127]. In addition, exercise training induces browning and thermogenic response in rat PVAT, which is associated with increased eNOS expression and reduced oxidative stress [137]. Sustained weight loss also increases eNOS expression and improves NO production in PVAT from rats [33]. In rats fed with a high-fat/high-sucrose diet, exercise significantly increases adiponectin levels compared with nonexercised controls, which is associated with increased eNOS phosphorylation in PVAT [136]. Increased GTP cyclohydrolase 1 expression, which is involved in the production of BH4, an essential cofactor for NO generation from eNOS, was reported after exercise training in obese rat thoracic PVAT [138]. Moreover, bariatric surgery improved NO bioavailability in PVAT of small subcutaneous arteries from severely obese individuals [139]. These beneficial effects of exercise training and weight loss may be attributed to the restoration of eNOS activity (Figure 2).

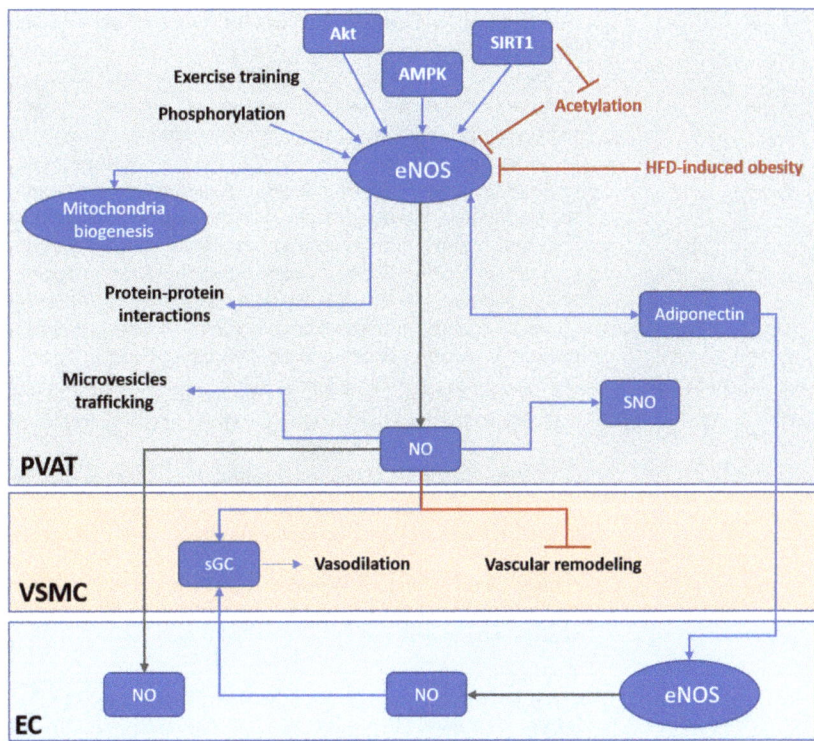

Figure 2. PVAT eNOS is an important modulator of vascular functions. Under HFD-induced obesity, the activity and expression of PVAT eNOS is significantly downregulated. PVAT eNOS may be even more important than endothelium eNOS in obesity-induced vascular dysfunction. Under normal condition, PVAT eNOS has multiple roles in regulating PVAT and vascular functions. PVAT eNOS can generate NO and regulate vasodilation via endothelium-dependent and endothelium-independent mechanisms. NO generated from PVAT eNOS can diffuse to the endothelium and activate EC, or directly activate sGC in the VSMC to evoke vasodilation. NO generated from PVAT eNOS can prevent vascular remodeling and stiffening via inhibiting VSMC proliferation and differentiation. PVAT eNOS is also responsible for modulating mitochondria biogenesis and browning of adipocytes in PVAT. In addition, NO generated from PVAT eNOS may regulate protein activities via SNO modification. Moreover, eNOS may, via protein–protein interactions and NO production, modulate miRNA-encapsulated microvesicles trafficking across PVAT. PVAT eNOS have a bidirectional regulation with adiponectin. Adiponectin is an important adipokine that modulates vascular functions via activating eNOS in both PVAT and EC. Current therapeutic strategies targeting PVAT eNOS include enhancing eNOS activity by phosphorylation, promoting deacetylation of eNOS via activation of SIRT1, activation of upstream kinase of eNOS (Akt, AMPK), and exercise training. AMPK, AMP-activated protein kinase; eNOS, endothelial nitric oxide synthase; EC, endothelial cell; HFD, high fat diet; NO, nitric oxide; PVAT, perivascular adipose tissue; sGC, soluble guanylyl cyclase; SNO, S-nitrosylation; VSMC, vascular smooth muscle cell.

8. Conclusions and Future Directions

PVAT has a unique role in the modulation of vascular functions due to its very close proximity to the vasculature. Important to note is also the significance of PVAT in modulating cardiovascular complications. In metabolic and cardiovascular diseases, adipose tissue dysfunction has a notable contribution to the associated vascular dysfunction. Recent evidence from different studies suggests that eNOS in PVAT, rather than eNOS in the vascular wall, plays a critical role in protection against obesity-induced vascular dysfunction (Figure 2). Conventional in vitro vascular experiments are mainly performed with PVAT-denuded vessels, which does not reflect the vascular function of in vivo conditions. In this regard, the study of PVAT functions and the unique role of eNOS in PVAT becomes extremely important for the investigation of metabolic and cardiovascular diseases and the research for pharmacological interventions. In order to have a better understanding of the unique role of eNOS in PVAT, there is an urgent need for a suitable animal model, i.e., a PVAT-specific eNOS knockout or overexpression mouse model. Nevertheless, due to the highly heterogenous origin and histological and functional variations among PVAT in different regions of the vascular bed, designing an ideal model for studying the specific functions of eNOS PVAT is a challenge. On the other hand, current understanding of eNOS functions in PVAT is based on the understanding of eNOS from endothelial cells, global knockout, or disease models. PVAT-specific gene knockout or overexpression animal models may help to answer the following questions:

o   What is the exact of role of PVAT eNOS in PVAT functions?
o   What are the exact expression levels of eNOS in different regions of PVAT and/or in different cells in PVAT?
o   What is the relative contribution of endothelial eNOS and PVAT eNOS to vascular function under physiological and pathological conditions?
o   Are there any specific functions of eNOS in PVAT but not in endothelial cells?

Author Contributions: A.W.C.M. wrote the initial draft of the manuscript. Y.Z., N.X. and H.L. critically reviewed and edited the manuscript. All authors have read and agreed to the published version of the manuscript.

Funding: Original works from the authors' laboratory contributing to this review were supported by grants LI-1042/1-1, LI-1042/3-1, LI-1042/5-1, and XI 139/2-1 from the Deutsche Forschungsgemeinschaft (DFG), Bonn, Germany. H.L. and N.X. were supported by a research grant from the Boehringer Ingelheim Foundation for the collaborative research consortium "Novel and neglected cardiovascular risk factors: molecular mechanisms and therapeutic implications".

Institutional Review Board Statement: Not applicable.

Informed Consent Statement: Not applicable.

Data Availability Statement: Not applicable.

Conflicts of Interest: The authors declare no conflict of interest.

References

1. Xia, N.; Li, H. The role of perivascular adipose tissue in obesity-induced vascular dysfunction. *Br. J. Pharmacol.* **2017**, *174*, 3425–3442. [CrossRef]
2. Soltis, E.E.; Cassis, L.A. Influence of Perivascular Adipose Tissue on Rat Aortic Smooth Muscle Responsiveness. *Clin. Exp. Hypertens. Part A Theory Pract.* **1991**, *13*, 277–296. [CrossRef]
3. Gao, Y.-J.; Zeng, Z.-H.; Teoh, K.; Sharma, A.M.; Abouzahr, L.; Cybulsky, I.; Lamy, A.; Semelhago, L.; Lee, R.M. Perivascular adipose tissue modulates vascular function in the human internal thoracic artery. *J. Thorac. Cardiovasc. Surg.* **2005**, *130*, 1130–1136. [CrossRef]
4. Greenstein, A.S.; Khavandi, K.; Withers, S.B.; Sonoyama, K.; Clancy, O.; Jeziorska, M.; Laing, I.; Yates, A.P.; Pemberton, P.W.; Malik, R.A.; et al. Local Inflammation and Hypoxia Abolish the Protective Anticontractile Properties of Perivascular Fat in Obese Patients. *Circulation* **2009**, *119*, 1661–1670. [CrossRef]
5. Loesch, A.; Dashwood, M.R. Saphenous Vein Vasa Vasorum as a Potential Target for Perivascular Fat-Derived Factors. *Braz. J. Cardiovasc. Surg.* **2020**, *35*, 964–969. [CrossRef]
6. Xia, N.; Horke, S.; Habermeier, A.; Closs, E.I.; Reifenberg, G.; Gericke, A.; Mikhed, Y.; Münzel, T.; Daiber, A.; Förstermann, U.; et al. Uncoupling of Endothelial Nitric Oxide Synthase in Perivascular Adipose Tissue of Diet-Induced Obese Mice. *Arterioscler. Thromb. Vasc. Biol.* **2016**, *36*, 78–85. [CrossRef]
7. Man, A.W.; Wang, Y. Age-Associated Arterial Remodelling. *EC Cardiol.* **2017**, *4*, 137–164.
8. Gil-Ortega, M.; Somoza, B.; Huang, Y.; Gollasch, M.; Fernández-Alfonso, M.S. Regional differences in perivascular adipose tissue impacting vascular homeostasis. *Trends Endocrinol. Metab.* **2015**, *26*, 367–375. [CrossRef]
9. Brown, N.K.; Zhou, Z.; Zhang, J.; Zeng, R.; Wu, J.; Eitzman, D.T.; Chen, Y.E.; Chang, L. Perivascular Adipose Tissue in Vascular Function and Disease. *Arter. Thromb. Vasc. Biol.* **2014**, *34*, 1621–1630. [CrossRef]

10. Miao, C.-Y.; Li, Z.-Y. The role of perivascular adipose tissue in vascular smooth muscle cell growth. *J. Cereb. Blood Flow Metab.* **2012**, *165*, 643–658. [CrossRef]
11. Fitzgibbons, T.P.; Kogan, S.; Aouadi, M.; Hendricks, G.M.; Straubhaar, J.; Czech, M.P. Similarity of mouse perivascular and brown adipose tissues and their resistance to diet-induced inflammation. *Am. J. Physiol. Heart Circ. Physiol.* **2011**, *301*, H1425–H1437. [CrossRef]
12. Drosos, I.; Chalikias, G.; Pavlaki, M.; Kareli, D.; Epitropou, G.; Bougioukas, G.; Mikroulis, D.; Konstantinou, F.; Giatromanolaki, A.; Ritis, K.; et al. Differences between perivascular adipose tissue surrounding the heart and the internal mammary artery: Possible role for the leptin-inflammation-fibrosis-hypoxia axis. *Clin. Res. Cardiol.* **2016**, *105*, 887–900. [CrossRef]
13. Victorio, J.A.; Fontes, M.T.; Rossoni, L.V.; Davel, A.P. Different Anti-Contractile Function and Nitric Oxide Production of Thoracic and Abdominal Perivascular Adipose Tissues. *Front. Physiol.* **2016**, *7*, 295. [CrossRef]
14. Gálvez-Prieto, B.; Bolbrinker, J.; Stucchi, P.; de Las Heras, A.I.; Merino, B.; Arribas, S.; Ruiz-Gayo, M.; Huber, M.; Wehland, M.; Kreutz, R.; et al. Comparative expression analysis of the renin–angiotensin system components between white and brown perivascular adipose tissue. *J. Endocrinol.* **2008**, *197*, 55–64. [CrossRef]
15. Tchkonia, T.; Lenburg, M.; Thomou, T.; Giorgadze, N.; Frampton, G.; Pirtskhalava, T.; Cartwright, A.; Cartwright, M.; Flanagan, J.; Karagiannides, I.; et al. Identification of depot-specific human fat cell progenitors through distinct expression profiles and developmental gene patterns. *Am. J. Physiol. Metab.* **2007**, *292*, E298–E307. [CrossRef]
16. Tran, K.-V.; Fitzgibbons, T.; Min, S.Y.; DeSouza, T.; Corvera, S. Distinct adipocyte progenitor cells are associated with regional phenotypes of perivascular aortic fat in mice. *Mol. Metab.* **2018**, *9*, 199–206. [CrossRef]
17. Hepler, C.; Vishvanath, L.; Gupta, R.K. Sorting out adipocyte precursors and their role in physiology and disease. *Genes Dev.* **2017**, *31*, 127–140. [CrossRef]
18. Fu, M.; Xu, L.; Chen, X.; Han, W.; Ruan, C.; Li, J.; Cai, C.; Ye, M.; Gao, P. Neural Crest Cells Differentiate Into Brown Adipocytes and Contribute to Periaortic Arch Adipose Tissue Formation. *Arter. Thromb. Vasc. Biol.* **2019**, *39*, 1629–1644. [CrossRef]
19. Ye, M.; Ruan, C.-C.; Fu, M.; Xu, L.; Chen, D.; Zhu, M.; Zhu, D.; Gao, P. Developmental and functional characteristics of the thoracic aorta perivascular adipocyte. *Cell Mol. Life Sci.* **2019**, *76*, 777–789. [CrossRef]
20. Kaviani, M.; Azarpira, N.; Aghdaie, M.H.; Esfandiari, E.; Geramizadeh, B.; Nikeghbalian, S.; Dehghani, M. Comparison of Human Mesenchymal Stem Cells Derived from Various Compartments of Human Adipose Tissue and Tunica Adventitia Layer of the Arteries Subsequent to Organ Donation. *Int. J. Organ Transplant. Med.* **2019**, *10*, 65–73.
21. Angueira, A.R.; Sakers, A.P.; Holman, C.D.; Cheng, L.; Arbocco, M.N.; Shamsi, F.; Lynes, M.D.; Shrestha, R.; Okada, C.; Batmanov, K.; et al. Defining the lineage of thermogenic perivascular adipose tissue. *Nat. Metab.* **2021**, *3*, 469–484. [CrossRef]
22. Chang, L.; Villacorta, L.; Li, R.; Hamblin, M.; Xu, W.; Dou, C.; Zhang, J.; Wu, J.; Zeng, R.; Chen, Y.E. Loss of Perivascular Adipose Tissue on Peroxisome Proliferator–Activated Receptor-γ Deletion in Smooth Muscle Cells Impairs Intravascular Thermoregulation and Enhances Atherosclerosis. *Circulation* **2012**, *126*, 1067–1078. [CrossRef]
23. Chau, Y.-Y.; Bandiera, R.; Serrels, A.; Estrada, O.M.M.; Qing, W.; Lee, M.; Slight, J.; Thornburn, A.; Berry, R.; McHaffie, S.; et al. Visceral and subcutaneous fat have different origins and evidence supports a mesothelial source. *Nat. Cell Biol.* **2014**, *16*, 367–375. [CrossRef]
24. Contreras, G.A.; Thelen, K.; Ayala-Lopez, N.; Watts, S.W. The distribution and adipogenic potential of perivascular adipose tissue adipocyte progenitors is dependent on sexual dimorphism and vessel location. *Physiol. Rep.* **2016**, *4*, e12993. [CrossRef]
25. Lehr, S.; Hartwig, S.; Lamers, D.; Famulla, S.; Müller, S.; Hanisch, F.-G.; Cuvelier, C.; Ruige, J.; Eckardt, K.; Ouwens, D.M.; et al. Identification and Validation of Novel Adipokines Released from Primary Human Adipocytes. *Mol. Cell. Proteom.* **2012**, *11*, M111.010504. [CrossRef]
26. Löhn, M.; Dubrovska, G.; Lauterbach, B.; Luft, F.C.; Gollasch, M.; Sharma, A.M. Periadventitial fat releases a vascular relaxing factor. *FASEB J.* **2002**, *16*, 1057–1063. [CrossRef]
27. Xia, N.; Förstermann, U.; Li, H. Effects of resveratrol on eNOS in the endothelium and the perivascular adipose tissue. *Ann. New York Acad. Sci.* **2017**, *1403*, 132–141. [CrossRef]
28. Man, A.W.C.; Zhou, Y.; Xia, N.; Li, H. Perivascular Adipose Tissue as a Target for Antioxidant Therapy for Cardiovascular Complications. *Antioxidants* **2020**, *9*, 574. [CrossRef]
29. Chang, L.; Garcia-Barrio, M.T.; Chen, Y.E. Perivascular Adipose Tissue Regulates Vascular Function by Targeting Vascular Smooth Muscle Cells. *Arter. Thromb. Vasc. Biol.* **2020**, *40*, 1094–1109. [CrossRef]
30. Kim, H.W.; Shi, H.; Winkler, M.A.; Lee, R.; Weintraub, N.L. Perivascular Adipose Tissue and Vascular Perturbation/Atherosclerosis. *Arter. Thromb. Vasc. Biol.* **2020**, *40*, 2569–2576. [CrossRef]
31. Stanek, A.; Brożyna-Tkaczyk, K.; Myśliński, W. The Role of Obesity-Induced Perivascular Adipose Tissue (PVAT) Dysfunction in Vascular Homeostasis. *Nutrients* **2021**, *13*, 3843. [CrossRef]
32. Omar, A.; Chatterjee, T.K.; Tang, Y.; Hui, D.Y.; Weintraub, N.L. Proinflammatory Phenotype of Perivascular Adipocytes. *Arter. Thromb. Vasc. Biol.* **2014**, *34*, 1631–1636. [CrossRef]
33. Bussey, C.E.; Withers, S.B.; Aldous, R.G.; Edwards, G.; Heagerty, A.M. Obesity-Related Perivascular Adipose Tissue Damage Is Reversed by Sustained Weight Loss in the Rat. *Arter. Thromb. Vasc. Biol.* **2016**, *36*, 1377–1385. [CrossRef]
34. Ketonen, J.; Shi, J.; Martonen, E.; Mervaala, E. Periadventitial Adipose Tissue Promotes Endothelial Dysfunction via Oxidative Stress in Diet-Induced Obese C57Bl/6 Mice. *Circ. J.* **2010**, *74*, 1479–1487. [CrossRef]

35. Xia, N.; Reifenberg, G.; Schirra, C.; Li, H. The Involvement of Sirtuin 1 Dysfunction in High-Fat Diet-Induced Vascular Dysfunction in Mice. *Antioxidants* **2022**, *11*, 541. [CrossRef]
36. Sowka, A.; Dobrzyn, P. Role of Perivascular Adipose Tissue-Derived Adiponectin in Vascular Homeostasis. *Cells* **2021**, *10*, 1485. [CrossRef]
37. Takaoka, M.; Nagata, D.; Kihara, S.; Shimomura, I.; Kimura, Y.; Tabata, Y.; Saito, Y.; Nagai, R.; Sata, M. Periadventitial Adipose Tissue Plays a Critical Role in Vascular Remodeling. *Circ. Res.* **2009**, *105*, 906–911. [CrossRef]
38. Chang, L.; Zhao, X.; Garcia-Barrio, M.; Zhang, J.; Chen, Y.E. MitoNEET in Perivascular Adipose Tissue Prevents Arterial Stiffness in Aging Mice. *Cardiovasc. Drugs Ther.* **2018**, *32*, 531–539. [CrossRef]
39. Chang, L.; Milton, H.; Eitzman, D.T.; Chen, Y.E. Paradoxical Roles of Perivascular Adipose Tissue in Atherosclerosis and Hypertension. *Circ. J.* **2013**, *77*, 11–18. [CrossRef]
40. Fésüs, G.; Dubrovska, G.; Gorzelniak, K.; Kluge, R.; Huang, Y.; Luft, F.C.; Gollasch, M. Adiponectin is a novel humoral vasodilator. *Cardiovasc. Res.* **2007**, *75*, 719–727. [CrossRef]
41. Wójcicka, G.; Jamroz-Wiśniewska, A.; Atanasova, P.; Chaldakov, G.N.; Chylińska-Kula, B.; Bełtowski, J. Differential effects of statins on endogenous H2S formation in perivascular adipose tissue. *Pharmacol. Res.* **2011**, *63*, 68–76. [CrossRef]
42. Zaborska, K.E.; Wareing, M.; Austin, C. Comparisons between perivascular adipose tissue and the endothelium in their modulation of vascular tone. *Br. J. Pharmacol.* **2017**, *174*, 3388–3397. [CrossRef]
43. Awata, W.M.; Gonzaga, N.A.; Borges, V.F.; Silva, C.B.; Tanus-Santos, J.E.; Cunha, F.Q.; Tirapelli, C.R. Perivascular adipose tissue contributes to lethal sepsis-induced vasoplegia in rats. *Eur. J. Pharmacol.* **2019**, *863*, 172706. [CrossRef]
44. Ozen, G.; Topal, G.; Gomez, I.; Ghorreshi, A.; Boukais, K.; Benyahia, C.; Kanyinda, L.; Longrois, D.; Teskin, O.; Uydes-Dogan, B.S.; et al. Control of human vascular tone by prostanoids derived from perivascular adipose tissue. *Prostaglandins Other Lipid Mediat.* **2013**, *107*, 13–17. [CrossRef]
45. Gao, Y.-J.; Lu, C.; Su, L.-Y.; Sharma, A.M.; Lee, R.M.K.W. Modulation of vascular function by perivascular adipose tissue: The role of endothelium and hydrogen peroxide. *J. Cereb. Blood Flow Metab.* **2007**, *151*, 323–331. [CrossRef]
46. Lee, R.M.K.W.; Lu, C.; Su, L.-Y.; Gao, Y.-J. Endothelium-dependent relaxation factor released by perivascular adipose tissue. *J. Hypertens.* **2009**, *27*, 782–790. [CrossRef]
47. Chang, L.; Xiong, W.; Zhao, X.; Fan, Y.; Guo, Y.; Garcia-Barrio, M.; Zhang, J.; Jiang, Z.; Lin, J.D.; Chen, Y.E. Bmal1 in Perivascular Adipose Tissue Regulates Resting-Phase Blood Pressure Through Transcriptional Regulation of Angiotensinogen. *Circulation* **2018**, *138*, 67–79. [CrossRef]
48. Alberti, K.; Eckel, R.H.; Grundy, S.M.; Zimmet, P.Z.; Cleeman, J.I.; Donato, K.A.; Fruchart, J.-C.; James, W.P.T.; Loria, C.M.; Smith, S.C., Jr. Harmonizing the metabolic syndrome: A joint interim statement of the international diabetes federation task force on epidemiology and prevention; national heart, lung, and blood institute; American heart association; world heart federation; international atherosclerosis society; and international association for the study of obesity. *Circulation* **2009**, *120*, 1640–1645.
49. Kumar, R.K.; Darios, E.S.; Burnett, R.; Thompson, J.M.; Watts, S.W. Fenfluramine-induced PVAT-dependent contraction depends on norepinephrine and not serotonin. *Pharmacol. Res.* **2018**, *140*, 43–49. [CrossRef]
50. Watts, S.W.; Dorrance, A.M.; Penfold, M.E.; Rourke, J.L.; Sinal, C.J.; Seitz, B.; Sullivan, T.J.; Charvat, T.T.; Thompson, J.M.; Burnett, R.; et al. Chemerin Connects Fat to Arterial Contraction. *Arter. Thromb. Vasc. Biol.* **2013**, *33*, 1320–1328. [CrossRef]
51. Owen, M.K.; Witzmann, F.A.; McKenney, M.L.; Lai, X.; Berwick, Z.C.; Moberly, S.P.; Alloosh, M.; Sturek, M.; Tune, J.D. Perivascular adipose tissue potentiates contraction of coronary vascular smooth muscle: Influence of obesity. *Circulation* **2013**, *128*, 9–18. [CrossRef] [PubMed]
52. Ayala-Lopez, N.; Martini, M.; Jackson, W.F.; Darios, E.; Burnett, R.; Seitz, B.; Fink, G.D.; Watts, S.W. Perivascular adipose tissue contains functional catecholamines. *Pharmacol. Res. Perspect.* **2014**, *2*, e00041. [CrossRef] [PubMed]
53. Gao, Y.-J.; Takemori, K.; Su, L.-Y.; An, W.-S.; Lu, C.; Sharma, A.M.; Lee, R.M. Perivascular adipose tissue promotes vasoconstriction: The role of superoxide anion. *Cardiovasc. Res.* **2006**, *71*, 363–373. [CrossRef] [PubMed]
54. Darios, E.S.; Winner, B.M.; Charvat, T.; Krasinksi, A.; Punna, S.; Watts, S.W. The adipokine chemerin amplifies electrical field-stimulated contraction in the isolated rat superior mesenteric artery. *Am. J. Physiol. Circ. Physiol.* **2016**, *311*, H498–H507. [CrossRef] [PubMed]
55. Costa, R.M.; Filgueira, F.P.; Tostes, R.C.; Carvalho, M.H.C.; Akamine, E.H.; Lobato, N.S. H_2O_2 generated from mitochondrial electron transport chain in thoracic perivascular adipose tissue is crucial for modulation of vascular smooth muscle contraction. *Vasc. Pharmacol.* **2016**, *84*, 28–37. [CrossRef] [PubMed]
56. Cacanyiova, S.; Majzunova, M.; Golas, S.; Berenyiova, A. The role of perivascular adipose tissue and endogenous hydrogen sulfide in vasoactive responses of isolated mesenteric arteries in normotensive and spontaneously hypertensive rats. *J. Physiol. Pharmacol.* **2019**, *70*, 295–306. [CrossRef]
57. Gálvez-Prieto, B.; Somoza, B.; Gil-Ortega, M.; García-Prieto, C.F.; de las Heras, A.I.; González, M.C.; Arribas, S.; Aranguez, I.; Bolbrinker, J.; Kreutz, R.; et al. Anticontractile Effect of Perivascular Adipose Tissue and Leptin are Reduced in Hypertension. *Front. Pharmacol.* **2012**, *3*, 103. [CrossRef]
58. Fang, L.; Zhao, J.; Chen, Y.; Ma, T.; Xu, G.; Tang, C.; Liu, X.; Geng, B. Hydrogen sulfide derived from periadventitial adipose tissue is a vasodilator. *J. Hypertens.* **2009**, *27*, 2174–2185. [CrossRef]

59. Payne, G.A.; Borbouse, L.; Kumar, S.; Neeb, Z.; Alloosh, M.; Sturek, M.; Tune, J.D. Epicardial Perivascular Adipose-Derived Leptin Exacerbates Coronary Endothelial Dysfunction in Metabolic Syndrome via a Protein Kinase C-β Pathway. *Arter. Thromb. Vasc. Biol.* **2010**, *30*, 1711–1717. [CrossRef]
60. Noblet, J.N.; Goodwill, A.; Sassoon, D.; Kiel, A.; Tune, J.D. Leptin augments coronary vasoconstriction and smooth muscle proliferation via a Rho-kinase-dependent pathway. *Basic Res. Cardiol.* **2016**, *111*, 25. [CrossRef]
61. Mendizábal, Y.; Llorens, S.; Nava, E. Vasoactive effects of prostaglandins from the perivascular fat of mesenteric resistance arteries in WKY and SHROB rats. *Life Sci.* **2013**, *93*, 1023–1032. [CrossRef] [PubMed]
62. Ayala-Lopez, N.; Thompson, J.M.; Watts, S.W. Perivascular Adipose Tissue's Impact on Norepinephrine-Induced Contraction of Mesenteric Resistance Arteries. *Front. Physiol.* **2017**, *8*, 37. [CrossRef] [PubMed]
63. Saxton, S.N.; Ryding, K.E.; Aldous, R.G.; Withers, S.B.; Ohanian, J.; Heagerty, A.M. Role of Sympathetic Nerves and Adipocyte Catecholamine Uptake in the Vasorelaxant Function of Perivascular Adipose Tissue. *Arter. Thromb. Vasc. Biol.* **2018**, *38*, 880–891. [CrossRef]
64. Jackson, W.F. Myogenic Tone in Peripheral Resistance Arteries and Arterioles: The Pressure Is On! *Front. Physiol.* **2021**, *12*, 699517. [CrossRef] [PubMed]
65. Schmidt, K.; De Wit, C. Endothelium-Derived Hyperpolarizing Factor and Myoendothelial Coupling: The In Vivo Perspective. *Front. Physiol.* **2020**, *11*, 602930. [CrossRef] [PubMed]
66. Watts, S.W.; Flood, E.D.; Garver, H.; Fink, G.D.; Roccabianca, S. A New Function for Perivascular Adipose Tissue (PVAT): Assistance of Arterial Stress Relaxation. *Sci. Rep.* **2020**, *10*, 1807. [CrossRef]
67. Miron, T.R.; Flood, E.D.; Tykocki, N.R.; Thompson, J.M.; Watts, S.W. Identification of Piezo1 channels in perivascular adipose tissue (PVAT) and their potential role in vascular function. *Pharmacol. Res.* **2021**, *175*, 105995. [CrossRef]
68. Ahmadieh, S.; Kim, H.W.; Weintraub, N.L. Potential role of perivascular adipose tissue in modulating atherosclerosis. *Clin. Sci.* **2020**, *134*, 3–13. [CrossRef]
69. Hu, H.; Garcia-Barrio, M.; Jiang, Z.-S.; Chen, Y.E.; Chang, L. Roles of Perivascular Adipose Tissue in Hypertension and Atherosclerosis. *Antioxidants Redox Signal.* **2021**, *34*, 736–749. [CrossRef]
70. Farias-Itao, D.S.; Pasqualucci, C.A.; de Andrade, R.A.; da Silva, L.F.F.; Yahagi-Estevam, M.; Lage, S.H.G.; Leite, R.E.P.; Campo, A.B.; Suemoto, C.K. Macrophage Polarization in the Perivascular Fat Was Associated with Coronary Atherosclerosis. *J. Am. Hear. Assoc.* **2022**, *11*, e023274. [CrossRef]
71. Irie, D.; Kawahito, H.; Wakana, N.; Kato, T.; Kishida, S.; Kikai, M.; Ogata, T.; Ikeda, K.; Ueyama, T.; Matoba, S.; et al. Transplantation of periaortic adipose tissue from angiotensin receptor blocker-treated mice markedly ameliorates atherosclerosis development in apoE$^{-/-}$ mice. *J. Renin-Angiotensin-Aldosterone Syst.* **2014**, *16*, 67–78. [CrossRef] [PubMed]
72. Li, X.; Ballantyne, L.L.; Yu, Y.; Funk, C.D. Perivascular adipose tissue–derived extracellular vesicle miR-221-3p mediates vascular remodeling. *FASEB J.* **2019**, *33*, 12704–12722. [CrossRef] [PubMed]
73. Ogawa, R.; Tanaka, C.; Sato, M.; Nagasaki, H.; Sugimura, K.; Okumura, K.; Nakagawa, Y.; Aoki, N. Adipocyte-derived microvesicles contain RNA that is transported into macrophages and might be secreted into blood circulation. *Biochem. Biophys. Res. Commun.* **2010**, *398*, 723–729. [CrossRef] [PubMed]
74. Van Niel, G.; D'Angelo, G.; Raposo, G. Shedding light on the cell biology of extracellular vesicles. *Nat. Rev. Mol. Cell Biol.* **2018**, *19*, 213–228. [CrossRef]
75. Thomou, T.; Mori, M.A.; Dreyfuss, J.M.; Konishi, M.; Sakaguchi, M.; Wolfrum, C.; Rao, T.N.; Winnay, J.N.; Garcia-Martin, R.; Grinspoon, S.K.; et al. Adipose-derived circulating miRNAs regulate gene expression in other tissues. *Nature* **2017**, *542*, 450–455. [CrossRef]
76. Liu, Y.; Sun, Y.; Lin, X.; Zhang, D.; Hu, C.; Liu, J.; Zhu, Y.; Gao, A.; Han, H.; Chai, M.; et al. Perivascular adipose-derived exosomes reduce macrophage foam cell formation through miR-382-5p and the BMP4-PPARγ-ABCA1/ABCG1 pathways. *Vasc. Pharmacol.* **2022**, *143*, 106968. [CrossRef]
77. Förstermann, U.; Sessa, W.C. Nitric oxide synthases: Regulation and function. *Eur. Heart J.* **2012**, *33*, 829–837. [CrossRef]
78. Caviedes, A.; Varas-Godoy, M.; Lafourcade, C.; Sandoval, S.; Bravo-Alegria, J.; Kaehne, T.; Massmann, A.; Figueroa, J.P.; Nualart, F.; Wyneken, U. Endothelial Nitric Oxide Synthase Is Present in Dendritic Spines of Neurons in Primary Cultures. *Front. Cell. Neurosci.* **2017**, *11*, 180. [CrossRef]
79. Crewe, C.; Joffin, N.; Rutkowski, J.M.; Kim, M.; Zhang, F.; Towler, D.A.; Gordillo, R.; Scherer, P.E. An Endothelial-to-Adipocyte Extracellular Vesicle Axis Governed by Metabolic State. *Cell* **2018**, *175*, 695–708.e13. [CrossRef]
80. Bendall, J.K.; Alp, N.J.; Warrick, N.; Cai, S.; Adlam, D.; Rockett, K.; Yokoyama, M.; Kawashima, S.; Channon, K.M. Stoichiometric Relationships Between Endothelial Tetrahydrobiopterin, Endothelial NO Synthase (eNOS) Activity, and eNOS Coupling in Vivo. *Circ. Res.* **2005**, *97*, 864–871. [CrossRef]
81. Leo, F.; Suvorava, T.; Heuser, S.K.; Li, J.; LoBue, A.; Barbarino, F.; Piragine, E.; Schneckmann, R.; Hutzler, B.; Good, M.E.; et al. Red Blood Cell and Endothelial eNOS Independently Regulate Circulating Nitric Oxide Metabolites and Blood Pressure. *Circulation* **2021**, *144*, 870–889. [CrossRef]
82. Nakladal, D.; Sijbesma, J.; Visser, L.; Tietge, U.; Slart, R.; Deelman, L.; Henning, R.; Hillebrands, J.; Buikema, H. Perivascular adipose tissue-derived nitric oxide compensates endothelial dysfunction in aged pre-atherosclerotic apolipoprotein E-deficient rats. *Vasc. Pharmacol.* **2021**, *142*, 106945. [CrossRef] [PubMed]

83. Nava, E.; Llorens, S. The Local Regulation of Vascular Function: From an Inside-Outside to an Outside-Inside Model. *Front. Physiol.* **2019**, *10*, 729. [CrossRef] [PubMed]
84. Baltieri, N.; Guizoni, D.M.; Victório, J.A.; Davel, A.P. Protective Role of Perivascular Adipose Tissue in Endothelial Dysfunction and Insulin-Induced Vasodilatation of Hypercholesterolemic LDL Receptor-Deficient Mice. *Front. Physiol.* **2018**, *9*, 229. [CrossRef] [PubMed]
85. Dashwood, M.R.; Dooley, A.; Shi-Wen, X.; Abraham, D.J.; Souza, D.S. Does Periadventitial Fat-Derived Nitric Oxide Play a Role in Improved Saphenous Vein Graft Patency in Patients Undergoing Coronary Artery Bypass Surgery? *J. Vasc. Res.* **2007**, *44*, 175–181. [CrossRef] [PubMed]
86. Gil-Ortega, M.; Stucchi, P.; Guzmán-Ruiz, R.; Cano, V.; Arribas, S.; González, M.C.; Ruiz-Gayo, M.; Fernández-Alfonso, M.S.; Somoza, B. Adaptative Nitric Oxide Overproduction in Perivascular Adipose Tissue during Early Diet-Induced Obesity. *Endocrinology* **2010**, *151*, 3299–3306. [CrossRef]
87. Förstermann, U.; Closs, E.I.; Pollock, J.S.; Nakane, M.; Schwarz, P.; Gath, I.; Kleinert, H. Nitric oxide synthase isozymes. Characterization, purification, molecular cloning, and functions. *Hypertension* **1994**, *23*, 1121–1131. [CrossRef]
88. Weston, A.H.; Egner, I.; Dong, Y.; Porter, E.L.; Heagerty, A.M.; Edwards, G. Stimulated release of a hyperpolarizing factor (ADHF) from mesenteric artery perivascular adipose tissue: Involvement of myocyte BK_{Ca} channels and adiponectin. *J. Cereb. Blood Flow Metab.* **2013**, *169*, 1500–1509. [CrossRef]
89. Virdis, A.; Duranti, E.; Rossi, C.; Dell'Agnello, U.; Santini, E.; Anselmino, M.; Chiarugi, M.; Taddei, S.; Solini, A. Tumour necrosis factor-alpha participates on the endothelin-1/nitric oxide imbalance in small arteries from obese patients: Role of perivascular adipose tissue. *Eur. Hear. J.* **2014**, *36*, 784–794. [CrossRef]
90. Aghamohammadzadeh, R.; Unwin, R.D.; Greenstein, A.S.; Heagerty, A.M. Effects of Obesity on Perivascular Adipose Tissue Vasorelaxant Function: Nitric Oxide, Inflammation and Elevated Systemic Blood Pressure. *J. Vasc. Res.* **2015**, *52*, 299–305. [CrossRef]
91. Saito, T.; Kurazumi, H.; Suzuki, R.; Matsunaga, K.; Tsubone, S.; Lv, B.; Kobayashi, S.; Nagase, T.; Mizoguchi, T.; Samura, M.; et al. Perivascular Adipose Tissue Is a Major Source of Nitric Oxide in Saphenous Vein Grafts Harvested via the No-Touch Technique. *J. Am. Hear. Assoc.* **2022**, *11*, e020637. [CrossRef] [PubMed]
92. Qi, X.-Y.; Qu, S.-L.; Xiong, W.-H.; Rom, O.; Chang, L.; Jiang, Z.-S. Perivascular adipose tissue (PVAT) in atherosclerosis: A double-edged sword. *Cardiovasc. Diabetol.* **2018**, *17*, 134. [CrossRef] [PubMed]
93. Barandier, C.; Montani, J.-P.; Yang, Z. Mature adipocytes and perivascular adipose tissue stimulate vascular smooth muscle cell proliferation: Effects of aging and obesity. *Am. J. Physiol. Circ. Physiol.* **2005**, *289*, H1807–H1813. [CrossRef] [PubMed]
94. Matsuzawa, Y. Adiponectin: A Key Player in Obesity Related Disorders. *Curr. Pharm. Des.* **2010**, *16*, 1896–1901. [CrossRef]
95. Koh, E.H.; Kim, M.; Ranjan, K.C.; Kim, H.S.; Park, H.-S.; Oh, K.S.; Park, I.-S.; Lee, W.J.; Kim, M.-S.; Park, J.-Y.; et al. eNOS plays a major role in adiponectin synthesis in adipocytes. *Am. J. Physiol. Metab.* **2010**, *298*, E846–E853. [CrossRef]
96. Sena, C.M.; Pereira, A.; Fernandes, R.; Letra, L.; Seiça, R.M. Adiponectin improves endothelial function in mesenteric arteries of rats fed a high-fat diet: Role of perivascular adipose tissue. *J. Cereb. Blood Flow Metab.* **2017**, *174*, 3514–3526. [CrossRef]
97. Lemecha, M.; Morino, K.; Imamura, T.; Iwasaki, H.; Ohashi, N.; Ida, S.; Sato, D.; Sekine, O.; Ugi, S.; Maegawa, H. MiR-494-3p regulates mitochondrial biogenesis and thermogenesis through PGC1-α signalling in beige adipocytes. *Sci. Rep.* **2018**, *8*, 15096. [CrossRef]
98. Kong, L.-R.; Zhou, Y.-P.; Chen, D.-R.; Ruan, C.-C.; Gao, P.-J. Decrease of Perivascular Adipose Tissue Browning Is Associated With Vascular Dysfunction in Spontaneous Hypertensive Rats During Aging. *Front. Physiol.* **2018**, *9*, 400. [CrossRef]
99. Hofseth, L.J.; Robles, A.I.; Espey, M.G.; Harris, C.C. Nitric Oxide Is a Signaling Molecule that Regulates Gene Expression. *Methods Enzymol.* **2005**, *396*, 326–340. [CrossRef]
100. Socco, S.; Bovee, R.C.; Palczewski, M.B.; Hickok, J.R.; Thomas, D.D. Epigenetics: The third pillar of nitric oxide signaling. *Pharmacol. Res.* **2017**, *121*, 52–58. [CrossRef]
101. Vasudevan, D.; Hickok, J.R.; Bovee, R.C.; Pham, V.; Mantell, L.L.; Bahroos, N.; Kanabar, P.; Cao, X.-J.; Maienschein-Cline, M.; Garcia, B.A.; et al. Nitric Oxide Regulates Gene Expression in Cancers by Controlling Histone Posttranslational Modifications. *Cancer Res.* **2015**, *75*, 5299–5308. [CrossRef]
102. Barp, C.G.; Benedet, P.O.; Assreuy, J. Perivascular adipose tissue phenotype and sepsis vascular dysfunction: Differential contribution of NO, ROS and beta 3-adrenergic receptor. *Life Sci.* **2020**, *254*, 117819. [CrossRef] [PubMed]
103. Jia, G.; Aroor, A.R.; Martinez-Lemus, L.A.; Sowers, J.R. Overnutrition, mTOR signaling, and cardiovascular diseases. *Am. J. Physiol. Integr. Comp. Physiol.* **2014**, *307*, R1198–R1206. [CrossRef] [PubMed]
104. Jia, G.; DeMarco, V.; Sowers, J.R. Insulin resistance and hyperinsulinaemia in diabetic cardiomyopathy. *Nat. Rev. Endocrinol.* **2015**, *12*, 144–153. [CrossRef] [PubMed]
105. Jia, G.; Habibi, J.; Aroor, A.R.; Martinez-Lemus, L.A.; DeMarco, V.G.; Ramirez-Perez, F.I.; Sun, Z.; Hayden, M.R.; Meininger, G.A.; Mueller, K.B.; et al. Endothelial Mineralocorticoid Receptor Mediates Diet-Induced Aortic Stiffness in Females. *Circ. Res.* **2016**, *118*, 935–943. [CrossRef] [PubMed]
106. Tajadura, V.; Hansen, M.H.; Smith, J.; Charles, H.; Rickman, M.; Farrell-Dillon, K.; Claro, V.; Warboys, C.; Ferro, A. β-catenin promotes endothelial survival by regulating eNOS activity and flow-dependent anti-apoptotic gene expression. *Cell Death Dis.* **2020**, *11*, 493. [CrossRef]

107. Cohen, A.W.; Hnasko, R.; Schubert, W.; Lisanti, M.P. Role of Caveolae and Caveolins in Health and Disease. *Physiol. Rev.* **2004**, *84*, 1341–1379. [CrossRef]
108. Lee, M.H.-H.; Chen, S.-J.; Tsao, C.-M.; Wu, C.-C. Perivascular Adipose Tissue Inhibits Endothelial Function of Rat Aortas via Caveolin-1. *PLoS ONE* **2014**, *9*, e99947. [CrossRef]
109. Chen, Z.; Oliveira, S.D.; Zimnicka, A.M.; Jiang, Y.; Sharma, T.; Chen, S.; Lazarov, O.; Bonini, M.G.; Haus, J.M.; Minshall, R.D. Reciprocal regulation of eNOS and caveolin-1 functions in endothelial cells. *Mol. Biol. Cell* **2018**, *29*, 1190–1202. [CrossRef]
110. Korda, M.; Kubant, R.; Patton, S.; Malinski, T. Leptin-induced endothelial dysfunction in obesity. *Am. J. Physiol. Circ. Physiol.* **2008**, *295*, H1514–H1521. [CrossRef]
111. Xia, N.; Weisenburger, S.; Koch, E.; Burkart, M.; Reifenberg, G.; Förstermann, U.; Li, H. Restoration of perivascular adipose tissue function in diet-induced obese mice without changing bodyweight. *Br. J. Pharmacol.* **2017**, *174*, 3443–3453. [CrossRef]
112. Gil-Ortega, M.; Condezo-Hoyos, L.; García-Prieto, C.F.; Arribas, S.M.; Gonzalez-Garcia, M.C.; Aranguez, I.; Ruiz-Gayo, M.; Somoza, B.; Fernandez-Alfonso, M.S. Imbalance between Pro and Anti-Oxidant Mechanisms in Perivascular Adipose Tissue Aggravates Long-Term High-Fat Diet-Derived Endothelial Dysfunction. *PLoS ONE* **2014**, *9*, e95312. [CrossRef] [PubMed]
113. Marchesi, C.; Ebrahimian, T.; Angulo, O.; Paradis, P.; Schiffrin, E.L. Endothelial Nitric Oxide Synthase Uncoupling and Perivascular Adipose Oxidative Stress and Inflammation Contribute to Vascular Dysfunction in a Rodent Model of Metabolic Syndrome. *Hypertension* **2009**, *54*, 1384–1392. [CrossRef] [PubMed]
114. Eyang, Z.; Eming, X.-F. Arginase: The Emerging Therapeutic Target for Vascular Oxidative Stress and Inflammation. *Front. Immunol.* **2013**, *4*, 149. [CrossRef]
115. Heiss, E.H.; Dirsch, V.M. Regulation of eNOS enzyme activity by posttranslational modification. *Curr. Pharm. Des.* **2014**, *20*, 3503–3513. [CrossRef] [PubMed]
116. Mattagajasingh, I.; Kim, C.-S.; Naqvi, A.; Yamamori, T.; Hoffman, T.A.; Jung, S.-B.; DeRicco, J.; Kasuno, K.; Irani, K. SIRT1 promotes endothelium-dependent vascular relaxation by activating endothelial nitric oxide synthase. *Proc. Natl. Acad. Sci. USA* **2007**, *104*, 14855–14860. [CrossRef]
117. da Costa, R.M.; Silva, J.F.d.; Alves, J.V.; Dias, T.B.; Rassi, D.M.; Garcia, L.V.; Lobato, N.d.S.; Tostes, R.C. Increased O-GlcNAcylation of endothelial nitric oxide synthase compromises the anti-contractile properties of perivascular adipose tissue in metabolic syndrome. *Front. Physiol.* **2018**, *9*, 341. [CrossRef]
118. Yu, Y.; Rajapakse, A.G.; Montani, J.-P.; Yang, Z.; Ming, X.-F. p38 mitogen-activated protein kinase is involved in arginase-II-mediated eNOS-Uncoupling in Obesity. *Cardiovasc. Diabetol.* **2014**, *13*, 113. [CrossRef]
119. Flood, E.D.; Watts, S.W. Endogenous Chemerin from PVAT Amplifies Electrical Field-Stimulated Arterial Contraction: Use of the Chemerin Knockout Rat. *Int. J. Mol. Sci.* **2020**, *21*, 6392. [CrossRef]
120. Neves, K.B.; Lobato, N.S.; Lopes, R.A.M.; Filgueira, F.P.; Zanotto, C.Z.; Oliveira, A.M.; Tostes, R.C. Chemerin reduces vascular nitric oxide/cGMP signalling in rat aorta: A link to vascular dysfunction in obesity? *Clin. Sci.* **2014**, *127*, 111–122. [CrossRef]
121. Neves, K.B.; Cat, A.N.D.; Lopes, R.A.M.; Rios, F.J.; Anagnostopoulou, A.; Lobato, N.S.; de Oliveira, A.M.; Tostes, R.C.; Montezano, A.C.; Touyz, R.M. Chemerin Regulates Crosstalk Between Adipocytes and Vascular Cells Through Nox. *Hypertension* **2015**, *66*, 657–666. [CrossRef]
122. Gómez-Serrano, M.; Camafeita, E.; López, J.A.; Rubio, M.A.; Bretón, I.; García-Consuegra, I.; García-Santos, E.; Lago, J.; Sánchez-Pernaute, A.; Torres, A.; et al. Differential proteomic and oxidative profiles unveil dysfunctional protein import to adipocyte mitochondria in obesity-associated aging and diabetes. *Redox Biol.* **2016**, *11*, 415–428. [CrossRef]
123. Bailey-Downs, L.C.; Tucsek, Z.; Toth, P.; Sosnowska, D.; Gautam, T.; Sonntag, W.E.; Csiszar, A.; Ungvari, Z. Aging exacerbates obesity-induced oxidative stress and inflammation in perivascular adipose tissue in mice: A paracrine mechanism contributing to vascular redox dysregulation and inflammation. *J. Gerontol. Ser. A Biomed. Sci. Med Sci.* **2013**, *68*, 780–792. [CrossRef] [PubMed]
124. Guo, X.; Zhang, Y.; Zheng, L.; Zheng, C.; Song, J.; Zhang, Q.; Kang, B.; Liu, Z.; Jin, L.; Xing, R.; et al. Global characterization of T cells in non-small-cell lung cancer by single-cell sequencing. *Nat. Med.* **2018**, *24*, 978–985. [CrossRef] [PubMed]
125. Yang, Y.-M.; Huang, A.; Kaley, G.; Sun, D. eNOS uncoupling and endothelial dysfunction in aged vessels. *Am. J. Physiol. Circ. Physiol.* **2009**, *297*, H1829–H1836. [CrossRef]
126. Sousa, A.S.; Sponton, A.C.d.S.; Trifone, C.B.; Delbin, M.A. Aerobic exercise training prevents perivascular adipose tissue (PVAT)-induced endothelial dysfunction in thoracic aorta of obese mice. *Front. Physiol.* **2019**, *10*, 1009. [CrossRef]
127. You, T.; Arsenis, N.C.; Disanzo, B.L.; LaMonte, M.J. Effects of Exercise Training on Chronic Inflammation in Obesity. *Sports Med.* **2013**, *43*, 243–256. [CrossRef] [PubMed]
128. Gu, P.; Hui, H.; Vanhoutte, P.; Lam, K.; Xu, A. Deletion of SIRT1 in perivascular adipose tissue accelerates obesity-induced endothelial dysfunction. In Proceedings of the 1st ASCEPT-BPS Joint Scientific Meeting, Hong Kong, China, 19–21 May 2015.
129. Nemoto, S.; Fergusson, M.M.; Finkel, T. SIRT1 Functionally Interacts with the Metabolic Regulator and Transcriptional Coactivator PGC-1α. *J. Biol. Chem.* **2005**, *280*, 16456–16460. [CrossRef]
130. Qiang, L.; Wang, H.; Farmer, S.R. Adiponectin Secretion Is Regulated by SIRT1 and the Endoplasmic Reticulum Oxidoreductase Ero1-Lα. *Mol. Cell. Biol.* **2007**, *27*, 4698–4707. [CrossRef]
131. Sun, Y.; Li, J.; Xiao, N.; Wang, M.; Kou, J.; Qi, L.; Huang, F.; Liu, B.; Liu, K. Pharmacological activation of AMPK ameliorates perivascular adipose/endothelial dysfunction in a manner interdependent on AMPK and SIRT1. *Pharmacol. Res.* **2014**, *89*, 19–28. [CrossRef]

132. Chen, Y.; Xu, X.; Zhang, Y.; Liu, K.; Huang, F.; Liu, B.; Kou, J. Diosgenin regulates adipokine expression in perivascular adipose tissue and ameliorates endothelial dysfunction via regulation of AMPK. *J. Steroid Biochem. Mol. Biol.* **2016**, *155*, 155–165. [CrossRef]
133. Dimmeler, S.; Fleming, I.; Fisslthaler, B.; Hermann, C.; Busse, R.; Zeiher, A.M. Activation of nitric oxide synthase in endothelial cells by Akt-dependent phosphorylation. *Nature* **1999**, *399*, 601–605. [CrossRef] [PubMed]
134. Bijland, S.; Mancini, S.J.; Salt, I.P. Role of AMP-activated protein kinase in adipose tissue metabolism and inflammation. *Clin. Sci.* **2013**, *124*, 491–507. [CrossRef] [PubMed]
135. Thors, B.; Halldórsson, H.; Thorgeirsson, G. eNOS activation mediated by AMPK after stimulation of endothelial cells with histamine or thrombin is dependent on LKB1. *Biochim. Et Biophys. Acta* **2011**, *1813*, 322–331. [CrossRef] [PubMed]
136. Meziat, C.; Boulghobra, D.; Strock, E.; Battault, S.; Bornard, I.; Walther, G.; Reboul, C. Exercise training restores eNOS activation in the perivascular adipose tissue of obese rats: Impact on vascular function. *Nitric Oxide* **2019**, *86*, 63–67. [CrossRef] [PubMed]
137. Aldiss, P.; Lewis, J.E.; Lupini, I.; Boocock, D.J.; Miles, A.K.; Ebling, F.J.; Budge, H.; Symonds, M.E. Exercise does not induce browning of WAT at thermoneutrality and induces an oxidative, myogenic signature in BAT. *bioRxiv* **2019**, 649061. [CrossRef]
138. DeVallance, E.; Branyan, K.W.; Lemaster, K.C.; Anderson, R.; Marshall, K.L.; Olfert, I.M.; Smith, D.M.; Kelley, E.E.; Bryner, R.W.; Frisbee, J.C.; et al. Exercise training prevents the perivascular adipose tissue-induced aortic dysfunction with metabolic syndrome. *Redox Biol.* **2019**, *26*, 101285. [CrossRef]
139. Aghamohammadzadeh, R.; Greenstein, A.S.; Yadav, R.; Jeziorska, M.; Hama, S.; Soltani, F.; Pemberton, P.W.; Ammori, B.; Malik, R.A.; Soran, H.; et al. Effects of Bariatric Surgery on Human Small Artery Function: Evidence for Reduction in Perivascular Adipocyte Inflammation, and the Restoration of Normal Anticontractile Activity Despite Persistent Obesity. *J. Am. Coll. Cardiol.* **2013**, *62*, 128–135. [CrossRef]

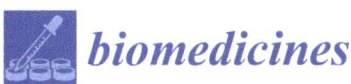

Review

Therapeutic Effects of Inhaled Nitric Oxide Therapy in COVID-19 Patients

Nikolay O. Kamenshchikov [1,*], Lorenzo Berra [2,3] and Ryan W. Carroll [3,4]

1. Cardiology Research Institute, Tomsk National Research Medical Center, Russian Academy of Sciences, 634012 Tomsk, Russia
2. Department of Anaesthesia, Critical Care and Pain Medicine, Massachusetts General Hospital, Boston, MA 02114, USA; lberra@mgh.harvard.edu
3. Department of Anaesthesia, Harvard Medical School, Boston, MA 02115, USA; rcarroll4@mgh.harvard.edu
4. Division of Pediatric Critical Care Medicine, Massachusetts General Hospital, Boston, MA 02114, USA
* Correspondence: cardio@cardio-tomsk.ru

Abstract: The global COVID-19 pandemic has become the largest public health challenge of recent years. The incidence of COVID-19-related acute hypoxemic respiratory failure (AHRF) occurs in up to 15% of hospitalized patients. Antiviral drugs currently available to clinicians have little to no effect on mortality, length of in-hospital stay, the need for mechanical ventilation, or long-term effects. Inhaled nitric oxide (iNO) administration is a promising new non-standard approach to directly treat viral burden while enhancing oxygenation. Along with its putative antiviral affect in COVID-19 patients, iNO can reduce inflammatory cell-mediated lung injury by inhibiting neutrophil activation, lowering pulmonary vascular resistance and decreasing edema in the alveolar spaces, collectively enhancing ventilation/perfusion matching. This narrative review article presents recent literature on the iNO therapy use for COVID-19 patients. The authors suggest that early administration of the iNO therapy may be a safe and promising approach for the treatment of COVID-19 patients. The authors also discuss unconventional approaches to treatment, continuous versus intermittent high-dose iNO therapy, timing of initiation of therapy (early versus late), and novel delivery systems. Future laboratory and clinical research is required to define the role of iNO as an adjunct therapy against bacterial, viral, and fungal infections.

Keywords: nitric oxide; COVID-19; acute respiratory syndrome coronavirus 2; inhaled nitric oxide therapy; endothelium

1. Introduction

The global Coronavirus Disease 2019 (COVID-19) pandemic has become the deadliest respiratory infection since the Spanish Flu in 1918–1920. COVID-19 is a respiratory infection that spans from mild involvement of the upper respiratory tract to severe pneumonia leading to respiratory failure, shock, and death [1].

COVID-19-associated complications are multifactorial and involve endothelial cell dysfunction, local hyperinflammation, intravascular coagulation, and microthrombosis [2–4]. This constellation of systemic and organ endotheliopathy has been proposed to explain phenotypic variants associated with COVID-19 [5–9]. A decrease in the angiotensin-converting enzyme 2 (ACE2) activity, caused by its interaction with the SARS-CoV-2 virus and endocytosis of the viral complex and downregulation, leads to an increase in vasoconstriction, pro-coagulation, pro-inflammation, and pro-oxidant angiotensin II effects. These effects, in turn, potentiate inflammation, trigger the release of injury-associated molecules, and cause viral damage to the lung. Specific viral and cytokine storm-induced endothelial damage is called SARS-CoV-2-associated endotheliitis, reflecting COVID-19 microangiopathy in the lungs, and other organs, coupled with the development of thrombosis due to vasculitis.

A respiratory treatment that halts the progression of disease could substantially improve both saved lives and spared hospital resources. At this time, treatment with dexamethasone (a systemic steroid) has been shown to reduce the 28-day mortality in patients requiring mechanical ventilation or oxygen but has no effect on the early progression of the disease [10]. Thus far, no inhaled treatment has been shown to be beneficial to both respiratory and systemic pathophysiology, the endothelium, and viral load, with the potential to halt progression of disease [11].

Antiviral drugs, such as molnupiravir and remdesivir, demonstrated an improvement on mortality, length of in-hospital stay, and the need for mechanical ventilation in specific subpopulations of hospitalized patients only [12]. Despite these advancements in therapeutics, an intervention that readily combines the improvement of clinical symptoms, including hypoxia, and the reduction of endothelial dysfunction is still lacking. High-dose inhaled nitric oxide (iNO) holds promise as an intervention that fulfills these goals.

We present here a review of published studies and ongoing trials on the therapeutic effects of iNO for COVID-19.

2. Historical Benefits of NO: iNO as Selective Pulmonary Vasodilator Improving Ventilation/Perfusion Matching

iNO gas is a therapy currently approved for the treatment of pulmonary hypertension in newborns and is also used as a rescue therapy in patients with ARDS [13,14]. Type 3 pulmonary hypertension (due to pulmonary pathology and/or hypoxia) occurs in 40–75% of patients admitted to the ICU with pneumonia, and up to 50% of patients with ARDS [15]. In 21% of ARDS cases, patients develop acute RV failure and acute pulmonary heart disease, associated with an increase in pulmonary vascular resistance [16,17]. During the current COVID-19 pandemic, elevated pulmonary artery systolic pressure has been identified as a hemodynamic parameter associated with a fatal outcome [18]. These data support the use of preventive interventions for RV failure as therapeutic targets and a reframing of therapy for ARDS, adding 'RV protective' strategies to the well-established 'lung protective' ventilation strategy [17,19].

An ideal medication that optimizes hemodynamics and pulmonary gas exchange should result in improved hypoxemia while positively affecting the underlying pathophysiological mechanisms, thereby preventing fatal complications (reduction of pulmonary hypertension and right ventricular dysfunction). In such a case, targeted antiviral therapy could be coupled with adjuvant pathogenetic therapy directed against the mechanisms that directly lead to mortality. iNO holds promise as an all-encompassing therapy for COVID-19 patients. It is a selective pulmonary vasodilator with known beneficial physiological effects for use in patients with ARDS, potentially reducing the acute RV failure associated with high mortality due to COVID-19 pneumonia, influences the mechanisms that enhance V/Q matching and reduce shunt alteration, and has direct anti-viral effects based on in vitro evidence [20]. The available data on the effect of iNO as a possible adjuvant agent for respiratory treatment in patients with COVID-19 are inconclusive. However, high-quality evidence from past pandemics suggests that iNO use in ARDS, due to SARS-CoV, results in improved arterial oxygenation, decreased pulmonary hypertension, and reduced spread and density of lung infiltrates [21]. However, iNO use has failed to reduce mechanical ventilation days and overall mortality in ARDS patients [21–24]. Considering the phenotype of intrapulmonary vascular architecture abnormalities found in COVID-19, there is a deep adaptive pathophysiological rationale for the favorable iNO-mediated changes in pulmonary hemodynamics. In COVID-19, an increase in the V/Q ratio is observed in well-aerated, intact sections due to angiotensin II-mediated vasoconstriction, endothelial dysfunction, vasculitis, and thrombosis [25]. Therefore, lung lesions in COVID-19 are not homogenous and occur due to the alternation of the alveolar shunt and alveolar dead space compartments [26,27]. The SARS-CoV-2 virus uses the angiotensin-converting enzyme 2 (ACE2) receptor to enter the cell, which leads to a decrease in its activity, through a negative feedback mechanism, while the levels of plasma angiotensin II increase and angiotensin

(1–7) decrease [28]. In this case, a specific pulmonary vasoconstrictor, pro-inflammatory, procoagulant phenotype is formed, mediated by angiotensin II [29,30]. This was confirmed by Santamarina MG et al., who showed that the pathophysiology of moderate to severe respiratory failure in COVID-19 is based on a severe ventilation/perfusion (V/Q) mismatch [8,9]. The authors demonstrated a decrease in the V/Q ratio in areas of the lung parenchyma with ground-glass nodules or consolidation due to an increase in perfusion in poorly ventilated areas. These areas are the morphological basis of the alveolar shunt in conditions of secondary loss of compensatory hypoxic pulmonary vasoconstriction [31].

At the same time, an increase in the V/Q ratio is observed in well-aerated intact sections due to angiotensin II-mediated vasoconstriction, endothelial dysfunction, vasculitis, and thrombosis [25]. Therefore, lung lesions in COVID-19 are inhomogeneous and occur due to the alternation of the alveolar shunt and alveolar dead space compartments [27]. Mechanical ventilation and other respiratory support strategies (non-invasive ventilation and high-flow oxygen therapy) do not affect the V/Q ratio in intact ventilation and perfusion pathology, while the positive effects of prone position on oxygenation can be explained by the gravitational redistribution of blood flow to intact areas with high V/Q ratio and a cumulative V/Q optimization in general. At the same time the increase in alveolar dead space is independently associated with mortality in ARDS [32]. This pathophysiological theory supports the early use of pulmonary vasodilators, such as iNO (Figure 1) [8,9]. To this end, there is evidence that iNO may be the most effective in patients with COVID-19 respiratory failure and concomitant pulmonary hypertension [33,34].

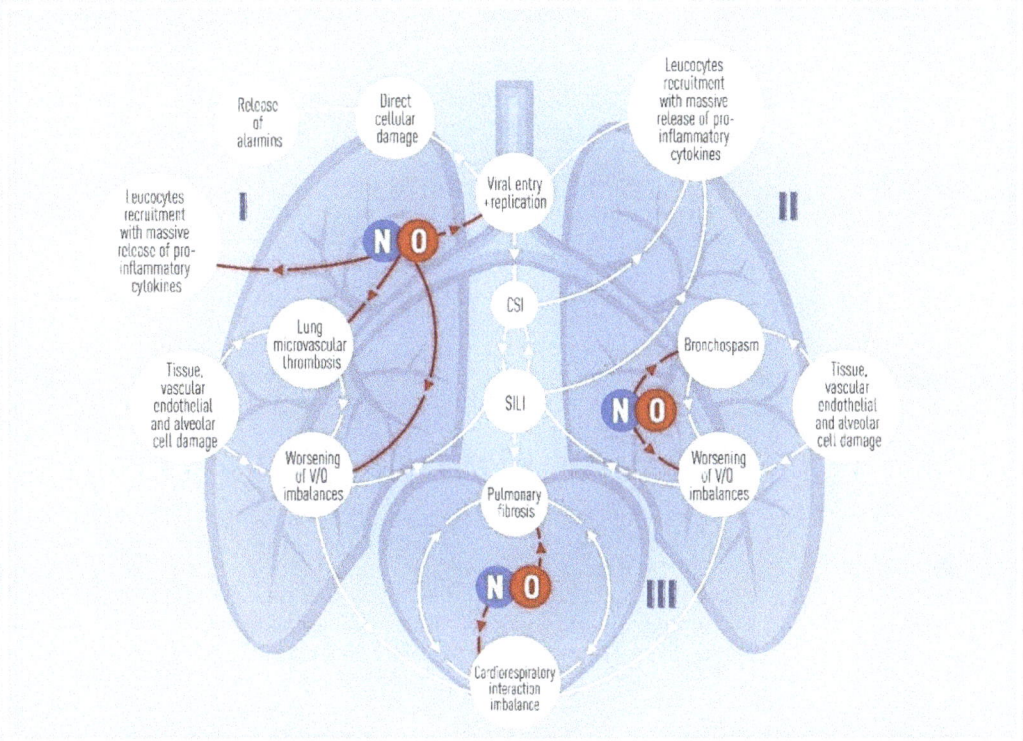

Figure 1. Illustrates the continuum of intrapulmonary pathophysiology at the early stages of COVID-19 pneumonia, highlighting the putative beneficial effects of NO. Part I. The effects of iNO are etiopathogenetic.

iNO may reduce viral load while halting the intrapulmonary cascade of inflammation, decreasing alveolar dead space, and thus optimizing ventilation-perfusion. In addition, a decrease in respiratory rate, improvement of gas exchange, and enhanced respiratory comfort may prevent the development of self-induced lung injury (SILI). iNO may also prevent co- and superinfection (CSI), including those involving hospital antibiotic-resistant flora. To this end, it is important to consider administering iNO therapy at the early stage of disease, before the development of irreversible changes in the lungs. Part II. Persistent SILI and CSI contribute to transition of disease into a self-maintaining and self-sustained process. The continuum of intrapulmonary pathophysiology is mediated by local and systemic hyper-inflammatory reactions, even after virus elimination. There is an increase in elastance and a decrease in aerated lung, an increase in intra-alveolar exudation, a transition to low compliance phenotype, mirroring the known pathogenesis ARDS. The NO-mediated impact at this stage is aimed at optimizing V/Q matching. Considering the transition of functional changes in the lungs to morphological changes, therapeutic effects of iNO would be quite limited, represent last-resort treatment, and do not consistently result in improved outcomes. Part III. iNO-mediated cardio-respiratory interactions to reduce the risk of right ventricular failure. Prevention of acute cor pulmonale development by reducing right ventricular afterload. Prevention of group 3 pulmonary hypertension due to prolonged antifibrotic effects of iNO in the lungs.

3. Burgeoning Antimicrobial Effects of iNO-Therapy: Viral, Bacterial, Fungal

The clinical role of NO in COVID-19 patients may be relevant due to in-vitro evidence of NO antiviral activity, specifically against the SARS coronavirus [35,36]. Preclinical and clinical evidence suggests that iNO has a viricidal effect, including the family of Coronaviridae. Moreover, in vitro studies demonstrate that the use of NO-donor compound S-nitroso-N-acetylpenicillamine leads to an increased survival rate of in vitro mammalian cells infected with SARS-CoV. SARS-CoV and SARS-CoV-2 share the same subgenus within the family Coronaviridae. Recent studies have confirmed that NO can inhibit SARS-CoV-2 replication, and the main viral protease for targeted NO therapy has also been identified [37].

Similar therapeutic effects of NO can be expected in patients with COVID-19 due to the genetic similarities between the two viruses. The literature seems to point towards nonspecific rather than pathogen-specific antimicrobial effects of NO. Thus, the role of exogenous iNO as an antiviral agent during a COVID-19 infection could be hypothesized [38].

NO-dependent virus elimination is most likely mediated by inhibiting viral replication with genetic modification [39–53]. Antiviral defense mechanisms involve the deactivation of viral proteins essential for viral replication: viral proteases, reverse transcriptases, transcription factors, etc. mediated by S-nitrosylation of essential thiol groups [54]. Dinitrosyl iron complexes with thiol ligands in lung and airway tissues, created by high-dose iNO therapy due to the prolonged release of nitrosonium cation (NO+) donors can suppress various metabolic processes utilized by a coronavirus that are responsible for penetration into cells as well as replication [55,56]. A. F. Vanin et al., using an experimental model and healthy volunteers, demonstrated that the inhalation of high-dose NO could be followed by the absorption of a large portion of the agent in the lung and respiratory tissues as dinitrosyl iron complexes with thiol ligands [57]. Systemic side effects did not occur. The authors concluded that a high concentration of NO donors are the main sites that host coronavirus in the human body as a result of the contact with a high-concentration of iNO and, therefore, could be of great use during eradication of a coronavirus [57]. High-concentrations of NO have been found to be microbicidal but still safe in spontaneously breathing subjects in a phase I trial [58]. However, the optimal therapeutic regimens and the efficacy of NO gas in reducing viral load while improving oxygenation in hypoxemic COVID-19 patients have not yet been tested. A pilot study showed that low-dose iNO (max 30 ppm) could shorten the time of ventilatory support for patients infected with SARS-CoV [21].

The antimicrobial and antifungal effects of iNO, convincingly shown in a number of studies, can improve the clinical course of COVID-19 in conditions of co- and superinfection [59,60]. The detection rate of atypical respiratory pathogens and viral co-infections in the general population of hospitalized patients with COVID-19 has reached 15.6–20.7% [61,62]. Despite the low incidence of bacterial co-infection upon admission to the hospital, 14–100% of patients admitted to ICUs demonstrate a co-infection, including bacterial co- and superinfection [63,64], while the frequency of ventilator-associated pneumonia (VAP) in a SARS-CoV-2 infection has been reported to be 50.5% [65]. VAP is associated with an increased 28-day mortality rate and longer duration of mechanical ventilation and ICU length of stay in SARS-CoV-2 patients [66]. Fungal invasion is also a major problem in the management of COVID-19 patients, which, together with bacterial infections, can significantly increase therapy costs and possibly worsen outcomes [67]. Thus, the incidence of secondary infections in patients hospitalized with COVID-19, especially in the ICU, may not be as low as that in early reports, and the iNO therapy may be able to improve outcomes by expanding the anti-infective spectrum of therapy regardless of the etiologic agent.

The type of escalation therapy, aimed at a wide range of pathogens, is especially promising in conditions of scarcity of resources for accurate verification of an infectious agent and determination of its possible resistance to therapy, including antibiotic resistance. In addition, the current principles of therapy for a complicated disease course of a SARS-CoV-2 infection prescribe immunosuppressive drugs as therapy for the "cytokine storm", which can lead not only to secondary infections, but also contribute to the long-term persistence of the virus in the body, and increase the frequency of its mutations and the likelihood of emerging new strains. In this regard, the early use of iNO as a universal direct-acting antiviral agent also seems reasonable. It could reduce viral load and attenuate the direct damaging effect of the virus on the lungs. The adjuvant antibacterial and antifungal effects of iNO could prevent the development of secondary infections of the respiratory tract, which is especially important in conditions of the multidrug-resistant bacteria commonly found in the ICU.

At the time being, iNO adjuvant therapy is recommended by a number of researchers as an effective strategy for the treatment of COVID-19 [68–70].

4. Other Benefits of iNO-Therapy: Endothelial Stability, Improving Inflammation, Biofilm Dispersion

Systemic and organ endotheliopathy in COVID-19 is likely multifactorial and involves direct viral invasion, endothelial cell dysfunction, local hyperinflammation, intravascular coagulation, and microthrombosis [2–4]. iNO therapy may reduce endothelial pulmonary syndrome with microvascular thrombosis. Possible favorable systemic actions of iNO treatment include antiplatelet, leukocyte antiadhesive, and anti-inflammatory effects, which can potentially prevent a cytokine storm and reduce the risk of extrapulmonary organ complications [71]. Moreover, the presence of a reserve pool of NO in extrapulmonary tissues due to the S-nitrosylation mechanism leads to a decrease in vascular tone and reduces the risk of thrombosis and leukocyte adhesion to the systemic vascular endothelium [72]. Severe forms of COVID-19 are associated with exaggerated and persistent injury to the endothelium of pulmonary microvasculature [73], endothelial apoptotic bodies were also observed during an autopsy in other organs [74]. In addition to bronchial epithelial cells and pulmonary type II cells, the SARS-CoV-2 virus has a tropism for endothelial cells leading to cell apoptosis and a decrease of endothelial NO production [75]. A significant decrease in endothelium-dependent synthesis has been demonstrated in patients with COVID-19, especially in complicated cases [76], which led to the hypothesis that NO imbalance is associated with lung damage [77]. Researchers put forth more pathways for the formation of NO deficiency in an infection caused by SARS-CoV-2: NO imbalance, reactive oxygen species associated with dysregulation of angiotensin II-angiotensin (1–7) [78], systemic inflammation, tissue inflammation, mitochondrial dysfunction, and changes to vascular tones by increasing intracellular calcium concentration and reducing the bioavailability of NO [79]. Hypertension, diabetes, and cardiovascular diseases significantly aggravate the course of COVID-19 and are associated with endothelial dysfunction and decreased endothelial NO production and bioavailability [80].

The mechanism for increasing the bioavailability of NO upon its exogenous administration is protein S-nitrosylation and an increase in the concentration of serum NO-NOx metabolites (nitrates, nitrites, S-nitrosothiol, N-nitrosamine, etc.), which serve as reserve NO donors in the body [81,82]. Extrapulmonary accumulation of these metabolites in target organs can realize the distant organ protective effects of exogenous NO [83]. Exposure and stabilization of endothelium function with iNO therapy can reduce COVID-associated distant complications such as AKI [84,85].

In addition, NO has a whole range of important pathogenetic effects: NO can reduce inflammatory cell-mediated lung injury by inhibiting neutrophil activation and local pro-inflammatory cytokine release, leading to a decrease edema in the alveolar spaces [71]. iNO is considered a pharmacological tool for monitoring the excessive inflammatory response of the host organism and overcoming the "cytokine storm" associated with viral diseases [86]. Progressive immunothrombosis in COVID-19 is associated with NO deficiency [87]. Endogenous NO, produced in the paranasal sinuses, and exogenous iNO have bronchodilatory effects and activate mucociliary clearance [88–92]. The enterosalivary nitrate–nitrite–NO pathway, as a storage pool plays an essential role in the prevention of ischaemic cardiovascular and septic events, and deficiency of a synthase-dependent pathway generating NO may be associated with sepsis, organ failure, and an increased mortality rate [92]. Thus, a number of researchers suggest that iNO is essential for sanogenesis of the respiratory tract in various pathological processes, including infections [93–95].

Increased salivary and serum NO levels are associated with survival in ARDS caused by the H1N1 virus [96]. There is an alternative point of view suggesting that the NO signaling pathway does not only fail to improve the outcomes of viral infections but can also be an independent damaging factor and/or a marker of the severity of lung damage in some cases [97–100].

At present, most data highlighting the antimicrobial efficacy of iNO were obtained on the culture of planktonic free forms of bacteria associated with the dispersed phase of the life cycle, which is necessary for the expansive colonization of new habitats. However, in nature, most bacteria live mainly in the heterogeneous multicellular communities of biofilms. The biofilm matrix reduces the degree of penetration of antibiotics, accumulating factors of specific and nonspecific resistance to cells of the immune system and biocides [101–103]. In biofilms, there is a modification of the native genetic material and post-transcriptional changes in the phenotype caused by the commensal community [104]. This gives bacterial colonies significant resistance to external factors, forms antibiotic resistance, and allows the avoidance of immune surveillance [105]. Moreover, some antibiotics can cause increased biofilm formation [106].

The proportion of infections associated with biofilm formation in clinical practice reaches 80% [107]. This is associated with resistance and chronicity of pathological process, an increase in morbidity and mortality [108]. Currently, iNO is being viewed as a novel therapeutic strategy for controlling and overcoming biofilm resistance [105]. The use of low doses of NO stimulates the transition to the dispersion phase of the cycle, which leads to the restoration of the sensitivity of biofilms and free bacteria to the action of antimicrobial drugs and increases the efficacy of antibiotic therapy [109], and an increase in exposure time inhibits biofilm formation [110–112]. At the same time, the intermittent effect of high concentrations of NO has a direct destructive effect on biofilms of gram-negative and gram-positive bacteria, including nosocomial pathogens [113–115]. Clinical studies of iNO use in biofilm-related infections have demonstrated significant reductions in the number of bacterial biofilm aggregates and improvement in lung function, suggesting that the use of iNO as adjunctive therapy may be very beneficial [116]. Widespread adoption of iNO therapy could provide unprecedented control and treatment of biofilms in the current pandemic, improve short-term outcomes for COVID-19 patients, and reduce the probability of "chronic critical illness" and post COVID-19 long-term antibiotic resistance substrate formation [117].

5. iNO and COVID-19 Specific Data

An effective etiological treatment for COVID-19 has not yet been developed. The large mortality rates in COVID-19 patients requiring mechanical ventilation are prompting clinicians and scientists to seek new technologies and pharmacological interventions that can improve outcomes. Researchers and clinicians consider iNO therapy promising for patients with COVID-19 and respiratory failure [38,71], supported by in vitro research from Akaberi et al. [37]. In 2003, during the SARS epidemic in China, a small observational study of patients with SARS pneumonia receiving non-invasive support, biphasic positive airway pressure (BiPAP), were treated with NO gas which improved oxygenation, accelerated the resolution of chest X-ray infiltrates, reduced the need for intubation, and led to a more rapid and sustained ARDS resolution and improved overall clinical outcomes [21]. In the current global pandemic, iNO therapy is accepted by the societies of critical care medicine as a temporary measure to maintain or improve oxygenation in mechanically ventilated patients [118,119]. In healthcare practice, about 30% of patients with severe C-ARDS have received iNO as a life-saving therapy [120,121]. However, the results of published randomized trials and clinical observations are highly controversial. Small cohort studies have not demonstrated a significant improvement in oxygenation and clinical outcomes with iNO therapy [122]. On the other hand, the frequency of responders ranges from 25% to 40% with a tendency of a more pronounced effect on gas exchange in patients with right ventricular dysfunction. The percentage of iNO responders is much lower than in patients with non-C-ARDS [123,124].

Several trials tested the efficacy of iNO therapy aimed at improving the outcomes in COVID-19 patients. A retrospective observational study showed that NO gas is useful in improving the oxygenation in spontaneously breathing patients with COVID-19 pneumonia [125]. High-dose nitric oxide (160 ppm) was safely administered to pregnant females with severe COVID-19 pneumonia [126] and as a rescue therapy to spontaneously breathing patients with COVID-19 and hypoxemic respiratory failure [127]. A recent trial non-invasively treating patients with moderate COVID-19 hypoxia demonstrated that iNO-therapy produced an acute improvement of systemic oxygenation in hypoxemic patients and reduced the respiratory rate [128]. Furthermore, data demonstrate that the administration of iNO improves functional status in ambulatory patients [33,34].

Preliminary data support the iNO-mediated improvement of oxygenation in mechanically ventilated patients and spontaneously breathing patients with COVID-19 [129]. However, the optimal therapeutic regimen of iNO administration in spontaneously breathing hypoxemic patients has not been identified.

Another strategy for iNO administration in COVID-19 involves the potential for selective pulmonary vasodilation to optimize ventilation/perfusion matching by reducing pulmonary vascular resistance and decreasing alveolar dead space. The drug intervention scheme herein assumes administration of a long-term, constant NO insufflation at low doses, in contrast to the pulse therapy, aimed directly at the elimination of the viral agent from the respiratory tract. Prolonged iNO therapy can also have an independent moderate antiviral effect, and, due to prolonged exposure, it can reduce inflammatory cell-mediated lung injury by inhibiting neutrophil activation and subsequent pro-inflammatory cytokine release. The study of iNO treatment in spontaneously breathing COVID-19 patients demonstrates not only an increase in oxygenation in all non-intubated patients, but also provides evidence that iNO therapy may have a role in preventing progression of hypoxemic respiratory failure [125].

6. Modality of iNO Therapy: Timing of iNO Administration

Hypoxemia in the early stages of COVID-19 is caused by a dysregulated pulmonary perfusion [130,131]. Changes in pulmonary biomechanics demonstrate that at an early, well-defined stage of COVID-19 disease (between the admission to the high-dependency unit to the time of healing or admission to the ICU), the lung weight in C-ARDS was approximately half of what has been described in a typical ARDS. The C-ARDS gas-volume was two times greater than what has been consistently described in the typical ARDS [132]. Thus, in the early stages, C-ARDS is fundamentally atypical, as the severity of hypoxemia is unrelated to the severity of the anatomical lung pathology. Moreover, the authors do not exclude that other viral pneumonias present similar characteristics [132]. In all of the studies that did not show improvement in oxygenation and/or clinical outcomes, attention was drawn to a significant time delay from patient intubation to initiation of iNO therapy, which is largely due to the behavioral despair paradigm of utilizing selective pulmonary vasodilators in severe hypoxemic respiratory failure. The median time from intubation to initiation of iNO, reported by different clinics, ranged from 3.6 days to 6.5 days in studies where iNO was used as a second-line pulmonary vasodilator [122,133]. It is noteworthy that in these cases, the frequency of response to iNO was 64%. Data from other authors indicate a response to iNO therapy in more than 65% of patients with C-ARDS, manifested in a significant increase in the PaO_2/FiO_2 ratio reduction in the oxygenation index and a reduction in the dead space fraction, associated with higher baseline BNP and troponin values. The authors put forward a hypothesis about a specific pulmonary vascular phenotype in iNO responders and a special role of pulmonary vascular function in COVID-19 pathophysiology [134,135]. A potential cause of the mentioned dissonance in the obtained data can be the severity and irreversibility of morphological changes both in the lung parenchyma and in the capillary bed of the pulmonary microcirculation at the late stages of the disease: pulmonary oedema and pulmonary consolidation prevent from alveolar supply with iNO; intravascular coagulation and organized thrombosis do not allow the effects of iNO in ventilated alveoli to reduce dead space in severe C-ARDS [25]. Thus, considering the pathogenesis of lung capillary injury and extrapulmonary complications in COVID-19, the use of iNO can be promising at the early stages of the disease when the disorders are potentially reversible or "functional" in nature [136]. De Grado et al. [133] observed a trend towards higher tidal volume and compliance in individuals who responded to inhaled vasodilators therapy, which led the authors to suggest that inhaled vasodilators therapy would be more effective in patients with a sufficient volume of functioning alveoli, possibly at the early stages of the disease before the evolution to late stage ARDS with low-compliance [27], while other authors suggest concentrating on the "vasocentric" nature of this disease [137]. We support the idea of tailoring the initiation of iNO therapy, which must be correlated with the stages of the progression of the disease-related intrapulmonary aberrations. Early initiation of iNO therapy may alter the dramatic development of COVID-19 pneumonia pathophysiology.

Figure 1 illustrates the evolution of COVID-19 from early to late stages and demonstrates the points of application of iNO (Part I: early stage; Part II: late stage; Part III: interaction in the lung-heart system).

The use of iNO in the early stages of the disease has pluripotent effects and can help eliminate the pathogen, stabilize and reduce pulmonary stress associated with changes in transpulmonary pressure in dyspnea, improve gas exchange, and prevent a secondary infection. Ultimately, this may prevent disease progression, and iNO should be considered as an intervention with self-healing potential. The use of iNO in the late stages of COVID-19 at severe extensive morphological changes in the lung parenchyma (usually consolidation) is an exclusively temporary measure to maintain gas exchange before escalation therapy (for example, transition to ECMO). In terms of cardio-respiratory interactions, the use of iNO may reflect the new concept of 'RV protective' strategies for respiratory therapy in the short and long term (prevention of acute cor pulmonale and chronic group 3 pulmonary hypertension).

7. Modality of iNO Therapy: Dosage Mode (Continuous versus Intermittent iNO Administration)

The idea of intermittent dosing of high-dose iNO to combat a SARS-CoV-2 infection appeared after analyzing data on COVID-19 cases among smokers in different countries: the incidence of COVID-19 patients among smokers was lower than in the general population [138–140]. While the toxic effects of smoking are devastating, it is worthy to note here for the purpose of this review that NO ranges in each puff from 250–1350 ppm, which is much higher than the medical use of iNO, generally no more than 80 ppm [141,142], suggesting that iNO dosed in short bursts and at high concentrations may protect against COVID-19 [143].

High doses of NO have been shown to be safe and well tolerated (160 ppm for 30 min, 5 times a day for 5 days) in healthy volunteers [58]. The original system for the high-dose iNO delivery for hospitalized patients was developed by Gianni S et al. [144]. It was easy to use and safe in clinical practice. A small group of pregnant patients ($n = 6$) with severe and critical COVID-19 received NO inhalation by mask twice a day at a high dose (160–200 ppm) for 30 min [126]. The authors explain the reasoning for this compassionate-use intermittent therapy, including its potential antiviral, anti-inflammatory, and mild bronchodilatory effects, in addition to selective pulmonary vasodilation, which may improve maternal and fetal oxygenation. Furthermore, iNO therapy was shown to be well-tolerated and associated with improved oxygenation, respiratory rate, cardiopulmonary system function in this population [126]. Moreover, in some patients, there was an association between intermittent high-dose iNO therapy and a decrease in markers of systemic inflammation [126]. Early adoption of this system contributes to a decrease in the respiratory rate, enhances patient respiratory comfort, and reduces the work of breathing. It might also prevent transpulmonary pressure variations and the progression of self-induced lung injury. iNO-mediated bronchodilation and the improvement of bronchial patency also prevent atelectasis formation, minimizing a decrease in lung compliance and progression to lung fibrosis. This hypothesis is supported by the encouraging results of clinical observations and studies carried out in spontaneously breathing patients with COVID-19-associated hypoxemic respiratory failure. Fakhr B.S. et al. demonstrated that the administration of iNO at 160 ppm for 30 min twice daily promptly improved the respiratory rate of tachypneic patients and systemic oxygenation of hypoxemic patients. No adverse events were observed [128]. None of the subjects were readmitted or had long-term COVID-19 sequelae [128]. Similar results were obtained in a group of COVID-19 patients at high risk for acute hypoxemic respiratory failure with worsening symptoms, despite the use of supplemental oxygen and/or awake proning, who were treated with high-dose iNO [127]. NO pulse therapy has been stated to be well-tolerated and used as an effective adjuvant rescue therapy for patients with COVID-19 [127]. Moreover, the authors suggest its effectiveness as an alternative to available antiviral drugs in cases when they may be contraindicated (pregnancy, drug intolerance, etc.)

Parikh et al. used the strategy for continuous iNO therapy in spontaneously breathing patients with COVID-19; at the same time, 54% did not require invasive mechanical ventilation after treatment with iNO [125]. If these findings are confirmed in larger studies, treatment with iNO, along with high-flow oxygen therapy and non-invasive ventilation may become the first respiratory treatment for this large cohort of patients.

A clinical trial titled "Nitric oxide therapy for COVID-19 patients with oxygen requirement (NICOR)" was registered with ClinicalTrials.gov (#NCT04476992). The trial aims to study the safety of intermittent versus continuous iNO in spontaneously breathing COVID-19 patients. Authors hypothesize that high-dose iNO with an adjunct of continuous low dose administration between the high-dose treatments can be safely administered in hypoxemic COVID-19 patients compared to the high dose treatment alone. The potential benefits of the prolonged administration may reduce the severity of disease and time to recovery in COVID-19 patients. Together, with a prolonged clinical effect on ventilation-perfusion matching, a prolonged regimen might increase antiviral activity (dose and time-dependent).

In this trial, the iNO spike therapy aims at suppressing replication and eliminating the virus. The constant iNO delivery aims to reduce pulmonary vasoconstriction and optimize V/Q matching. There is an observation that the mass of well-aerated lung tissue decreases over time, which makes it impossible to deliver iNO to the alveoli and thus underscores the importance of early therapy. Lung inhomogeneity manifests in mosaicism of areas of hyperperfusion, hypoperfusion, and consolidation, as a morphological substrate for a combination of continuous and intermittent iNO therapy. At the same time, it is necessary to emphasize the critical importance of early initiation of therapy during potentially reversible phases of lung injury, ideally before the consolidation occurs, which radically changes the current paradigm of the iNO application. Though essential, the study #NCT04476992 has some limitations as it is a single-center study on a limited population of patients of the same ethnicity. Patients enrolled in the study needed oxygen therapy but were without severe gas exchange abnormalities as they were treated in the hospital general medicine ward, and the proportion of older adults, comorbidity and frailty in the study were low. Patients with severe C-ARDS might have a different respiratory pattern and physiological response to iNO treatments. Nevertheless, this study has been the largest randomized analysis of different iNO treatment options in spontaneously breathing COVID-19 patients; it has now been completed and its results have been prepared for publication, but larger scale studies are required.

8. Special Consideration of Safety iNO in COVID-19

There are a number of areas of potential concern with iNO therapy, especially with high-dose regimens: (1) direct toxicity; (2) toxicity associated with the oxidative product; NO_2; (3) the formation of high concentrations of methemoglobin; (4) the possibility of rebound pulmonary hypertension; (5) systemic hemodynamic disorders; (6) decreased platelet activation and subsequent aggregation; and (7) increased risk of acute kidney injury [145].

Direct iNO toxicity may, in fact, contribute to bacterial death when high-dose iNO is used as an antimicrobial. Traditionally, the concern for direct iNO toxicity stems from high doses inhaled by the smoker population. As researchers investigate the benefits of high-dose iNO, one of the first steps will be to determine the least toxic, effective dose. Intertwined with determining the safety of high-dose iNO, there is a known potential of inhaling the byproduct of the interaction of NO with oxygen: nitrogen dioxide, NO_2. NO is highly reactogenic; in the presence of oxygen (O_2), it undergoes a chemical reaction with the formation of NO_2: $2NO + O_2 = 2NO_2$. NO_2 combines with water to become nitric acid, which can be caustic to tissues. NO_2 itself is a highly non-toxic gas with a maximum permissible level of 5 ppm as a short-term exposure and 3 ppm in an 8-h time-weighted average, and more conservative recommendations regulate a short-term exposure limit of 1 ppm [146]. The level of NO_2 in the gas mixture delivered to the patient must be monitored continuously throughout the entire period of NO therapy. The rate of NO_2 formation depends on the concentration of NO and O_2, the time during which the two gases come in contact, pressure, and temperature. This fact has important implications for NO delivery: sources with high concentrations of NO should be avoided, and NO and inspiratory O_2 should be used in minimal, clinically acceptable doses. Monitoring NO_2 during iNO therapy is absolutely essential, and the addition of "scrubbers" to the ventilator circuit can be used to absorb NO_2, including charcoal and lime soda [142,144]. Air, or N_2, may be used as a diluent and is required when high levels of NO are administered [147]. Available in stock iNO delivery systems are equipped with alarms when the level of NO_2 has reached upper limits.

NO oxidizes hemoglobin from the ferrous (Fe^{2+}) to the ferric (Fe^{3+}) form, rendering the hemoglobin incapable of attaching and delivering oxygen. Therefore, when delivering high-dose iNO, the level of methemoglobin (MetHb) in blood/plasma, invasively or non-invasively, should be monitored. The level of MetHb present during inhaled NO therapy depends on the amount of MetHb formed from oxidation and the amount eliminated by reduction within erythrocytes by the methemoglobin reductase enzyme. In most clinical situations, MetHb levels remain low during the NO therapy. The maximum level in clinical practice should be kept to less than 5% of the total hemoglobin concentration, while it can be monitored both discretely with blood sampling and/or continuously and non-invasively using pulse co-oximetry technology. MetHb monitoring is especially important in patients with hypoxemia and/or a suspected methemoglobin reductase enzyme defect. Prior studies using intermittent high-dose iNO have demonstrated safe metHb levels [126–128,148].

Abrupt discontinuation of iNO may be accompanied by rebound pulmonary hypertension, characterized by worsening oxygenation and hypoxemia, systemic hypotension, bradycardia, and acute right ventricular failure [149]. However, these phenomena were noted only after the discontinuation of long-term continuous therapy with iNO, and there have been no reports of this in the current pandemic; timely diagnosis of this condition comes down to careful monitoring of the patient. Earlier studies using high-dose NO have not demonstrated rebound pulmonary hypertension [148].

The danger of a decrease in platelet activation and subsequent aggregation during iNO therapy was not demonstrated in a randomized, controlled, blinded study on the hemostasis in healthy adults after being administered iNO [150], and in the case of COVID-19, earlier studies have not revealed a worsening of hemostasis [127–129].

A significant limitation to the widespread administration of iNO therapy could be the fear of an increased risk of acute kidney injury seen in patients with non-COVID ARDS [151], but our data does not confirm this, and in fact, refutes this notion [152]. Taking into consideration the uniqueness of the pathogenesis of organ complications in COVID-19, the data obtained may indicate the possibility of context-sensitive use of iNO in various clinical scenarios, in particular, to reduce microvascular damage and microcirculatory thrombosis, leading to systemic manifestations of infection and organ dysfunction [75]. iNO therapy may be the key to preventing angiocentric multi-organ injury, unique to COVID-19, caused by endothelial cell injury and the development of systemic "vascular disease" [153]. In systemic endothelial dysfunction, the deficiency of the synthase-dependent pathway of NO generation can be corrected by its exogenous supplementation. Recent studies reported a decreased total NO and its metabolites in hospitalized COVID-19 patients, as well as a decreased nitric oxide diffusion in around 40% of patients discharged from the hospital [154,155]. Other authors claim that reduced concentrations of NO metabolites may be potential biomarkers of long-term poor or irreversible outcomes after a SARS-CoV-2 infection and might serve as a predictor to track the health status of recovered COVID-19 patients [156].

However, to confirm or refute this hypothesis, further studies of NO homeostasis in COVID-19 are needed within the framework of the classical and non-enzymatic pathways of its synthesis and exchange. Endogenous NO metabolism and the role of endothelial and inducible NO synthases in COVID-19 require further research. It is especially important in the context of safety, since one of the mechanisms for the development of acute kidney injury during iNO therapy may be oxidative stress associated with overexpression of iNOS and the overproduction of endogenous NO in the case of non-COVID ARDS [157].

The unique nature of systemic inflammation and the cytokine profile in COVID-19 suggests a different pathway from classic non-COVID ARDS mechanisms of extra-pulmonary organ dysfunction. In particular, the level of cytokines, even in severe and critical COVID-19, is significantly lower than in other disorders associated with lung injury (hypo- and hyperinflammatory ARDS, sepsis, etc.) [158]. It will be important to better understand the imbalance of endogenous NO production in the context of C-ARDS.

In conclusion from a safety profile, a low and high dose of iNO can be safely implemented if continuous monitoring of metHb, NO_2, and O_2 levels, as well as the use of NO_2-scavengers, are diligently employed.

9. Challenges and Innovations: iNO Delivery Devices

The cost of iNO treatment is an essential factor to consider, especially when iNO is administered over days or in the context of high-dose therapy. The reported cost of the NO is $6/L [159], at the same time, the average cost of 1 h of therapy is approximately 100–150$ [160,161]. Annual clinic costs associated with iNO were reported approximately as high as $1.8-million, and nationwide, this could be approximately $200 million, with analysis only available for the neonatal patients [162]. Naturally, financial costs and logistical challenges make it impossible to widely implement iNO therapy to combat the current COVID-19 pandemic. In this regard, it is extremely important to introduce it into clinical practice using novel delivery devices. Currently, there is an active development of new iNO delivery devices that offer portability, stability, and on-demand NO generation. The essence of the development is to abandon traditional cylinder-based systems and switch to bedside NO synthesis and delivery technologies: electricity-generated NO systems, chemical-based NO systems, NO-releasing solutions, and nanoparticle NO technology. These devices are at different stages of development: from clinical testing to the start of sales in some countries. A detailed overview of the systems currently developed to administer inhaled NO for mechanically ventilated and non-intubated patients is presented by Gianni S, et al. [163]. It should be noted that a study on the comparison between high-dose nitric oxide delivered from pressurized cylinders and nitric oxide produced by an electric generator from air has already been carried out and demonstrated a high efficacy and safety of the technology [164]. Completion of the current clinical trials, FDA and European regulatory approval, and market entry into the commercial sector of these devices can revolutionize iNO delivery in medicine and, in particular, with COVID-19. For these purposes, an inhalation mask system to deliver high concentrations of iNO in spontaneously breathing subjects has already been developed [144,165].

10. Future Directions

Every year, new strains of viruses with pandemic potential appear in the world. Antibiotic resistance of known microorganisms increases. The planet's population is rapidly aging, and the population's polymorbidity is increasing. New pandemics are likely to await humanity, and in order to overcome them, healthcare systems need to develop a coordinated response strategy to face the significant uncertainty in the etiotropic therapy of pathogens and pathogenetic approaches. iNO can significantly change the trajectory of this response both in the current pandemic and in future scenarios. Clinicians' and researchers' efforts should be combined to define the antimicrobial activity of iNO. Possible prospects for further research are presented in Table 1.

Table 1. Prospects for further research investigating the beneficial effects of iNO.

Local Effects in the Lungs
Optimization of V/Q matching: electrical impedance tomography, CT angiography
Anti-inflammatory and antiproliferative effects: concentration of inflammatory mediators in bronchoalveolar lavage, pulmonary ultrasonography, CT scan
Antiviral effects: *viral load*, PCR cycle time
Effect of NO-therapy on the microbiome of the respiratory tract, frequency of superinfections and secondary infectious complications
Effect of NO-therapy to prevent disease progression: reduction in intubation frequency, reduction in duration and aggressiveness of respiratory therapy
Impact on long-term pulmonary function ("long COVID"): level of reducing fibrotic lung disease after C-ARDS

Table 1. *Cont.*

Systemic Effects (Nitrosylhem Formation)
Anti-inflammatory effect: concentration of interleukins and inflammatory markers in the peripheral blood, improvement of organ function
Antiplatelet effect: D-dimer, thromboelastography, thromboembolic burden, improvement of distal organ function (e.g., AKI, liver function)
Suppression of apoptosis: long-term improved organ functions, improved long-term clinical outcomes
Influence on the general functional state and the degree of frailty of patients in the long-term period after suffering from COVID-19: KATZ score
Individual and Population Effects
Expression of inducible and endothelial NO synthases and metabolism of endogenous NO in COVID-19 patients
NO-therapy in patients of various COVID-19 endotypes: thrombotic, immunopathic, adaptive
NO-therapy in specific categories of patients with COVID-19 and comorbidity, increasing the risk of a severe course of the disease: chronic lung disease; conditions associated with endothelial dysfunction: hypertension, diabetes mellitus, obesity, smoking
Optimal start time of NO-therapy and its variant (intermittent versus intermittent + continuous inhalation): optimization to the phase of the disease course and individual trajectory (possibly not only by clinical markers of hypoxemia development, but also by laboratory indicators of disease progression, for example, D-dimer)
The effect of adjuvant NO-therapy on mutagenic activity of the virus: sequestration of the virus genome in individuals and in the population
NO therapy and the development of antibiotic resistance in individuals and the population

11. Conclusions

The review of iNO impact on COVID-19 pathophysiology and approaches to iNO delivery suggest that the early administration of iNO therapy may be a safe and promising approach for treatment of COVID-19 patients and beyond. Future large studies focusing on safety and efficacy of iNO therapy regimens in patients with hypoxemic respiratory failure associated with COVID-19 or other viral infections, are required and should be based on the traditional safety paradigm of iNO therapy. For the widespread introduction of iNO therapy into clinical practice, fundamental studies of homeostasis, metabolism and bioavailability of endogenous NO in COVID-19 are needed. The evaluation of endothelial and inducible NO synthases is extremely important for the development of personalized therapeutic protocols, as well as risk stratification and prognosis of severe disease in COVID-19 positive patients.

Author Contributions: Conceptualization, N.O.K.; investigation, N.O.K., L.B. and R.W.C.; resources, L.B.; writing—original draft preparation, N.O.K.; writing—review and editing, L.B. and R.W.C.; supervision, L.B. and R.W.C. All authors have read and agreed to the published version of the manuscript.

Funding: This research received no external funding.

Institutional Review Board Statement: Not applicable.

Informed Consent Statement: Not applicable.

Data Availability Statement: The datasets used and/or analyzed during the current study are available from the corresponding author on reasonable request.

Acknowledgments: The authors would like to thank Katerina Tokareva, Nina Anfinogenova, and Elena Kim for their contribution to the editing of the manuscript. The authors would like to acknowledge the timeless contribution Warren M. Zapol made to translational research and clinical care by dedicating his life to the tireless pursuit of discovery and innovation, including the development of inhaled nitric oxide. We are grateful for his mentorship and friendship.

Conflicts of Interest: The authors declare no conflict of interest.

Abbreviations

AHRF	Acute Hypoxemic Respiratory Failure
iNO	Inhaled Nitric Oxide
ICU	Intensive Care Unit
ARDS	Acute Respiratory Distress Syndrome
RV	Right Ventricular; V/Q: Ventilation/Perfusion
ACE_2	Angiotensin-Converting Enzyme 2
AKI	Acute Kidney Injury
C-ARDS	COVID-Related Ards
PaO_2/FiO_2	Arterial Oxygen Partial Pressure/Fractional Inspired Oxygen
MetHb	Methemoglobin

References

1. Yang, X.; Yu, Y.; Xu, J.; Shu, H.; Xia, J.; Liu, H.; Wu, Y.; Zhang, L.; Yu, Z.; Fang, M.; et al. Clinical course and outcomes of critically ill patients with SARS-CoV-2 pneumonia in Wuhan, China: A single-centered, retrospective, observational study. *Lancet Respir. Med.* **2020**, *8*, 475–481. [CrossRef]
2. Batlle, D.; Soler, M.J.; Sparks, M.A.; Hiremath, S.; South, A.M.; Welling, P.A.; Swaminathan, S. Acute Kidney Injury in COVID-19: Emerging Evidence of a Distinct Pathophysiology. *J. Am. Soc. Nephrol.* **2020**, *31*, 1380–1383. [CrossRef] [PubMed]
3. Noris, M.; Benigni, A.; Remuzzi, G. The case of complement activation in COVID-19 multiorgan impact. *Kidney Int.* **2020**, *98*, 314–322. [CrossRef] [PubMed]
4. Helms, J.; Tacquard, C.; Severac, F.; Leonard-Lorant, I.; Ohana, M.; Delabranche, X.; Merdji, H.; Clere-Jehl, R.; Schenck, M.; Gandet, F.F.; et al. High risk of thrombosis in patients with severe SARS-CoV-2 infection: A multicenter prospective cohort study. *Intensive Care Med.* **2020**, *46*, 1089–1098. [CrossRef]
5. Ranjeva, S.; Pinciroli, R.; Hodell, E.; Mueller, A.; Hardin, C.C.; Thompson, B.T.; Berra, L. Identifying clinical and biochemical phenotypes in acute respiratory distress syndrome secondary to coronavirus disease-2019. *EClinicalMedicine* **2021**, *34*, 100829. [CrossRef]
6. Sinha, P.; Calfee, C.S.; Cherian, S.; Brealey, D.; Cutler, S.; King, C.; Killick, C.; Richards, O.; Cheema, Y.; Bailey, C.; et al. Prevalence of phenotypes of acute respiratory distress syndrome in critically ill patients with COVID-19: A prospective observational study. *Lancet Respir. Med.* **2020**, *8*, 1209–1218. [CrossRef]
7. Gutiérrez-Gutiérrez, B.; del Toro, M.D.; Borobia, A.M.; Carcas, A.; Jarrín, I.; Yllescas, M.; Ryan, P.; Pachón, J.; Carratalà, J.; Berenguer, J.; et al. Identification and validation of clinical phenotypes with prognostic implications in patients admitted to hospital with COVID-19: A multicentre cohort study. *Lancet Infect. Dis.* **2021**, *21*, 783–792. [CrossRef]
8. Santamarina, M.G.; Boisier, D.; Contreras, R.; Baque, M.; Volpacchio, M.; Beddings, I. COVID-19: A hypothesis regarding the ventilation-perfusion mismatch. *Crit. Care* **2020**, *24*, 395. [CrossRef]
9. Santamarina, M.G.; Riscal, D.B.; Beddings, I.; Contreras, R.; Baque, M.; Volpacchio, M.; Lomakin, F.M. COVID-19: What Iodine Maps from Perfusion CT can reveal—A Prospective Cohort Study. *Crit. Care* **2020**, *24*, 619. [CrossRef]
10. The RECOVERY Collaborative Group. Dexamethasone in Hospitalized Patients with COVID-19. *N. Engl. J. Med.* **2021**, *384*, 693–704. [CrossRef]
11. Ackermann, M.; Verleden, S.E.; Kuehnel, M.; Haverich, A.; Welte, T.; Laenger, F.; Vanstapel, A.; Werlein, C.; Stark, H.; Tzankov, A.; et al. Pulmonary Vascular Endothelialitis, Thrombosis, and Angiogenesis in COVID-19. *N. Engl. J. Med.* **2020**, *383*, 120–128. [CrossRef] [PubMed]
12. WHO Solidarity Trial Consortium. Repurposed Antiviral Drugs for COVID-19—Interim WHO Solidarity Trial Results. *N. Engl. J. Med.* **2021**, *384*, 497–511. [CrossRef] [PubMed]
13. Sherlock, L.G.; Wright, C.J.; Kinsella, J.P.; Delaney, C. Inhaled nitric oxide use in neonates: Balancing what is evidence-based and what is physiologically sound. *Nitric Oxide* **2019**, *95*, 12–16. [CrossRef] [PubMed]
14. Cherian, S.V.; Kumar, A.; Akasapu, K.; Ashton, R.W.; Aparnath, M.; Malhotra, A. Salvage therapies for refractory hypoxemia in ARDS. *Respir. Med.* **2018**, *141*, 150–158. [CrossRef]
15. Gómez, F.P.; Amado, V.M.; Roca, J.; Torres, A.; Nicolas, J.M.; Rodriguez-Roisin, R.; Barberà, J.A. Effect of nitric oxide inhalation on gas exchange in acute severe pneumonia. *Respir. Physiol. Neurobiol.* **2013**, *187*, 157–163. [CrossRef]
16. Saydain, G.; Awan, A.; Manickam, P.; Kleinow, P.; Badr, S. Pulmonary Hypertension an Independent Risk Factor for Death in Intensive Care Unit: Correlation of Hemodynamic Factors with Mortality. *Clin. Med. Insights Circ. Respir. Pulm. Med.* **2015**, *9*, 27–33. [CrossRef]
17. Sato, R.; Dugar, S.; Cheungpasitporn, W.; Schleicher, M.; Collier, P.; Vallabhajosyula, S.; Duggal, A. The impact of right ventricular injury on the mortality in patients with acute respiratory distress syndrome: A systematic review and meta-analysis. *Crit. Care* **2021**, *25*, 172. [CrossRef]
18. Gibson, L.E.; Di Fenza, R.; Lang, M.; Capriles, M.I.; Li, M.D.; Kalpathy-Cramer, J.; Little, B.P.; Arora, P.; Mueller, A.L.; Ichinose, F.; et al. Right Ventricular Strain Is Common in Intubated COVID-19 Patients and Does Not Reflect Severity of Respiratory Illness. *J. Intensive Care Med.* **2021**, *36*, 900–909. [CrossRef]

19. Dessap, A.M.; Boissier, F.; Charron, C.; Bégot, E.; Repessé, X.; Legras, A.; Brun-Buisson, C.; Vignon, P.; Vieillard-Baron, A. Acute corpulmonale during protective ventilation for acute respiratory distress syndrome: Prevalence, predictors, and clinical impact. *Intensive Care Med.* **2015**, *42*, 862–870. [CrossRef]
20. Ichinose, F.; Roberts, J.D., Jr.; Zapol, W.M. Inhaled nitric oxide: A selective pulmonary vasodilator: Current uses and therapeutic potential. *Circulation* **2004**, *109*, 3106–3111. [CrossRef]
21. Chen, L.; Liu, P.; Gao, H.; Sun, B.; Chao, D.; Wang, F.; Zhu, Y.; Hedenstierna, G.; Wang, C.G. Inhalation of nitric oxide in the treatment of severe acute respiratory syndrome: A rescue trial in Beijing. *Clin. Infect. Dis.* **2004**, *39*, 1531–1535. [CrossRef] [PubMed]
22. Gebistorf, F.; Karam, O.; Wetterslev, J.; Afshari, A. Inhaled nitric oxide for acute respiratory distress syndrome (ARDS) in children and adults. *Cochrane Database Syst. Rev.* **2016**, *2016*, CD002787. [CrossRef] [PubMed]
23. Dellinger, R.P.; Zimmerman, J.L.; Taylor, R.W. Effects of inhaled nitric oxide in patients with acute respiratory distress syndrome: Results of a randomized phase II trial. *Crit. Care Med.* **1998**, *26*, 15–23. [CrossRef] [PubMed]
24. Taylor, R.W.; Zimmerman, J.L.; Dellinger, R.P.; Straube, R.C.; Criner, G.J.; Davis, J.K.; Kelly, K.M.; Smith, T.C.; Small, R.J.; Inhaled Nitric Oxide in ARDS Study Group. Low-dose inhaled nitric oxide in patients with acute lung injury: A randomized controlled trial. *JAMA* **2004**, *291*, 1603–1609. [CrossRef]
25. Teuwen, L.-A.; Geldhof, V.; Pasut, A.; Carmeliet, P. COVID-19: The vasculature unleashed. *Nat. Rev. Immunol.* **2020**, *20*, 389–391. [CrossRef]
26. Patel, B.V.; Arachchillage, D.J.; Ridge, C.A.; Bianchi, P.; Doyle, J.F.; Garfield, B.; Ledot, S.; Morgan, C.; Passariello, M.; Price, S.; et al. Pulmonary angiopathy in severe COVID-19: Physiologic, imaging, and hematologic observations. *Am. J. Respir. Crit. Care Med.* **2020**, *202*, 690–699. [CrossRef]
27. Vasques, F.; Sanderson, B.; Formenti, F.; Shankar-Hari, M.; Camporota, L. Physiological dead space ventilation, disease severity and outcome in ventilated patients with hypoxaemic respiratory failure due to coronavirus disease 2019. *Intensive Care Med.* **2020**, *46*, 2092–2093. [CrossRef]
28. Vaduganathan, M.; Vardeny, O.; Michel, T.; McMurray, J.J.V.; Pfeffer, M.A.; Solomon, S.D. Renin–Angiotensin–Aldosterone System Inhibitors in Patients with COVID-19. *N. Engl. J. Med.* **2020**, *382*, 1653–1659. [CrossRef]
29. Liu, P.; Blet, A.; Smyth, D.; Li, H. The science underlying COVID-19: Implicationsfor the cardiovascular system. *Circulation* **2020**, *142*, 68–78. [CrossRef]
30. Zhang, H.; Baker, A. Recombinant human ACE2: Acing out angiotensin II in ARDS therapy. *Crit. Care* **2020**, *21*, 305. [CrossRef]
31. Reynolds, A.; Lee, A.G.; Renz, J.; DeSantis, K.; Liang, J.; Powell, C.A.; Ventetuolo, C.E.; Poor, H.D. Pulmonary Vascular Dilatation Detected by Automated Transcranial Doppler in COVID-19 Pneumonia. *Am. J. Respir. Crit. Care Med.* **2020**, *202*, 1037–1039. [CrossRef] [PubMed]
32. Lecompte-Osorio, P.; Pearson, S.D.; Pieroni, C.H.; Stutz, M.R.; Pohlman, A.S.; Lin, J.; Hall, J.B.; Htwe, Y.M.; Belvitch, P.G.; Dudek, S.M.; et al. Bedside estimates of dead space using end-tidal CO2 are independently associated with mortality in ARDS. *Crit. Care* **2021**, *25*, 333. [CrossRef] [PubMed]
33. Zamanian, R.T.; Pollack, C.V.; Gentile, M.A.; Rashid, M.; Fox, J.C.; Mahaffey, K.W.; Perez, V.D.J. Outpatient Inhaled Nitric Oxide in a Patient with Vasoreactive Idiopathic Pulmonary Arterial Hypertension and COVID-19 Infection. *Am. J. Respir. Crit. Care Med.* **2020**, *202*, 130–132. [CrossRef] [PubMed]
34. Alvarez, R.A.; Berra, L.; Gladwin, M.T. Home NO therapy for COVID-19. *Am. J. Respir. Crit. Care Med.* **2020**, *202*, 16–20. [CrossRef]
35. Keyaerts, E.; Vijgen, L.; Chen, L.; Maes, P.; Hedenstierna, G.; Van Ranst, M. Inhibition of SARS-coronavirus infection in vitro by S-nitroso-N-acetylpenicillamine, a nitric oxide donor compound. *Int. J. Infect. Dis.* **2004**, *8*, 223–226. [CrossRef]
36. Åkerström, S.; Mousavi-Jazi, M.; Klingström, J.; Leijon, M.; Lundkvist, A.; Mirazimi, A. Nitric Oxide Inhibits the Replication Cycle of Severe Acute Respiratory Syndrome Coronavirus. *J. Virol.* **2005**, *79*, 1966–1969. [CrossRef]
37. Akaberi, D.; Krambrich, J.; Ling, J.; Luni, C.; Hedenstierna, G.; Järhult, J.D.; Lennerstrand, J.; Lundkvist, Å. Mitigation of the replication of SARS-CoV-2 by nitric oxide in vitro. *Redox Biol.* **2020**, *37*, 101734. [CrossRef]
38. Ignarro, L. Inhaled nitric oxide and COVID-19. *Br. J. Pharmacol.* **2020**, *177*, 3848–3849. [CrossRef]
39. Stark, J.M.; Khan, A.M.; Chiappetta, C.L.; Xue, H.; Alcorn, J.L.; Colasurdo, G.N. Immune and Functional Role of Nitric Oxide in a Mouse Model of Respiratory Syncytial Virus Infection. *J. Infect. Dis.* **2005**, *191*, 387–395. [CrossRef]
40. Sanders, S.P.; Siekierski, E.S.; Porter, J.D.; Richards, S.M.; Proud, D. Nitric Oxide Inhibits Rhinovirus-Induced Cytokine Production and Viral Replication in a Human Respiratory Epithelial Cell Line. *J. Virol.* **1998**, *72*, 934–942. [CrossRef]
41. Karupiah, G.; Harris, N. Inhibition of viral replication by nitric oxide and its reversal by ferrous sulfate and tricarboxylic acid cycle metabolites. *J. Exp. Med.* **1995**, *181*, 2171–2179. [CrossRef]
42. Mehta, D.R.; Ashkar, A.; Mossman, K.L. The Nitric Oxide Pathway Provides Innate Antiviral Protection in Conjunction with the Type I Interferon Pathway in Fibroblasts. *PLoS ONE* **2012**, *7*, e31688. [CrossRef] [PubMed]
43. Rimmelzwaan, G.F.; Baars, M.M.J.W.; de Lijster, P.; Fouchier, R.; Osterhaus, A.D.M.E. Inhibition of Influenza Virus Replication by Nitric Oxide. *J. Virol.* **1999**, *73*, 8880–8883. [CrossRef] [PubMed]
44. Åkerström, S.; Gunalan, V.; Keng, C.T.; Tan, Y.-J.; Mirazimi, A. Dual effect of nitric oxide on SARS-CoV replication: Viral RNA production and palmitoylation of the S protein are affected. *Virology* **2009**, *395*, 1–9. [CrossRef] [PubMed]
45. Xu, W.; Zheng, S.; Dweik, R.A.; Erzurum, S.C. Role of epithelial nitric oxide in airway viral infection. *Free Radic. Biol. Med.* **2006**, *41*, 19–28. [CrossRef] [PubMed]

46. Croen, K.D. Evidence for antiviral effect of nitric oxide. Inhibition of herpes simplex virus type 1 replication. *J. Clin. Investig.* **1993**, *91*, 2446–2452. [CrossRef]
47. Kaul, P.; Singh, I.; Turner, R.B. Effect of Nitric Oxide on Rhinovirus Replication and Virus-Induced Interleukin-8 Elaboration. *Am. J. Respir. Crit. Care Med.* **1999**, *159*, 1193–1198. [CrossRef] [PubMed]
48. Klingstrom, J.; Åkerström, S.; Hardestam, J.; Stoltz, M.; Simon, M.; Falk, K.I.; Mirazimi, A.; Rottenberg, M.; Lundkvist, Å. Nitric oxide and peroxynitrite have different antiviral effects against hantavirus replication and free mature virions. *Eur. J. Immunol.* **2006**, *36*, 2649–2657. [CrossRef]
49. Saura, M.; Zaragoza, C.; McMillan, A.; Quick, R.A.; Hohenadl, C.; Lowenstein, J.M.; Lowenstein, C.J. An antiviral mechanism of nitric oxide: Inhibition of a viral protease. *Immunity* **1999**, *10*, 21–28. [CrossRef]
50. Lin, Y.L.; Huang, Y.L.; Ma, S.H.; Yeh, C.T.; Chiou, S.Y.; Chen, L.K.; Liao, C.L. Inhibition of Japanese encephalitis virus infection by nitric oxide: Antiviral effect of nitric oxide on RNA virus replication. *J. Virol.* **1997**, *71*, 5227–5235. [CrossRef]
51. Akarid, K.; Sinet, M.; Desforges, B.; A Gougerot-Pocidalo, M. Inhibitory effect of nitric oxide on the replication of a murine retrovirus in vitro and in vivo. *J. Virol.* **1995**, *69*, 7001–7005. [CrossRef] [PubMed]
52. Harris, N.; Buller, R.M.; Karupiah, G. Gamma interferon-induced, nitric oxide-mediated inhibition of vaccinia virus replication. *J. Virol.* **1995**, *69*, 910–915. [CrossRef] [PubMed]
53. Jung, K.; Gurnani, A.; Renukaradhya, G.J.; Saif, L.J. Nitric oxide is elicited and inhibits viral replication in pigs infected with porcine respiratory coronavirus but not porcine reproductive and respiratory syndrome virus. *Vet. Immunol. Immunopathol.* **2010**, *136*, 335–339. [CrossRef] [PubMed]
54. Uehara, E.U.; de Stefano Shida, B.; de Brito, C.A. The role of nitric oxide in immune responses against viruses is beyond microbicidal activity. *Inflamm. Res.* **2015**, *64*, 845–852. [CrossRef]
55. Vanin, A.F. Dinitrosyl iron complexes with thiolate ligands: Physico-chemistry, biochemistry and physiology. *Nitric Oxide* **2009**, *21*, 1–13. [CrossRef]
56. Vanin, A.F. *Dinitrosyl Iron Complexes as a "Working Form" of Nitric Oxide in Living Organisms*; Cambridge Scholars Publishing: Cambridge, UK, 2019.
57. Vanin, A.F. Dinitrosyl Iron Complexes with Thiol-Containing Ligands Can Suppress Viral Infections as Donors of the Nitrosonium Cation (Hypothesis). *Biophysics* **2020**, *65*, 698–702. [CrossRef]
58. Miller, C.; Miller, M.; McMullin, B.; Regev, G.; Serghides, L.; Kain, K.; Road, J.; Av-Gay, Y. A phase I clinical study of inhaled nitric oxide in healthy adults. *J. Cyst. Fibros.* **2012**, *11*, 324–331. [CrossRef]
59. Deppisch, C.; Herrmann, G.; Graepler-Mainka, U.; Wirtz, H.; Heyder, S.; Engel, C.; Marschal, M.; Miller, C.C.; Riethmüller, J. Gaseous nitric oxide to treat antibiotic resistant bacterial and fungal lung infections in patients with cystic fibrosis: A phase I clinical study. *Infection* **2016**, *44*, 513–520. [CrossRef]
60. Miller, C.; McMullin, B.; Ghaffari, A.; Stenzler, A.; Pick, N.; Roscoe, D.; Ghahary, A.; Road, J.; Av-Gay, Y. Gaseous nitric oxide bactericidal activity retained during intermittent high-dose short duration exposure. *Nitric Oxide* **2009**, *20*, 16–23. [CrossRef]
61. Ma, L.; Wang, W.; Le Grange, J.M.; Wang, X.; Du, S.; Li, C.; Wei, J.; Zhang, J.-N. Coinfection of SARS-CoV-2 and other respiratory pathogens. *Infect. Drug Resist.* **2020**, *13*, 3045–3053. [CrossRef]
62. Kim, D.; Quinn, J.; Pinsky, B.; Shah, N.H.; Brown, I. Rates of co-infection between SARS-CoV-2 and other respiratory pathogens. *JAMA* **2020**, *323*, 2085–2086. [CrossRef] [PubMed]
63. Lansbury, L.; Lim, B.; Baskaran, V.; Lim, W.S. Co-infections in people with COVID-19: A systematic review and meta-analysis. *J. Infect.* **2020**, *81*, 266–275. [CrossRef] [PubMed]
64. Sharifipour, E.; Shams, S.; Esmkhani, M.; Khodadadi, J.; Fotouhi-Ardakani, R.; Koohpaei, A.; Doosti, Z.; Golzari, S.E. Evaluation of bacterial co-infections of the respiratory tract in COVID-19 patients admitted to ICU. *BMC Infect. Dis.* **2020**, *20*, 646. [CrossRef] [PubMed]
65. Rouzé, A.; Martin-Loeches, I.; Povoa, P.; Makris, D.; Artigas, A.; Bouchereau, M.; Lambiotte, F.; Metzelard, M.; Cuchet, P.; Geronimi, C.B.; et al. Relationship between SARS-CoV-2 infection and the incidence of ventilator-associated lower respiratory tract infections: A European multicenter cohort study. *Intensive Care Med.* **2021**, *47*, 188–198. [CrossRef]
66. Nseir, S.; Martin-Loeches, I.; Povoa, P.; Metzelard, M.; Du Cheyron, D.; Lambiotte, F.; Tamion, F.; Labruyere, M.; Makris, D.; Geronimi, C.B.; et al. Relationship between ventilator-associated pneumonia and mortality in COVID-19 patients: A planned ancillary analysis of the coVAPid cohort. *Crit. Care* **2021**, *25*, 177.
67. Armstrong-James, D.; Youngs, J.; Bicanic, T.; Abdolrasouli, A.; Denning, D.W.; Johnson, E.; Mehra, V.; Pagliuca, T.; Patel, B.; Rhodes, J.; et al. Confronting and mitigating the risk of COVID-19 associated pulmonary aspergillosis. *Eur. Respir. J.* **2020**, *56*, 2002554. [CrossRef]
68. He, J.; Hu, L.; Huang, X.; Wang, C.; Zhang, Z.; Wang, Y.; Zhang, D.; Ye, W. Potential of coronavirus 3C-like protease inhibitors for the development of new anti-SARS-CoV-2 drugs: Insights from structures of protease and inhibitors. *Int. J. Antimicrob. Agents* **2020**, *56*, 106055. [CrossRef]
69. Stefano, G.B.; Esch, T.; Kream, R.M. Potential Immunoregulatory and Antiviral/SARS-CoV-2 Activities of Nitric Oxide. *Med. Sci. Monit.* **2020**, *26*, e925679-1. [CrossRef]
70. Andreou, A.; Trantza, S.; Filippou, D.; Sipsas, N.; Tsiodras, S. COVID-19: The potential role of copper and N-acetylcysteine (NAC) in a combination of candidate antiviral treatments against SARS-CoV-2. *In Vivo* **2020**, *34*, 1567–1588. [CrossRef]

71. Kobayashi, J.; Murata, I. Nitric oxide inhalation as an interventional rescue therapy for COVID-19-induced acute respiratory distress syndrome. *Ann. Intensive Care* **2020**, *10*, 61. [CrossRef]
72. McMahon, T.J.; Doctor, A. Extrapulmonary effects of inhaled nitric oxide: Role of reversible S-nitrosylation of erythrocytic hemoglobin. *Proc. Am. Thorac. Soc.* **2006**, *3*, 153–160. [CrossRef] [PubMed]
73. Fraser, D.D.; Patterson, E.K.; Slessarev, M.; Gill, S.E.; Martin, C.; Daley, M.; Miller, M.R.; Patel, M.A.; dos Santos, C.C.; Bosma, K.J.; et al. Endothelial Injury and Glycocalyx Degradation in Critically Ill Coronavirus Disease 2019 Patients: Implications for Microvascular Platelet Aggregation. *Crit. Care Explor.* **2020**, *2*, e0194. [CrossRef] [PubMed]
74. Becker, R.C. COVID-19 update: COVID-19-associated coagulopathy. *J. Thromb. Thrombolysis* **2020**, *50*, 54–67. [CrossRef] [PubMed]
75. Varga, Z.; Flammer, A.J.; Steiger, P.; Haberecker, M.; Andermatt, R.; Zinkernagel, A.S.; Mehra, M.R.; Schuepbach, R.A.; Ruschitzka, F.; Moch, H. Endothelial cell infection and endotheliitis in COVID-19. *Lancet* **2020**, *395*, 1417–1418. [CrossRef]
76. Ozdemir, B.; Yazici, A. Could the decrease in the endothelial nitric oxide (NO) production and NO bioavailability be the crucial cause of COVID-19 related deaths? *Med. Hypotheses* **2020**, *144*, 109970. [CrossRef]
77. Amraei, R.; Rahimi, N. COVID-19, renin-angiotensin system and endothelial dysfunction. *Cells* **2020**, *9*, 1652. [CrossRef]
78. Banu, N.; Panikar, S.S.; Leal, L.R.; Leal, A.R. Protective role of ACE2 and its downregulation in SARS-CoV-2 infection leading to Macrophage Activation Syndrome: Therapeutic implications. *Life Sci.* **2020**, *256*, 117905. [CrossRef]
79. Fang, W.; Jiang, J.; Su, L.; Shu, T.; Liu, H.; Lai, S.; Ghiladi, R.A.; Wang, J. The role of NO in COVID-19 and potential therapeutic strategies. *Free Radic. Biol. Med.* **2020**, *163*, 153–162. [CrossRef]
80. Bohlen, H.G. Nitric Oxide and the Cardiovascular System. *Compr. Physiol.* **2015**, *5*, 803–828. [CrossRef]
81. Piknova, B.; Gladwin, M.T.; Schechter, A.N.; Hogg, N. Electron Paramagnetic Resonance Analysis of Nitrosylhemoglobin in Humans during NO Inhalation. *J. Biol. Chem.* **2005**, *280*, 40583–40588. [CrossRef]
82. Gladwin, M.T.; Schechter, A.N.; Shelhamer, J.H.; Pannell, L.K.; Conway, D.A.; Hrinczenko, B.W.; Nichols, J.S.; Pease-Fye, M.E.; Noguchi, C.T.; Rodgers, G.P.; et al. Inhaled nitric oxide augments nitric oxide transport on sickle cell hemoglobin without affecting oxygen affinity. *J. Clin. Investig.* **1999**, *104*, 937–945. [CrossRef] [PubMed]
83. Nagasaka, Y.; Fernandez, B.O.; Steinbicker, A.U.; Spagnolli, E.; Malhotra, R.; Bloch, D.B.; Bloch, K.D.; Zapol, W.M.; Feelisch, M. Pharmacological preconditioning with inhaled nitric oxide (NO): Organ-specific differences in the lifetime of blood and tissue NO metabolites. *Nitric Oxide* **2018**, *80*, 52–60. [CrossRef] [PubMed]
84. Sardu, C.; Gambardella, J.; Morell, M.B.; Wang, X.; Marfella, R.; Santulli, G. Hypertension, thrombosis, kidney failure, and diabetes: Is COVID-19 an endothelial disease? A comprehensive evaluation of clinical and basic evidence. *J. Clin. Med.* **2020**, *9*, 1417. [CrossRef]
85. Marrazzo, F.; Spina, S.; Zadek, F.; Lama, T.; Xu, C.; Larson, G.; Rezoagli, E.; Malhotra, R.; Zheng, H.; A Bittner, E.; et al. Protocol of a randomised controlled trial in cardiac surgical patients with endothelial dysfunction aimed to prevent postoperative acute kidney injury by administering nitric oxide gas. *BMJ Open* **2019**, *9*, e026848. [CrossRef]
86. Guo, X.-Z.J.; Thomas, P.G. New fronts emerge in the influenza cytokine storm. *Semin. Immunopathol.* **2017**, *39*, 541–550. [CrossRef] [PubMed]
87. Martel, J.; Ko, Y.-F.; Young, J.D.; Ojcius, D.M. Could nasal nitric oxide help to mitigate the severity of COVID-19? *Microbes Infect.* **2020**, *22*, 168–171. [CrossRef]
88. Lundberg, J.O.N.; Farkas-Szallasi, T.; Weitzberg, E.; Rinder, J.; Lidholm, J.; Änggård, A.; Hökfelt, T.; Alving, K. High nitric oxide production in human paranasal sinuses. *Nat. Med.* **1995**, *1*, 370–373. [CrossRef]
89. Lundberg, J.O.N.; Weitzberg, E. Nasal nitric oxide in man. *Thorax* **1999**, *54*, 947–952. [CrossRef]
90. Lundberg, J.O. Nitric oxide and the paranasal sinuses. *Anat. Rec. Adv. Integr. Anat. Evol. Biol. Adv. Integr. Anat. Evol. Biol.* **2008**, *291*, 1479–1484. [CrossRef]
91. Myers, E.N.; Runer, T.; Cervin, A.; Lindberg, S.; Uddman, R. Nitric oxide is a regulator of mucociliary activity in the upper respiratory tract. *Otolaryngol.—Head Neck Surg.* **1998**, *119*, 278–287. [CrossRef]
92. Nagaki, M.; Shimura, S.; Irokawa, T.; Sasaki, T.; Shirato, K. Nitric oxide regulation of glycoconjugate secretion from feline and human airways in vitro. *Respir. Physiol.* **1995**, *102*, 89–95. [CrossRef]
93. Lundberg, J.O.; Nordvall, S.L.; Weitzberg, E.; Kollberg, H.; Alving, K. Exhaled nitric oxide in paediatric asthma and cystic fibrosis. *Arch. Dis. Child.* **1996**, *75*, 323–326. [CrossRef] [PubMed]
94. Karupiah, G.; Xie, Q.W.; Buller, R.M.; Nathan, C.; Duarte, C.; MacMicking, J.D. Inhibition of viral replication by interferon-gamma-induced nitric oxide synthase. *Science* **1993**, *261*, 1445–1448. [CrossRef] [PubMed]
95. Noda, S.; Tanaka, K.; Sawamura, S.-A.; Sasaki, M.; Matsumoto, T.; Mikami, K.; Aiba, Y.; Hasegawa, H.; Kawabe, N.; Koga, Y. Role of Nitric Oxide Synthase Type 2 in Acute Infection with Murine Cytomegalovirus. *J. Immunol.* **2001**, *166*, 3533–3541. [CrossRef]
96. Avnon, L.S.; Munteanu, D.; Smoliakov, A.; Jotkowitz, A.; Barski, L. Thromboembolic events in patients with severe pandemic influenza A/H1N1. *Eur. J. Intern. Med.* **2015**, *26*, 596–598. [CrossRef]
97. Darwish, I.; Miller, C.; Kain, K.; Liles, W.C. Inhaled Nitric Oxide Therapy Fails to Improve Outcome in Experimental Severe Influenza. *Int. J. Med. Sci.* **2012**, *9*, 157–162. [CrossRef]
98. Kharitonov, S.A.; Yates, D.; Barnes, P.J. Increased nitric oxide in exhaled air of normal human subjects with upper respiratory tract infections. *Eur. Respir. J.* **1995**, *8*, 295–297. [CrossRef]
99. Kharitonov, S.A.; Chung, K.F.; Evans, D.; O'Connor, B.J.; Barnes, P.J. Increased exhaled nitric oxide in asthma is mainly derived from the lower respiratory tract. *Am. J. Respir. Crit. Care Med.* **1996**, *153*, 1773–1780. [CrossRef]

100. Taylor, D.R.; Pijnenburg, M.W.; Smith, A.D.; Jongste, J.C.D. Exhaled nitric oxide measurements: Clinical application and interpretation. *Thorax* **2006**, *61*, 817–827. [CrossRef]
101. Høiby, N.; Bjarnsholt, T.; Givskov, M.; Molin, S.; Ciofu, O. Antibiotic resistance of bacterial biofilms. *Intern. J. Antimicrob. Agents* **2010**, *35*, 322–332. [CrossRef]
102. Mulcahy, H.; Charron-Mazenod, L.; Lewenza, S. Extracellular DNA chelates cations and induces antibiotic resistance in Pseudomonas aeruginosa biofilms. *PLoS Pathog.* **2008**, *4*, e1000213. [CrossRef] [PubMed]
103. Hassett, D.J.; Ma, J.-F.; Elkins, J.G.; McDermott, T.R.; Ochsner, U.A.; West, S.E.H.; Huang, C.-T.; Fredericks, J.; Burnett, S.; Stewart, P.; et al. Quorum sensing in Pseudomonas aeruginosa controls expression of catalase and superoxide dismutase genes and mediates biofilm susceptibility to hydrogen peroxide. *Mol. Microbiol.* **1999**, *34*, 1082–1093. [CrossRef] [PubMed]
104. Roberts, A.P.; Mullany, P. Oral biofilms: A reservoir of transferable, bacterial, antimicrobial resistance. *Expert Rev. Anti-infective Ther.* **2010**, *8*, 1441–1450. [CrossRef]
105. Barraud, N.; Kelso, M.; Rice, S.; Kjelleberg, S. Nitric Oxide: A Key Mediator of Biofilm Dispersal with Applications in Infectious Diseases. *Curr. Pharm. Des.* **2014**, *21*, 31–42. [CrossRef] [PubMed]
106. Kaplan, J.B. Antibiotic-Induced Biofilm Formation. *Int. J. Artif. Organs* **2011**, *34*, 737–751. [CrossRef]
107. Hall-Stoodley, L.; Costerton, J.W.; Stoodley, P. Bacterial biofilms: From the Natural environment to infectious diseases. *Nat. Rev. Genet.* **2004**, *2*, 95–108. [CrossRef] [PubMed]
108. Buckingham-Meyer, K.; Goeres, D.M.; Hamilton, M.A. Comparative evaluation of biofilm disinfectant efficacy tests. *J. Microbiol. Methods* **2007**, *70*, 236–244. [CrossRef] [PubMed]
109. Barraud, N.; Hassett, D.J.; Hwang, S.-H.; Rice, S.A.; Kjelleberg, S.; Webb, J. Involvement of Nitric Oxide in Biofilm Dispersal of Pseudomonas aeruginosa. *J. Bacteriol.* **2006**, *188*, 7344–7353. [CrossRef]
110. Schlag, S.; Nerz, C.; Birkenstock, T.A.; Altenberend, F.; Götz, F. Inhibition of Staphylococcal Biofilm Formation by Nitrite. *J. Bacteriol.* **2007**, *189*, 7911–7919. [CrossRef]
111. Schreiber, F.; Beutler, M.; Enning, D.; Lamprecht-Grandío, M.; Zafra, O.; González-Pastor, J.E.; De Beer, D. The role of nitric-oxide-synthase-derived nitric oxide in multicellular traits of Bacillus subtilis 3610: Biofilm formation, swarming, and dispersal. *BMC Microbiol.* **2011**, *11*, 111. [CrossRef]
112. Carlson, H.K.; Vance, R.E.; Marletta, M.A. H-NOX regulation of c-di-GMP metabolism and biofilm formation in Legionella pneumophila. *Mol. Microbiol.* **2010**, *77*, 930–942. [CrossRef] [PubMed]
113. Ghaffari, A.; Miller, C.C.; McMullin, B.; Ghahary, A. Potential application of gaseous nitric oxide as a topical antimicrobial agent. *Nitric Oxide Biol. Chem.* **2006**, *14*, 21–29. [CrossRef] [PubMed]
114. Shekhter, A.B.; Serezhenkov, V.A.; Rudenko, T.G.; Pekshev, A.V.; Vanin, A.F. Beneficial effect of gaseous nitric oxide on the healing of skin wounds. *Nitric Oxide* **2005**, *12*, 210–219. [CrossRef] [PubMed]
115. Sulemankhil, I.; Ganopolsky, J.G.; Dieni, C.A.; Dan, A.F.; Jones, M.L.; Prakash, S. Prevention and Treatment of Virulent Bacterial Biofilms with an Enzymatic Nitric Oxide-Releasing Dressing. *Antimicrob. Agents Chemother.* **2012**, *56*, 6095–6103. [CrossRef]
116. Cathie, K.; Howlin, R.; Carroll, M.; Clarke, S.; Connett, G.; Cornelius, V.; Daniels, T.; Duignan, C.; Hall-Stoodley, L.; Jefferies, J.; et al. G385 RATNO-Reducing Antibiotic Tolerance using Nitric Oxide in Cystic Fibrosis: Report of a proof of concept clinical trial. *Arch. Dis. Child.* **2014**, *99* (Suppl. S1), A159. [CrossRef]
117. Rawson, T.M.; Moore, L.; Castro-Sanchez, E.; Charani, E.; Davies, F.; Satta, G.; Ellington, M.J.; Holmes, A.H. COVID-19 and the potential long-term impact on antimicrobial resistance. *J. Antimicrob. Chemother.* **2020**, *75*, 1681–1684. [CrossRef]
118. Alhazzani, W.; Møller, M.H.; Arabi, Y.M.; Loeb, M.; Gong, M.N.; Fan, E.; Oczkowski, S.; Levy, M.M.; Derde, L.; Dzierba, A.; et al. Surviving Sepsis Campaign: Guidelines on the management of critically ill adults with Coronavirus Disease 2019 (COVID-19). *Intensive Care Med.* **2020**, *46*, 854–887. [CrossRef]
119. Bartlett, R.H.; Ogino, M.T.; Brodie, D.; McMullan, D.M.; Lorusso, R.; MacLaren, G.; Stead, C.M.; Rycus, P.; Fraser, J.F.; Belohlavek, J.; et al. Initial ELSO Guidance Document: ECMO for COVID-19 Patients with Severe Cardiopulmonary Failure. *ASAIO J.* **2020**, *66*, 472–474. [CrossRef]
120. Barbaro, R.P.; MacLaren, G.; Boonstra, P.S.; Iwashyna, T.J.; Slutsky, A.S.; Fan, E.; Bartlett, R.H.; E Tonna, J.; Hyslop, R.; Fanning, J.J.; et al. Extracorporeal membrane oxygenation support in COVID-19: An international cohort study of the Extracorporeal Life Support Organization registry. *Lancet* **2020**, *396*, 1071–1078. [CrossRef]
121. Falcoz, P.-E.; Monnier, A.; Puyraveau, M.; Perrier, S.; Ludes, P.-O.; Olland, A.; Mertes, P.-M.; Schneider, F.; Helms, J.; Meziani, F. Extracorporeal Membrane Oxygenation for Critically Ill Patients with COVID-19–related Acute Respiratory Distress Syndrome: Worth the Effort? *Am. J. Respir. Crit. Care Med.* **2020**, *202*, 460–463. [CrossRef]
122. Ferrari, M.; Santini, A.; Protti, A.; Andreis, D.T.; Iapichino, G.; Castellani, G.; Rendiniello, V.; Costantini, E.; Cecconi, M. Inhaled nitric oxide in mechanically ventilated patients with COVID-19. *J. Crit. Care* **2020**, *60*, 159–160. [CrossRef] [PubMed]
123. Tavazzi, G.; Pozzi, M.; Mongodi, S.; Dammassa, V.; Romito, G.; Mojoli, F. Inhaled nitric oxide in patients admitted to intensive care unit with COVID-19 pneumonia. *Crit. Care* **2020**, *24*, 508. [CrossRef]
124. Longobardo, A.; Montanari, C.; Shulman, R.; Benhalim, S.; Singer, M.; Arulkumaran, N. Inhaled nitric oxide minimally improves oxygenation in COVID-19 related acute respiratory distress syndrome. *Br. J. Anaesth.* **2020**, *126*, e44–e46. [CrossRef] [PubMed]
125. Parikh, R.; Wilson, C.; Weinberg, J.; Gavin, D.; Murphy, J.; Reardon, C.C. Inhaled nitric oxide treatment in spontaneously breathing COVID-19 patients. *Ther. Adv. Respir. Dis.* **2020**, *14*. Available online: https://pubmed.ncbi.nlm.nih.gov/32539647/ (accessed on 10 January 2022). [CrossRef]

126. Fakhr, B.S.; Wiegand, S.B.; Pinciroli, R.; Gianni, S.; Morais, C.C.A.; Ikeda, T.; Miyazaki, Y.; Marutani, E.; Di Fenza, R.; Larson, G.; et al. High Concentrations of Nitric Oxide Inhalation Therapy in Pregnant Patients With Severe Coronavirus Disease 2019 (COVID-19). *Obstet. Gynecol.* **2020**, *136*, 1109–1113. [CrossRef]
127. Wiegand, S.B.; Fakhr, B.S.; Carroll, R.W.; Zapol, W.M.; Kacmarek, R.M.; Berra, L. Rescue Treatment With High-Dose Gaseous Nitric Oxide in Spontaneously Breathing Patients With Severe Coronavirus Disease 2019. *Crit. Care Explor.* **2020**, *2*, e0277. [CrossRef]
128. Fakhr, B.S.; Di Fenza, R.; Gianni, S.; Wiegand, S.B.; Miyazaki, Y.; Morais, C.C.A.; Gibson, L.E.; Chang, M.G.; Mueller, A.L.; Rodriguez-Lopez, J.M.; et al. Inhaled high dose nitric oxide is a safe and effective respiratory treatment in spontaneous breathing hospitalized patients with COVID-19 pneumonia. *Nitric Oxide* **2021**, *116*, 7–13. [CrossRef]
129. Ziehr, D.R.; Alladina, J.; Wolf, M.E.; Brait, K.L.; Malhotra, A.; La Vita, C.; Berra, L.; Hibbert, K.A.; Hardin, C.C. Respiratory Physiology of Prone Positioning With and Without Inhaled Nitric Oxide Across the Coronavirus Disease 2019 Acute Respiratory Distress Syndrome Severity Spectrum. *Crit. Care Explor.* **2021**, *3*, e0471. [CrossRef]
130. Busana, M.; Giosa, L.; Cressoni, M.; Gasperetti, A.; Di Girolamo, L.; Martinelli, A.; Sonzogni, A.; Lorini, L.; Palumbo, M.M.; Romitti, F.; et al. The impact of ventilation–perfusion inequality in COVID-19: A computational model. *J. Appl. Physiol.* **2021**, *130*, 865–876. [CrossRef]
131. Ramos, C.D.; Fernandes, A.P.; Souza, S.P.M.; Fujiwara, M.; Tobar, N.; Dertkigil, S.S.J.; Takahashi, M.E.S.; Gonçales, E.S.L.; Trabasso, P.; Zantut-Wittmann, D.E. Simultaneous Imaging of Lung Perfusion and Glucose Metabolism in COVID-19 Pneumonia. *Am. J. Respir. Crit. Care Med.* **2021**, *203*, 1186–1187. [CrossRef]
132. Coppola, S.; Chiumello, D.; Busana, M.; Giola, E.; Palermo, P.; Pozzi, T.; Steinberg, I.; Roli, S.; Romitti, F.; Lazzari, S.; et al. Role of total lung stress on the progression of early COVID-19 pneumonia. *Intensive Care Med.* **2021**, *47*, 1130–1139. [CrossRef] [PubMed]
133. DeGrado, J.R.; Szumita, P.M.; Schuler, B.R.; Dube, K.M.; Lenox, J.; Kim, E.Y.; Weinhouse, G.L.; Massaro, A.F. Evaluation of the Efficacy and Safety of Inhaled Epoprostenol and Inhaled Nitric Oxide for Refractory Hypoxemia in Patients With Coronavirus Disease 2019. *Crit. Care Explor.* **2020**, *2*, e0259. [CrossRef] [PubMed]
134. Garfield, B.; McFadyen, C.; Briar, C.; Bleakley, C.; Vlachou, A.; Baldwin, M.; Lees, N.; Price, S.; Ledot, S.; McCabe, C.; et al. Potential for personalised application of inhaled nitric oxide in COVID-19 pneumonia. *Br. J. Anaesth.* **2020**, *126*, e72–e75. [CrossRef] [PubMed]
135. Bagate, F.; Tuffet, S.; Masi, P.; Perier, F.; Razazi, K.; De Prost, N.; Carteaux, G.; Payen, D.; Dessap, A.M. Rescue therapy with inhaled nitric oxide and almitrine in COVID-19 patients with severe acute respiratory distress syndrome. *Ann. Intensiv. Care* **2020**, *10*, 151. [CrossRef] [PubMed]
136. Rodríguez, C.; Luque, N.; Blanco, I.; Sebastian, L.; Barberà, J.A.; Peinado, V.I.; Tura-Ceide, O. Pulmonary Endothelial Dysfunction and Thrombotic Complications in Patients with COVID-19. *Am. J. Respir. Cell Mol. Biol.* **2021**, *64*, 407–415. [CrossRef]
137. Chiumello, D.; Busana, M.; Coppola, S.; Romitti, F.; Formenti, P.; Bonifazi, M.; Pozzi, T.; Palumbo, M.M.; Cressoni, M.; Herrmann, P.; et al. Physiological and quantitative CT-scan characterization of COVID-19 and typical ARDS: A matched cohort study. *Intensive Care Med.* **2020**, *46*, 2187–2196. [CrossRef]
138. Parascandola, M.; Xiao, L. Tobacco and the lung cancer epidemic in China. *Transl. Lung Cancer Res.* **2019**, *8* (Suppl. S1), S21–S30. [CrossRef]
139. Miyara, M.; Tubach, F.; Martinez, V.; Morelot-Panzini, C.; Pernet, J.; Haroche, J.; Lebbah, S.; Morawiec, E.; Gorochov, G.; Caumes, E.; et al. Low rate of daily smokers in patients with symptomatic COVID-19. *MedRxiv* **2020**. [CrossRef]
140. Goyal, P.; Choi, J.J.; Pinheiro, L.C.; Schenck, E.J.; Chen, R.; Jabri, A.; Satlin, M.J.; Campion, T.R., Jr.; Nahid, M.; Ringel, J.B.; et al. Clinical Characteristics of COVID-19 in New York City. *N. Engl. J. Med.* **2020**, *382*, 2372–2374. [CrossRef]
141. Adam, T.; Mitschke, S.; Streibel, T.; Baker, R.R.; Zimmermann, R. Quantitative Puff-by-Puff-Resolved Characterization of Selected Toxic Compounds in Cigarette Mainstream Smoke. *Chem. Res. Toxicol.* **2006**, *19*, 511–520. [CrossRef]
142. Branson, R.D.; Hess, D.R.; Campbell, R.S.; Johannigman, J.A. Inhaled Nitric Oxide: Delivery Systems and Monitoring. *Respir. Care* **1999**, *44*, 281–306.
143. Hedenstierna, G.; Chen, L.; Hedenstierna, M.; Lieberman, R.; Fine, H.D. Nitric oxide dosed in short bursts at high concentrations may protect against COVID 19. *Nitric Oxide* **2020**, *103*, 1–3. [CrossRef]
144. Gianni, S.; Morais, C.C.; Larson, G.; Pinciroli, R.; Carroll, R.; Yu, B.; Zapol, W.M.; Berra, L. Ideation and assessment of a nitric oxide delivery system for spontaneously breathing subjects. *Nitric Oxide* **2020**, *104–105*, 29–35. [CrossRef] [PubMed]
145. Weinberger, B.; Djerad, A.; Monier, C.; Houzé, P.; Borron, S.W.; Lefauconnier, J.-M.; Baud, F.J. The Toxicology of Inhaled Nitric Oxide. *Toxicol. Sci.* **2001**, *59*, 5–16. [CrossRef]
146. Available online: https://www.cdc.gov/niosh/npg/npgd0454.html (accessed on 10 January 2022).
147. Barnes, M.; Brisbois, E.J. Clinical use of inhaled nitric oxide: Local and systemic applications. *Free Radic. Biol. Med.* **2019**, *152*, 422–431. [CrossRef] [PubMed]
148. Bartley, B.L.; Gardner, K.; Spina, S.; Hurley, B.P.; Campeau, D.; Berra, L.; Yonker, L.M.; Carroll, R.W. High-Dose Inhaled Nitric Oxide as Adjunct Therapy in Cystic Fibrosis Targeting Burkholderia multivorans. *Case Rep. Pediatrics* **2020**, *2020*, 1536714. [CrossRef] [PubMed]
149. Atz, A.M.; Adatia, I.; Wessel, D.L. Rebound Pulmonary Hypertension After Inhalation of Nitric Oxide. *Ann. Thorac. Surg.* **1996**, *62*, 1759–1764. [CrossRef]

150. Goldstein, B.; Baldassarre, J.; Young, J.N. Effects of inhaled nitric oxide on hemostasis in healthy adults treated with heparin: A randomized, controlled, blinded crossover study. *Thromb. J.* **2012**, *10*, 1. [CrossRef]
151. Ruan, S.-Y.; Huang, T.-M.; Wu, H.-Y.; Wu, H.-D.; Yu, C.-J.; Lai, M.-S. Inhaled nitric oxide therapy and risk of renal dysfunction: A systematic review and meta-analysis of randomized trials. *Crit. Care* **2015**, *19*, 137. [CrossRef]
152. Kamenshchikov, N.O.; Anfinogenova, Y.J.; Kozlov, B.N.; Svirko, Y.S.; Pekarskiy, S.; Evtushenko, V.V.; Lugovsky, V.A.; Shipulin, V.M.; Lomivorotov, V.V.; Podoksenov, Y.K. Nitric oxide delivery during cardiopulmonary bypass reduces acute kidney injury: A randomized trial. *J. Thorac. Cardiovasc. Surg.* **2020**. Available online: https://pubmed.ncbi.nlm.nih.gov/32718702/ (accessed on 10 January 2022). [CrossRef]
153. Jonigk, D.; Märkl, B.; Helms, J. COVID-19: What the clinician should know about post-mortem findings. *Intensive Care Med.* **2020**, *47*, 86–89. [CrossRef] [PubMed]
154. Dominic, P.; Ahmad, J.; Bhandari, R.; Pardue, S.; Solorzano, J.; Jaisingh, K.; Watts, M.; Bailey, S.R.; Orr, A.W.; Kevil, C.G.; et al. Decreased availability of nitric oxide and hydrogen sulfide is a hallmark of COVID-19. *Redox Biol.* **2021**, *43*, 101982. [CrossRef]
155. Núñez-Fernández, M.; Ramos-Hernández, C.; García-Río, F.; Torres-Durán, M.; Nodar-Germiñas, A.; Tilve-Gómez, A.; Rodríguez-Fernández, P.; Valverde-Pérez, D.; Ruano-Raviña, A.; Fernández-Villar, A. Alterations in Respiratory Function Test Three Months after Hospitalisation for COVID-19 Pneumonia: Value of Determining Nitric Oxide Diffusion. *J. Clin. Med.* **2021**, *10*, 2119. [CrossRef] [PubMed]
156. Wang, J.; Mei, F.; Bai, L.; Zhou, S.; Liu, D.; Yao, L.; Ahluwalia, A.; Ghiladi, R.A.; Su, L.; Shu, T.; et al. Serum nitrite and nitrate: A potential biomarker for post-Covid-19 complications? *Free Radic. Biol. Med.* **2021**, *175*, 216–225. [CrossRef] [PubMed]
157. Guimarães, L.M.; Rossini, C.V.; Lameu, C. Implications of SARS-CoV-2 infection on eNOS and iNOS activity: Consequences for the respiratory and vascular systems. *Nitric Oxide* **2021**, *111–112*, 64–71. [CrossRef] [PubMed]
158. Leisman, D.E.; Ronner, L.; Pinotti, R.; Taylor, M.D.; Sinha, P.; Calfee, C.S.; Hirayama, A.V.; Mastroiani, F.; Turtle, C.J.; Harhay, M.O.; et al. Cytokine elevation in severe and critical COVID-19: A rapid systematic review, meta-analysis, and comparison with other inflammatory syndromes. *Lancet Respir. Med.* **2020**, *8*, 1233–1244. [CrossRef]
159. Yang, Y.; Qi, P.; Yang, Z.; Huang, N. Nitric oxide based strategies for applications of biomedical devices. *Biosurface Biotribol.* **2015**, *1*, 177–201. [CrossRef]
160. Tzanetos, D.R.T.; Housley, J.J.; Barr, F.E.; May, W.L.; Landers, C.D. Implementation of an Inhaled Nitric Oxide Protocol Decreases Direct Cost Associated With Its Use. *Respir. Care* **2015**, *60*, 644–650. [CrossRef]
161. Mahone, J.; Pavlichko, M.S. Inhaled nitric oxide: Expensive therapy or smart investment? *RT Decis. Mak. Respir. Care* **2013**, *26*, 12–16.
162. Carey, W.A.; Ellsworth, M.A.; Harris, M.N. Inhaled Nitric Oxide Use in the Neonatal Intensive Care Unit. *JAMA Pediatrics* **2016**, *170*, 639–640. [CrossRef]
163. Gianni, S.; Carroll, R.W.; Kacmarek, R.M.; Berra, L. Inhaled Nitric Oxide Delivery Systems for Mechanically Ventilated and Nonintubated Patients: A Review. *Respir. Care* **2021**, *66*, 1021–1028. [CrossRef] [PubMed]
164. Gianni, S.; Di Fenza, R.; Morais, C.C.A.; Fakhr, B.S.; Mueller, A.L.; Yu, B.; Carroll, R.W.; Ichinose, F.; Zapol, W.M.; Berra, L. High-Dose Nitric Oxide From Pressurized Cylinders and Nitric Oxide Produced by an Electric Generator From Air. *Respir. Care* **2021**, *67*, 201–208. [CrossRef] [PubMed]
165. Pinciroli, R.; Traeger, L.; Fischbach, A.; Gianni, S.; Morais, C.C.A.; Fakhr, B.S.; Di Fenza, R.; Robinson, D.; Carroll, R.; Zapol, W.M.; et al. A Novel Inhalation Mask System to Deliver High Concentrations of Nitric Oxide Gas in Spontaneously Breathing Subjects. *J. Vis. Exp. Jove* **2021**, e61769. [CrossRef] [PubMed]

MDPI AG
Grosspeteranlage 5
4052 Basel
Switzerland
Tel.: +41 61 683 77 34

Biomedicines Editorial Office
E-mail: biomedicines@mdpi.com
www.mdpi.com/journal/biomedicines

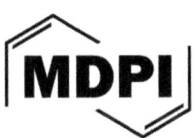

Disclaimer/Publisher's Note: The statements, opinions and data contained in all publications are solely those of the individual author(s) and contributor(s) and not of MDPI and/or the editor(s). MDPI and/or the editor(s) disclaim responsibility for any injury to people or property resulting from any ideas, methods, instructions or products referred to in the content.